THE H
HEALTH PROFESSIONAL EDUCATION

THE HIDDEN CURRICULUM IN HEALTH PROFESSIONAL EDUCATION

Edited by Frederic W. Hafferty and Joseph F. O'Donnell

Dartmouth College Press
HANOVER, NEW HAMPSHIRE

Dartmouth College Press
An imprint of University Press of New England
www.upne.com
© 2014 Trustees of Dartmouth College
Manufactured in the United States of America
Designed by Dean Bornstein
Typeset in Garamond Premier Pro by The Perpetua Press

For permission to reproduce any of the material in this book, contact Permissions, University Press of New England, One Court Street, Suite 250, Lebanon NH 03766; or visit www.upne.com

Library of Congress Cataloging-in-Publication Data

The hidden curriculum in health professional education / edited by Frederic W. Hafferty and Joseph F. O'Donnell.
        p. ; cm.
Includes bibliographical references and index.
ISBN 978-1-61168-659-3 (cloth : alk. paper)—ISBN 978-1-61168-660-9 (pbk. : alk. paper)—ISBN 978-1-61168-661-6 (ebook)
I. Hafferty, Frederic W., 1947– editor. II. O'Donnell, Joseph F.
[DNLM: 1. Curriculum. 2. Education, Professional. 3. Organizational Culture. 4. Teaching—methods. W 18]

R834
610.71—dc23

2014023650

5 4 3 2 1

Fred: To my loving family and network of colleagues who, over the years, have made my sociological walk on the wild side so intoxicating, to my buddy (Joe) who literally dreamed this book into existence, and to the best writing companion (Drover) a man could ask for. RIP D-man.

Joe: To my loving and patient wife of forty-one years, Janice, and my amazing children, Katie, Jenny, Beth, and Michael, and my grandchildren, Charlie and Max. It is also dedicated to a long and deep friendship and an enormous amount of respect for Fred Hafferty.

Contents

Foreword

DEWITT C. BALDWIN

Education is by nature and definition complex. Unfortunately, most people—even educators—don't think of it that way. They often view it as a relatively simple, linear, structured process leading to a clearly defined, predictable conclusion or end point that when properly attended to and followed results in an accepted standardized product.

Every so often a new term or concept enters the conversations of medical educators and is seemingly accorded immediate recognition and acceptance as an idea whose time has come. It is as if these concepts are attracted to empty educational receptor sites, where they attach and appear to offer a facile grasp or understanding of one or another of the ever-present issues facing medical education.

Within relatively recent memory, two such concepts have emerged. Each has created considerable discussion and early recognition without a great deal in the way of critical definition or empirical study. I refer to the concepts of *professionalism* and the *hidden curriculum*. In each case, there has been an instant, "aha" or "satori" of discovery and recognition. In each case, there was a similar pattern of instant, enthusiastic acceptance of a concept that has the appeal of suggesting some fresh new answers to the continuing puzzle of what really goes on (or awry) during the course of medical education and professional formation. In each case, most educators and researchers initially tended to follow medicine's well-entrenched deficit model of thinking, finding it easier to describe negative aspects of practitioner behaviors or curricular alignments.

The Initial framing of the hidden curriculum as something suspicious or even sinister, something that was deliberately concealed from the learners and aimed at intentionally molding, shaping, or warping the students' knowledge, attitudes, or behavior in ways that were untoward was not surprising—at least from a historical perspective. Much of this view can be seen in early literature on the subject, in which liberal educators and writers such as Paolo Freire in *Poverty of the Oppressed* (1970) viewed the state or governing establishment as fostering an educational system or curriculum designed to preserve the existing social structure and power of the "haves," while denying the rights of the "have-nots."

Since its re-introduction into the medical education literature in 1994 by Hafferty and Franks, the concept of a hidden curriculum has become an appealing and convenient heuristic for referring to a number of perceived barriers to a humane and effective learning environment. On the other hand, and as captured in this volume, certain framings have served to limit discussion and an understanding of the full complexity of its nature as a proxy of all the variables that will always remain at the edge or in the borderlands of one of the most complex human acts—that of participating in the education and formation of our young. Exploring those boundaries, the edges and borderlands of knowledge and meaning, lies at the heart of the human challenge. There will always be—indeed, must be—a hidden curriculum, if only to keep us aware of the human condition.

THE HIDDEN CURRICULUM IN HEALTH PROFESSIONAL EDUCATION

Introduction

The Hidden Curriculum—a Focus on Learning and Closing the Gap

The real voyage of discovery consists not in seeking new landscapes but in having new eyes.
—MARCEL PROUST

Periodically, there appears in the medical literature an article that wakes us up, changes the conversation, and causes us to "have new eyes." Such a watershed article appeared in the journal *Academic Medicine* in 1994. It was titled "The Hidden Curriculum, Ethics Teaching, and the Structure of Medical Education," and in it, the authors (re)introduced the notion that something called the hidden curriculum had a great deal to do with what students learned about the knowledge base, the appropriate behaviors, and the underlying values that signify what it means to be a good doctor (Hafferty and Franks 1994). Fred Hafferty had been sent by his dean to a conference about the Holocaust and the role of physicians in carrying out "medical experiments" on concentration camp inmates. Many of those speaking at the conference resolutely called upon medical educators to devote even more curricular time to teaching ethics to trainees to prevent such a moral calamity from ever happening again. Hafferty and Franks, however, pointed out that much of what students learn about "being ethical" was taking place not in the classroom or in formal bedside teaching, but on the shop floor of clinical settings; and that in these settings, they were learning "things" (knowledge, behaviors, and values) that sometimes were quite different from those being presented in required coursework and related formal teaching activities. Hafferty and Franks labeled the culprit the *hidden curriculum*, and asserted that in addition to what formally was being taught in the classroom and at the bedside, students were being shaped by a multitude of other learning opportunities taking place in the hallways, the on-call rooms, and the cafeteria, and even by the architecture and layout of the school itself. Although educational settings have always had a more hidden counterpart to their formal curriculum, identifying this new lens in the case of medical education came to be what Clayton Christensen called a disruptive force or innovation (Christensen 1997).

There was an almost immediate response within medical education circles: "Eureka. That's it!" Medical educators began to situate much that was bad within their training venues, or at least not going as intended, within this other space. These educators also began to recognize that much of the learning by their trainees was antithetical to what they and other faculty, the guardians of the profession, assumed students were learning through the school's meticulously planned courses, clerkships, learning objectives, and competencies. Suddenly, there was something to blame for things not working out as planned. The hidden curriculum became a scapegoat.

If the students weren't learning professional values, blame the hidden curriculum!

If the students on their clerkships weren't learning that death was imminent for some patients or that pain management was less than optimal, blame the hidden curriculum!

If the faculty were complaining about the ungrateful students only wanting to know "what will be on the test," blame the hidden curriculum!

In short order, the hidden curriculum became the usual suspect and the go-to explanation for a wide range of educational ills facing health science training—including a troubling ethical erosion; the loss of student idealism, patient-centeredness, empathy, and humanism; the rise of student burnout and cynicism; and the devastating impact of student abuse, harassment, and mistreatment. The hidden curriculum has been linked to the failure of the leaders to address problematic behavioral issues in students, and it has been linked to a host of educational challenges such as multiculturalism, cultural competency and cross-cultural care, end-of-life care, medical ethics, faculty development, resource allocation, conflict of interest and relations with industry, evidence-based medicine, mindful practice, self-awareness and relationship-centered care, clinical teaching, humanism and bedside manner, medical errors, duty hours, the impact of longitudinal training, and online learning. Its impact as an analytic tool keeps expanding as our eyes learn to see what, in the past, all too readily flew beneath our perceptual radar.

The introduction of the notion that there might be an alternative and more hidden dimension to educational practices spawned an enormous number of articles about the other-than-formal aspects of medical education. By using the keywords "hidden curriculum" to search PubMed or the Institute for Scientific Information (ISI) Web of Science, one uncovers more than 500 articles in journals covering a vast range including dentistry, dietetics education, ethics, nursing, psychiatry, evidence-based teaching, pediatrics, primary care, orthopedics, obstetrics/gynecology, anesthesia, urology orthopedics, physical therapy, internal medicine, oncology, emergency medicine, healthcare analysis, political science, urban studies, and architecture. The concept has appeared in literature from the United States, Canada, the United Kingdom, Australia, New Zealand, Europe, Scandinavia, India, Saudi Arabia, Sri Lanka, Qatar, and Japan. In the Association of American Medical Colleges' (AAMC) premier journal *Academic Medicine*, where the Hafferty and Franks article first appeared, their article is the fourth most frequently cited resource in *Academic Medicine*'s list of Citation Classics. Google Scholar lists more than 800 citations to this article. A subsequent and solo-authored article by Hafferty (1998) is the seventh most cited article in this list (with over 700 citations). A deep well had been tapped, and results were gushing.

Across such publications, one frequent focus has been on the topic of professionalism and professional formation—something that, until recently, had been conveyed primarily at a tacit and implied level, but now was becoming more explicit and codified within the formal curriculum. Indeed, it was the very formalization process that began to highlight (particularly for students) that there were disjunctions between what was currently being taught in the classroom and what had long been more tacitly conveyed on the wards and in the clinics. Thus, and somewhat ironically, the move to make professional formation more explicit helped uncover more of the places where other-than-professional values and behaviors were being transmitted. Let no good deed go unstoned.

Besides the formal medical literature, many popular books about medical training and the socialization of new recruits into healthcare—including both fictional and autobiographical accounts such as Samuel Shem's *The House of God*, *Intern* by Dr. X, and *Not an Entirely Benign Procedure* by Perri Klass; along with works by Fitzhugh Mullen, Danielle Ofri, Pauline Chen, Malcolm Connor, and many others—depict (without using the term) the hidden curriculum as part of the package of becoming a doctor.

Perhaps the most influential of all such books is Shem's 1972 classic, *The House of God*, which, along with Sinclair Lewis's *Arrowsmith*, has been called one of the two most influential books about medicine from the last century

(Kohn and Donley 2008). *The House of God* is full of clashes between implicit and explicit rules, organizational culture versus subcultures, differentials in power and status, protagonists "living the life," and the complicity of nurses and other healthcare allies. Its own counterculture resident, the Fat Man, has become an icon of rationality and resistance.

If books are one window into the hidden curriculum, so too are popular television shows and movies, such as *ER*, *Gray's Anatomy*, and *St. Elsewhere*, as well as the new genre of medical reality shows. They depict the "gritty reality" of life in the fast lane of medicine, with all of healthcare's mixed messages, contradictions, and challenges, along with vivid moments of compassion and competence.

And if medical literature, fiction, and television drama are not enough, real-life controversies—the Affordable Care Act, medical marijuana, death with dignity legislation, the wave of mergers, and the public's take on the big, bad insurers and those "greedy doctors" with their lapses of professionalism profiled in the media—all provide yet another layer of background context and windows into the inside story of medicine and medical education.

To make matters even more complex, there are many new challenges tied to our emerging technologies, such as how to apply what we've learned from the human genome project, the prospect of individualized or genomic medicine, the implications of the widespread use of social media, new tools in informatics, the role and place of the computer in the interface with patients, new learners who learn differently, the arrival of new learning technologies such as online learning and flipped classrooms, the potential of the cloud, and more. It has been said that the advent of electronic records, once predominantly aimed at billing, with their check-the-boxes-with-a-single-mouse-click formats, are becoming a huge source of fiction in medicine. Did that doctor who doesn't even have a reflex hammer really check your reflexes, as the chart says? Did that resident really do a status update, or did she merely cut and paste old information into the new record fields?

When you put on your hidden-curriculum lenses (your "new eyes"), you see that the other-than-formal aspects of organizational life and concurrent socialization practices really are *everywhere*, and the intriguing fact is that they always have been there. They just were less visible when our doctors seemed like heroes to be revered and trusted!

There have been national and international meetings about the hidden curriculum; efforts to measure it; and even a new undergraduate medical education accreditation standard (MS-31-A), adopted by the accrediting body, the Liaison Commission on Medical Education (LCME), designed to address the hidden curriculum and its impact on the learning environment. In 2010 the Association of Faculties of Medicine of Canada released a reform report (*Future of Medical Education in Canada*) listing ten key reform initiatives. "Addressing the hidden curriculum" was fifth on this list (Association of Faculties of Medicine of Canada 2013).

What an explosion of effort and implications. Nonetheless, all this activity also represents a new set of hidden curricular challenges for educators. How a hidden curriculum might operate in the shadow of the formal curriculum certainly is better understood than it was ten years ago, but how do we mold our emerging understandings for the good rather than simply identify the bad? Such challenges are the major reason for this book. We hope you will consider the range of topics covered here as a form of one-stop shopping to facilitate your journey into discovering, evaluating, understanding, and modifying this space called the hidden curriculum.

What Is the Hidden Curriculum?

When one reads the literature, it becomes clear that not every author has the same definition for, or way of thinking about, the hidden curriculum. For the purposes of this book, and as an overarching framework, we harken back to one of the earliest uses of the term and think of the hidden curriculum as "that which the school teaches without, in general, intending or being aware that it is taught" (Cowell 1972).

This definition is rooted in the distinction between intention and act, including the difference between what formally is depicted as being done versus what actually does take place during the course of everyday events. A parallel way to frame this distinction is what is listed in the course catalog versus what actually takes place on the educational shop floor. Sometimes, all parties (faculty, students, staff, administration) agree that what was learned by students was both explicitly stated and intended by faculty. But at other times, there may be no such agreement. Faculty may claim that they are teaching a great deal about a particular subject and doing so via very specific learning objectives or competencies. *Systems-based practice* (an Accreditation Council for Graduate Medical Education [ACGME] competency) might be one such example. However, students may not see the fruits of these efforts quite as clearly as faculty do, or they may feel that they are learning a lot of quite specific information never mentioned in the course syllabus.

A curriculum is a very complex thing, and, as we will see across the chapters of this book, it contains many dimensions or parts. Even the label *hidden curriculum* itself is more aptly framed as a pluralistic rather than a monolithic entity. Too often, and particularly when educators gather to undertake what they call "curricular reform"—they unfortunately limit their efforts to what we term the formal curriculum. Yet, there are lots of places where learning goes on outside this space. Throughout this book, we will encounter a variety of rather distinct curricular spaces, including the formal, the informal, the hidden, and what Flinders and colleagues (1986) have called the *null curriculum*—a space identified by what is *not* taught. Although the actual labels used, and sometimes the definitions employed, may vary for each of these spaces, the editors of this book feel that there are good analytic reasons to routinely draw upon at least four distinctions.

Types of Curricula

The formal curricular space also has been called the intended curriculum, the espoused curriculum, the written curriculum, the curriculum-on-paper, the planned curriculum, the codified curriculum, the official curriculum, the manifest curriculum, and the stated curriculum. This space is where curricular planners and reformers spend the bulk of their time revising, renewing, and reforming. This space is populated with course objectives, syllabi, competencies, and now even subcomponents ("entrustable professional activities") of those competencies. The formal curriculum also contains a second or parallel space within which students formally are evaluated—although it is important to note that even though we are still talking about testing as "stated and intended," if students are told they are responsible for a certain set of knowledge, skills, or values, and yet are assessed on other things, then we do have a hidden curriculum at work. Nonetheless, if someone asks what you teach (or evaluate) at your school (or in your course or clerkship), the response, whether it comes from the school or a given faculty member, is the formal curriculum.

In contrast to the formal curriculum, a second type of learning space focuses less on things (for example, course content, or goal-specific and sanctioned educational activities) and more on the interpersonal dynamics that populate the learning environment. This space has been called the actual curriculum, the curriculum-in-action, the experiential curriculum, the informal curriculum, the latent curriculum, and the peripheral curriculum. Though the terms just listed for the formal curriculum are fairly synonymous, the concept labels for these more ad hoc and serendipitous domains of learning house different nuances in meaning and therefore different implications for learning.

The informal curricular space refers to the idiosyncratic, sporadic, and happenstance learning that occurs when a student asks questions after class or has a conversation in the cafeteria, dorm room, elevator, or on-call room, or in the corridor outside the patient's room with a peer or teacher. There are countless places where informal learning can occur. It is an education on the fly, and thus often is unscripted and highly particular to time and place. Role modeling, both good and bad, is a very important source of informal learning—particularly given the fact that role models need not even be aware of their modeling status. As with the formal curriculum, it is important not to link or tie the informal curriculum to particular settings, places, or people. If a faculty member (role-model status or not) formally is charged with delivering specific content—and does so—then he or she is functioning as an agent of the formal curriculum. Some of the informal curriculum reinforces what is said in the classroom, but it may just as often contradict or undermine the intended and stated curriculum. This informal space is very hard or even impossible to control, but we may be able to modify its impact or at least point out inconsistencies.

A third space is the hidden curricular space. This space lies at the level of organizational culture. This is the place where one learns, often tacitly, "how things work around here." When anthropologists study a culture, they often try to distinguish among *artifacts* (cultural products such as tools, written documents, pictures or other wall decorations, the layout and organization of space, and so on); *espoused values* (mission statements, written documents, and so on); and *underlying assumptions*, the unstated, taken-for-granted, and sometimes unconscious group understandings about how things are done within the group (Schein 2004). It is in this last area where culture fundamentally exists, and just as "a fish cannot know water," so too, group members often cannot tell you why they do what they do in the way they do it. Cultures are broad, deep, stable, and very difficult to change. The culture of an organization, for example, forms an ethos in which learning goes on, and it includes such things as the architecture of the building; the power differentials between the players; and the messages about who or what is cool or valued, including what gets included and left out of awards ceremonies, who gets to be chief resident and why, who gets paid the most, who really controls the dean's budget versus who does the menial jobs, who and what types of behavior are tolerated, and who is forced to take the lecture time right after lunch. This space is neither formal nor idiosyncratic, but it does send messages to community members.

One important attribute of the hidden curriculum is that although it certainly is social and relational in nature (and thus is a product of social interactions), it also can operate devoid of people. For instance, we often can tell a great deal about how learning occurs at a school by just doing a walk-through, noticing the artifacts such as the award plaques, the space each department occupies, or even the relative distribution of large-group lecture spaces with their chairs in fixed rows and seats bolted to the floor versus more flexible small-group learning spaces. We can look at class pictures or the printed materials to see where matriculates come from or where graduates go for their residencies. We can observe how many women or minorities are in positions of power, or whether a course or material is listed as required or elective. All of these observations (and therefore lessons) can take place without ever talking to another person. Nonetheless, the information gleaned can be very informative.

In the case of education in general, and health professions education in particular, the hidden curriculum comprises the organizational contexts and cultural subtexts that shape the way students make sense of their learning environments. Examples include the more subterranean forces of organizational life, such as the structure of power and privilege, the forces of organizational culture, and the architectural layout of work and learning environments.

The hidden curriculum can be quite pervasive, and often it is hard to appreciate or fathom exactly how much is happening just beneath the surface of organizational life. Some have used the metaphor of an iceberg to describe the difference between the formal and the hidden curriculum. Students learn that there are things just under the formally stated that they also must understand or master if they are to succeed, and that many of these things differ from what they have been formally taught that they are supposed to know or do.

Finally, there is the additional challenge of noticing the null curriculum—what is not said or attended to. Here, we are talking about lessons that are conspicuous by their absence, and thus are voids that, over time, become more obvious or apparent to community members—even if they do so at a largely unconscious level. For instance, if nothing is said within the formal curriculum about social justice or teamwork, then students may conclude that these are unimportant issues, and that a whole range of related topics— such as health disparities or collaboration with other health professionals— really is not all that important or relevant to becoming a "good doctor."

An "Outside" Example

One concrete example of the role played by other-than-formal understandings in shaping social action happens in everyday driving. Although one must learn a broad array of formal rules in order to pass one's driving test and acquire a license to operate a motor vehicle, including the meaning of speed-limit signs, one also learns that many of these rules are "paper rules," and that actual driving behaviors are governed by other understandings. Virtually all roads have posted speed limits (think formal curriculum), yet virtually all drivers come to know that the "real" speed limit (at which you are allowed to drive) is something different from the posted one. This same type of street knowledge becomes significant as health professions students begin to navigate the various learning environments that make up their training. Students quickly learn (and without being formally taught) that what one teacher puts forth as core knowledge or essential skills, or what it means to "be a professional," can differ greatly from what is being put forth by another attending or on a different clinical service. Learning that much of medical education is grounded in "it depends" lessons can be very unsettling to students, many of whom signed up for what they thought would be an objective, evidence-based, scientific undertaking to learn to become a good doctor.

Hidden Agendas

An important lexiconic distinction to keep in mind as one probes the presence and impact of these four domains of learning, along with their interactions and interdependencies, is the distinction between the hidden curriculum and *hidden agendas*. Hidden agendas, by definition, imply duplicity and intentionality. Conversely, and in most cases, the hidden curriculum truly is hidden to both the purveyors and its subjects. We will speak more about hidden agendas in chapter 21, but our focus in this book is on the contrast between what is formal and intended (the formal curriculum) versus the possibility that other-than-formal factors may be influencing learning; our focus is not on how one set of actors (faculty, students, administrators) may be trying to dupe or manipulate others in the environment. There certainly may be surreptitious agendas operating within a given setting. Moreover, identifying such a presence may be valuable to understanding the full scope of factors influencing what is taking place in the learning environment. Nonetheless, the presence of guile or hypocrisy, at least at the level of those responsible for the structural integrity of the learning environment, represents a layer of social action not covered within the hidden curriculum framework.

Mastering the Hidden Curriculum

As noted by Benson Snyder more than forty years ago, the most successful students (medical or otherwise) are not those who are the brightest, but those who learn what the system really wants of them (Snyder 1971). Students spend a lot of time trying to figure out the expected versus the stated. They often get angry when there is a large gap or when they find it difficult to untangle this difference. Students also spend a lot of time engaged in what sociologists call *image management*, the putting on of masks (for example, other-than-authentic expressions or appearances) as they adapt to what they think their teachers want. They become situational chameleons, and often practice what in twelve-step programs is called "faking it until you make it."

Although such social posturings may be seen merely as situational coping mechanisms, there is a range of negative consequences, including student fears that they are losing who they "really are," along with the feeling of being unsafe or having no place to be vulnerable. What often happens in the face of these disjunctures is that students band together against what they see as the malevolent intentions of the faculty and the institution.

These other-than-formal curricular spaces should be a place for change or remediation. In a classic paper in the literature of medical education, Samuel Bloom focused on the role of structure and ideology in medical schools and their resistance to change. When we focus our remedial lens only on the formal curriculum, we doom ourselves to engineering what Bloom termed "reform without change" (Bloom 1988, 295).

A Brief History of the Hidden Curriculum in the Sociology, Education, and Medical Literature

The hidden curriculum, as a conceptual tool, first surfaced in the 1960s within the fields of sociology and education. But its roots go back even farther, at least to the time of Cotton Mather and the founders of Harvard College, who recognized the "collegiate way of living" had important implications for student learning. The hidden curriculum has many conceptual forerunners, including John Dewey's reference to *collateral learning* (the learning that takes place outside the classroom). It also has a variety of conceptual cousins, such as the sociological distinction between formal and informal norms; Robert Merton's concept of unintended consequences, and his delineation between concepts of manifest and latent functions (1957); as well as the broader educational distinctions between explicit/implicit and deep/superficial learning. Much of the early educational literature on the hidden curriculum focused on how schools (the primary focus was on elementary school education) functioned to reproduce societal values, including notions of obedience to authority and existing class structures. Those writing about this worried about the stifling of dissent or creativity.

Although there are frequent references within the hidden curriculum literature to Philip Jackson's 1968 *Life in Classrooms*, which does reference the concept within a broader discussion of student socialization in an elementary school context, a more conceptually focused work is Snyder's 1971 tome *The Hidden Curriculum*. Snyder, a physician and psychotherapist, compared student life at Wellesley College and Massachusetts Institute of Technology. He focused on the space between a school's formal expectations and real requirements versus what was "actually expected of students" (Snyder 1971, 9). As a psychiatrist, Snyder was interested in the effects of context on students, what he called the "emotional and social surround of the formal curriculum" (4). He found that the difference between the expected and its real requirements produced considerable dissonance among the students and resulted in cynicism, scorn, and hypocrisy within both student bodies. Snyder also found students engaging in a great deal of gamesmanship as they worked to figure out what the faculty really wanted, and the most successful students were the best at navigating this gap. He identified a covert student subculture in both of these learning environments and, in an important and often underappreciated distinction, he found that minority students had more difficulty in these turbulent waters.

The initial application of this concept to medical school education came in 1986 via work by Canadian sociologists Jack Haas and William Shaffir. They were interested in exploring professional socialization within the context of a newly minted problem-based learning curriculum at McMaster University (Haas and Shaffir 1986). They titled their paper "Ritual Evaluation of Competence: The Hidden Curriculum of Professionalization in an Innovative Medical School Program." Even though the article title marques the concept, the article itself only briefly references the term *hidden curriculum* and does so more as a reference label than as a point of conceptual development. Unfortunately, the article had no traceable impact on the medical education literature, perhaps related to the fact that it was published in a sociology journal or the possibility that the medical education world was not ready for a discussion about the other-than-formal aspects of medical school training. Instead, the deep dive would have to wait until 1994, when Hafferty and Franks published their opening salvo in *Academic Medicine*. As noted in my opening comments in this chapter, the implications of this work have been profound.

I want to highlight two other early and seminal works on the hidden curriculum and medical education. Edward Hundert, while dean of student affairs at Harvard, conducted a study in which all interns and residents in a general surgery program tape-recorded conversations that took place in small-group classroom settings, on-call rooms, apartments, the cafeteria ... essentially every place they went. After analyzing themes from hundreds of hours of recordings, Hundert and his colleague, Darleen Douglas-Steele, concluded that professional and moral development was more likely to occur among these trainees when faculty were *not* present, and that the informal curriculum was informal in name only (Douglas-Steele and Hundert 1996). They found that peer-influenced learning was quite rule bound in tightly governed ways and that there was an unwritten, but very evident code of behavior that was readily passed along to novitiates about how to act. Hundert suggested that "teaching hospitals" shift their moniker to a more accurate "learning hospitals," and he reflects on his journey in understanding the hidden curriculum in chapter 2.

The second important work was David Stern's PhD dissertation (Stanford University, Graduate School of Education) titled "Hanging Out: Teaching Values in Medical Education" (Stern 1996). Stern already had completed his medical training before beginning his PhD work, and he used the hidden curriculum as an analytic lens to better understand the process of professional formation within medicine. Like Douglas-Steele and Hundert, Stern found that values most often were learned when attendings were not present, late at night, and when on call. Some recommended values (for example, accountability) were displayed frequently, while others (for example, integrity) were displayed rarely. Some, such as interprofessional relationships, were learned in ways contradictory to medical school recommendations; but others, such as industry and efficiency, were learned in the absence of recommendations to do so. The learning of values, via what Stern termed *values excerpts*, took the form of jokes, quips, and narratives. The most striking finding by Stern was that the majority of values learning occurred not as dichotomous events (for example, the choice between being honest and being dishonest), but instead as a conflict between two, often equally meritorious values, such as integrity and efficiency. Both Hundert and Stern reflect in Part I on the role the hidden curriculum has played in their own understandings of medical education.

To summarize, the hidden curriculum asks observers to begin with what schools or organizations *say* they are teaching or doing (for example, their formal practices and curriculum—and as captured in documents such as course curricula, student and faculty handbooks, mission statements, and so on) and then move to the other-than-formal aspects of organizational life in order to ask, "What else is going on? What other kinds of learning are taking place?"

Some Lessons to Begin with as You Read This Book

1. The most important thing to remember about the hidden curriculum is that it is hidden. Even when certain aspects of that curriculum are "outed," vestiges are still left behind, and new configurations of hidden curricula may emerge in response to new permutations of the formal curriculum. In short, the hidden curriculum always is there and always will be.

2. The hidden curriculum is everywhere and touches everything. It is highly intertwined with and interdependent on other types of curricula, such as the formal and informal. As such, the hidden curriculum is present in the classroom, in the clinic, and at the bedside as much as it is in the

hallways, the cafeteria, and the living spaces of students. Think about the classroom and the way basic scientists teach a different version of science to graduate students versus medical students. Graduate students receive a version of science that is far more probabilistic and uncertain—with mysteries yet to be solved—than the science medical students receive. Even something as formally structured as the OSCE (Objective Structured Clinical Evaluations) can harbor a range of subterrestrial messages via the body language of different evaluators or what students are instructed to "skip" as time runs short in the later stations. The possibilities for more subterrestrial forms of learning are endless.

3. Insiders (within the system) often have a harder time "seeing" the hidden curriculum than do outsiders. Often, gaps or disjunctures between the other-than-formal curricula are most apparent to newcomers whose view of things has yet to be influenced by the "way things are supposed to be." A related opportunity for new eyes can come at points of transitions: the first days of a clerkship, internship, or new training experience. Even for those well within the system, encountering new settings and expectations can disrupt the taken-for-granted nature of everyday social life that so often hides or camouflages the hidden curriculum.

4. The hidden curriculum is extremely complex. In a classic paper, Glouberman and Zimmerman note that there are three types of problems: those that are simple, those that are complicated, and those that are complex (Glouberman and Zimmerman 2002). For complicated problems, solutions often lie with external knowledge gained from sources external to the system (for example, the space program and putting a human on the moon, with each step relying on learning done from prior space shots). For complex problems, solutions often lie with knowledge gained from within the current system (the example the coauthors mentioned was raising a child, when the experience from raising a prior child can be helpful, but often is insufficient as a guide). Hidden curricular problems may have complicated parts, but we would argue that they are best approached as complex social entities.

5. The things that happen because of the hidden curriculum are not always bad. Sometimes good learning, such as learning to be a good doctor, nurse, or pharmacist, happens in this space. Sometimes, structures or culture are in alignment with formally stated goals and objects, so the hidden curriculum is not always considered "evil" or negative.

6. Efforts to out the hidden curriculum may lead to untoward or unantic-

ipated outcomes. Witness the whole outing of professionalism for an enterprise (medicine) that seems to have lost its way. All the attention gained by taking something that largely had functioned on a tacit and implied level, and reframing it (via codes, definitions, decrees, evaluation standards, and so on) into something that now is explicit, has unintentionally fomented a situation in which students resist messages they consider more nostalgic than "real," and reject certain vehicles of education ("stop lecturing us to death about this") by their elders or their institutions, both having provided students with numerous examples of unprofessional conduct. The result has been a moving baseline about this whole concept (Hafferty 2009).

7. The hidden curriculum is very hard to address and change. Cultures are deep, wide, stable, and meant to be this way. Which is easier: to add a course on ethics or professionalism, or to change the ethical behaviors of clinical role models and mentors?

8. Much, if not most, of the focus on the effects of the hidden curriculum has targeted individuals. However, the greatest influence may be in changing the behavior of organizations. We are only at the very beginning of trying to do this effectively. Organizations are, as was said in the 1960s, "part of the problem," and therefore should be part of the solution.

9. Ignoring the hidden curriculum as we try to revise curriculum will continue to risk reform without change . . . the equivalent of moving the deck chairs around on the Titanic.

10. Finally, whatever is done to improve or close the gap between what is supposed to be learned and what is really being learned on the clinical shop floor will most certainly be difficult, but it also will have a huge impact. Closing the gap may help reduce the cynicism, burnout, dissatisfaction, unrest, and other ills that plague medicine and medical education today. Doing this may play a major role in creating the kind of safe, effective, efficient, equitable, timely, high-quality, and patient- and family-centered system—and at more reasonable costs—that we all desire.

Most of what has been written to date on the hidden curriculum has focused on noticing, describing, or defining it within the context of the educational spaces, decrying its power and influence, and advising about possible change strategies. There are several (but not many) articles about evaluating it. Most of these articles come from medicine and examine the hidden curriculum's effects on students. There also is a small but growing literature about its effects on, and between, the other health professions and on faculty, now including other players on the field, such as administrators and those in the area of human resources.

This is why we wrote this book. It is a compilation of ideas from those who have wrestled with this concept in the past and have written numerous thoughtful pieces about the hidden curriculum. As mentioned earlier, one goal for this book is that it might function as a great place for one-stop shopping about the hidden curriculum and thus a venue that covers theory, methods, and applications. There is still so much to do and to learn about this topic. This volume is meant to be a launching point, and it is up to readers to take the next step and try to harness the hidden curriculum, shape its use for good (better) outcomes, and create what we all long for, innovation *with* change.

About the Book and Its Structure

This volume has brought together, for the first time, selected essays on a diverse range of hidden curriculum topics in health professions education. The book is organized around six parts or themes:

I. Working within the Framework: Some Personal and System-Level Journeys into the Field, in which two long-time education scholars analyze the role played by the hidden curriculum in their own work, followed by a look at educational reform at a national (Canadian) level driven in part by a focus on the hidden curriculum

II. Theoretical Considerations, both descriptively (What is the hidden curriculum?) and critically (How has it been used—and not—to analyze medical education?)

III. Methodological and Assessment Approaches (How do you biopsy the hidden curriculum, and what do you do with this knowledge once you have done so?)

IV. The Hidden Curriculum and Health Professions Education (What does the hidden curriculum look like within the different domains of health professions education?)

V. Special Topics and Applications (research training, cross-national perspectives, and professional formation)

In the concluding section, the editors present their thoughts on the next generation of work to be done on the hidden curriculum.

Overall, the book contains twenty-one chapters. All but three of the chapter authors having previously published on hidden curriculum issues. The three non–hidden curriculum authors bring the concept to areas in which they have expertise, but where no hidden curriculum literature currently exists. Each author was asked to take a topic or area around which he or she had previously published, and either expand on that work or apply the hidden curriculum to a new topic or area of interest. All chapters capture new insights into the field of health professions education. The authors also were placed under rather restrictive word and page limits, and many could have gone into far greater detail about their topics. If any discussion appears overly truncated, it is the fault of the editors, not the chapter authors.

This volume is the first of its kind. No other volume on the hidden curriculum and health professions education has been published, nor is there any other volume (regardless of the academic discipline or focus) that combines theory, methods, and application into a single resource.

Some Final Thoughts

As we move into the body of the book, I want to close this introduction with three stories. Taken together, I believe they capture both the challenges and opportunities inherent in viewing health professions education through a hidden curriculum lens.

The first is my challenge story. At my school, we are in the throes of curricular reform. I am on the steering group charged with orchestrating this reform—something often characterized within this group as a "curricular overhaul." As my perceptual antenna became newly energized by this book, I found myself becoming a tireless promoter (some might say obnoxiously so) for talking about the hidden curriculum every chance I got. My goal was to get people thinking about reform *with* change. My good intentions notwithstanding, some colleagues have taken to rolling their eyes, and one even told me to stop sidetracking the group: "We don't want to go there!" I am at once bemused and befuddled. Why does this topic meet with such resistance? A book I once reviewed likened the subject of death to that of the sun. You can't stare at it too long. Does the hidden curriculum produce a similar threat? Do people really believe they will go blind if they try to fathom its depths? Whatever the case, the not-so-hidden message I have received from my colleagues is that faculty feel more at home reengineering the formal curriculum than they do redesigning the learning environments that make up, in this case, the medical school experience. As such, I fear we will endlessly revisit Bloom's reform without change.

My second story reinforces the reform-without-change theme while, I believe, pointing to the hidden curriculum as a way out. In addition to curricular reform, I recently had to weather a "space reform," and move out of an office I had occupied for many years. In cleaning out my files, I came across a poster summarizing a curricular renewal process we had undergone in 1996. The principles outlined on this poster were unnervingly similar to those produced in 2013! The principles and strategies we are seeing as visionary and cutting edge today are virtually indistinguishable from our cutting-edge "visionizing" of almost twenty years previously. It was as if all the changes we had made in the interim—and there were real changes, by the way—had become hidden over time. What is going on? Why this invisibility? Why this organizational blindness?

As I pondered this 1996 poster and its implications, I also came to realize another aspect of our dilemma: unless something was formally labeled with a name, it did not exist. For example, in 1996 we intentionally began to design student learning exercises that were integrated across a variety of courses and learning environments. In doing so, we unintentionally—but also unknowingly—made these exercises largely invisible to both students and faculty. Then, when one of our current students began to complain about the lack of current ethics teaching, something we had doggedly worked to integrate into a range of course settings and formats in 1996, I realized that ethics was recognized by students as "ethics" only when we labeled it as such. No label—no ethics.

We had a similar conundrum with the issue of feedback. For many students, feedback had become something that took place only when a session formally was identified as a "feedback session." It was as if someone had to get up on a chair at the front of the room and announce, "This is a feedback session" for students to take what was being said as feedback. Otherwise, it was viewed either as something else, or worse, as something bad—perhaps criticism, or worse yet, "student bashing."

By embedding educational initiatives within larger curricular settings, but without the labels, we unknowingly had created an invisible curriculum. This same form of evanescence could be seen among faculty as well.

During our recent LCME self-study, and in an effort to identify content, we did a lot of "curricular mapping." However, my new hidden-curriculum eyes made me realize that some of the things we had intentionally integrated during our previous reform efforts were nowhere to be seen on this new map. The topics had become unintentionally invisible. A lot really had changed in the ensuing two decades, but it seemed that those of us who had lived through the changes had become more like the proverbial frog immersed in the slowly bubbling pot of hot water than sentient beings mindfully attuned to changes in our environment (much of which we had created).

My third story is another wake-up for me on how far the concept of the hidden curriculum has become embedded in even more of what we do than my pre-book eyes had even imagined. One of the signature activities at my school is the production of the *Dartmouth Atlas of Healthcare*. Even though I now see that this atlas is loaded with "hidden" hidden curricular issues (see chapter 21 for more on this distinction), only recently have atlas-related publications begun to out some of these invisibilities. For example, a recent publication from the *Dartmouth Atlas* specifically refers to the hidden curriculum in terms of the culture of training sites (and the way they go about doing their work), and it gives advice to students applying to these schools to be aware of hidden curricular issues at these sites. Here is a quote from this publication:

> It is also important to know that each teaching hospital has its own style and culture of practice that represents a hidden training curriculum. This *Dartmouth Atlas* report will help you understand these less visible hospital characteristics that can have profound effects on how you care for patients. The report first provides background on health care variation and then presents information about specific teaching hospitals. When you read the report, we would encourage you to consider the current problems and future opportunities in health care, and how your training can help you become a leader in tomorrow's health care system. (Aurora and True 2012)

When I run into publications like this, I realize that the hidden curriculum has come into its own as a key concept in how we approach all kinds of things, not only in medical education but in medical practice as well. It is an emerging theme within the quality of care and the patient safety literature. There even are funding sources to study it! The Arnold P. Gold Foundation recently announced a hidden curriculum initiative for graduate medical education and is soliciting proposals from ACGME-accredited residency programs for educational interventions that seek to mitigate the negative consequences of the hidden curriculum on the delivery of compassionate, patient-centered care.

Now, the hidden curriculum, at least as it applies to health professions education, has its own book! We hope you will enjoy our attempt to produce a place for one-stop shopping.

PART I

WORKING WITHIN THE FRAMEWORK

Some Personal and System-Level Journeys into the Field

Our opening section provides readers with an overview of the field, first by calling upon two of the earliest writers on the hidden curriculum, followed by a contemporary journey into educational reform using this concept as a conceptual fulcrum. The three chapters in part 1 represent an overview that covers where-have-we-come-from and where-might-we-be-going. Both David Stern (chapter 1) and Ed Hundert (chapter 2) played key roles in applying the hidden curriculum to medical education; and we, as editors, asked both authors to look back on their early work and appraise the current state of the field from that vantage point.

Hundert's work, undertaken in the early 1990s while he was at Harvard, was the earliest large-scale effort to systematically examine the other-than-formal aspects of medical learning at both the medical school and residency levels. In what was then a relatively radical finding, Hundert and his colleagues discovered that the most important influences on trainee moral and professional development took place outside the scope of the formal curriculum and within conversations where no faculty were present. Meanwhile, 3,000 miles to the west, in Palo Alto, California, Stern was adding a PhD in education to his MD degree by applying this concept to his study of medical students, residents, and attendings on an inpatient ward. Like Hundert, Stern found that key occupational values were being taught most frequently during times (late at night, on-call rooms) when attendings were not present. We also were struck by Hundert's observation that after an extended period of time away from using the hidden curriculum as a conceptual lens, he found, as Jean-Batiste Alphonse Karr wrote in 1849, *Plus ça change, plus c'est la meme chose* (The more things change, the more they remain the same).

Our third chapter in part 1 is by Brian Hodges and Ayelet Kuper. They stake out a more contemporary arena by examining how the hidden curriculum became a key tool in a national Canadian effort to reform medical education. Although, as noted by the authors, the hidden curriculum had "entered the everyday discourse of medical education" by the twenty-first century, there still was no overarching framework for situating this concept within large-scale educational reform—an effort the authors capture in their chapter. This chapter also highlights a theme that surfaces throughout this book, most notably in chapter 4, by Janelle Taylor and Claire Wendland, which opens part 2. Although the hidden curriculum is grounded in the conceptual frameworks of culture and context, there has been a disconcerting tendency among medical education reformers over the past twenty years to seek solutions at the level of individuals (for example, students and faculty) or, in the words of Hodges and Kuper, through "simplistic curricular interventions" rather than via a more fundamental redesign of those structures and culture. This tendency—some might say perversion—is itself a product of medicine's "culture of no culture" (Taylor 2003) and, as noted by Taylor and Wendland in chapter 4, represents one of the primary reasons that the hidden curriculum remains hidden.

1: A Hidden Narrative

DAVID T. STERN

When Fred and Joe invited me to write this opening chapter, I was both honored and intimidated. Since the first moment I learned about the concept of the hidden curriculum, it has been the single most influential idea in my research on professional behavior in medicine. As often happens with discoveries, both Fred and I were thinking about the hidden in the early 1990s, and we have lived with the idea through our professional careers. For that reason, we decided to open this book on the hidden curriculum with a personal narrative of my experience with the hidden (which tracks the narrative of the hidden curriculum in medical education). This chapter begins with how I first understood when, where, and how the hidden curriculum operated in the context of medical education. I will discuss some unique ways that teachers teach in the hidden, and then describe how I believe we can most effectively use our understanding of the hidden curriculum to influence the professional formation of physicians.

Finding the Hidden

In the fall of 1992, having recently completed an intense internal medicine residency, I was enjoying the relatively diastolic life of a graduate student at Stanford Graduate School of Education. I selected courses based on faculty popularity rather than content per se, which explains how I found myself sitting in the back row of a course on curriculum theory. The attraction here was Professor Elliot Eisner, an art educator by training, who cares as much about beautiful ideas as he does about the aesthetics of how they are communicated.

My self-appointed task was to absorb the educational theories expounded for this roomful of elementary and secondary school teachers and interpret them within the context of medical education. In one class, Professor Eisner spoke about the three curricula that all schools teach: the *explicit*, the *implicit*, and the *null* (Eisner 1985). The explicit seemed easiest to understand. It is all the content intentionally taught by teachers. It includes the philosophy of a school, the course objectives, syllabi, lecture notes, slides, activities, and even examinations that form the explicit learning content of the school.

The null curriculum is that which is intentionally not taught. Eisner's mission had been to demonstrate how the lack of art education in schools not only creates a society ignorant of aesthetic perspective, but also (by failing to include it in the curriculum) a society that fails to see the value of art. The first example that came to mind was a historical one. Ethicists in the 1970s and 1980s had been fighting for legitimacy in the traditional curriculum dominated by the basic sciences. Most medical schools in the 1970s had no formal ethics curriculum, leaving it to the null domain (Eisner 1985; Flinders et al. 1986). Students did not simply fail to learn the utility of applying ethical concepts to the practice of medicine, they also learned (by its intentional absence) that their deans and teachers believed ethics to be irrelevant in comparison to the explanatory power of physiology and pharmacology. Through its absence, students learned that ethics had no place in medicine. By the early 1990s, the tide had turned. Medical schools had adopted medical ethics as a core competency, and accrediting organizations ensured that ethics permanently moved from the null to the explicit curriculum (Hutzler 2012).

An example of something that remains in the null curriculum for many allopathic medical schools is the (lack of) teaching about the use of chiropractic as a therapy for back pain. By not teaching manipulation techniques, allopathic medical schools not only fail to provide physicians with those skills (for better or worse), but also teach (by avoiding teaching) that chiropractic is valueless or even harmful. If manipulation had any value, medical students reason, of course we would have been taught how to use—or at least when to refer for—these techniques.

It was, however, the implicit curriculum that most held my attention. Eisner prefers the term *implicit* to *hidden* for a variety of reasons, not the least of which is that it forms a pleasantly parallel construct alongside the explicit and null. The idea of the implicit (hereafter referred to as hidden) derives from educational theory at least as far back as Dewey (1938, 49), who preferred the term *collateral learning*:

> Perhaps the greatest of all pedagogical fallacies is the notion that a person learns only the particular thing he is studying at the time. Collateral

learning in the way of formation of enduring attitudes, of likes and dislikes, may be and often is much more important than the spelling lesson or lesson in geography or history that is learned.

A vibrant example to consider is the 1968 book by Philip Jackson reporting on his sabbatical year observing in elementary school classrooms. In his analysis, there was more happening in the classroom than the items listed in the daily lesson planner. "The other curriculum might be described as unofficial or perhaps even hidden. . . . This hidden curriculum can also be represented by the three R's, but not the familiar one of reading, 'riting, and 'rithmetic. It is, instead, the curriculum of rules, regulations, and routines, of things teachers and students must learn if they are to make their way with minimum pain in the social institution called the school" (Jackson 1968, 145–6).

Remember being in first and second grade and the teacher asked, "What's 2 plus 2?" If you blurted out the answer "4" you were likely chastised. Only after properly raising your hand, waiting to be called upon, and then providing the answer were you praised for correctness. School is not just about learning the right answers—it is about learning normative behavior in a civil society.

It was a very short cognitive step for me to consider the "normative behaviors" we try to teach in medical education. The values of the profession, like the values of a civil society, have been a core part of the profession since its inception. Although much work was under way in the 1970s considering how doctors learn clinical reasoning and clinical skills (Elstein et al. 1978; Harden et al. 1975), few considered how professional values and behaviors were taught, learned, or evaluated in medical education.

So when—and where and how—are these values taught? Where is the hidden curriculum in medical training? To find out, I designed my dissertation in education, in part, after the work of Jackson to observe medical school "classrooms" and look for the hidden teaching of values (Stern 1996). Except that in medical training, the classrooms are actually hospital wards, call rooms, conference rooms, cafeterias, and elevators. In these early studies, I found that at least two-thirds of the "teaching" of professional behavior was done during the non-explicit or hidden part of the curriculum of clinical education in medicine. Professional behaviors were sometimes taught in formal settings such as noon conferences or teaching rounds, but were more often taught in what I call the "interstitial fluid of the day," walking in the hallway, in the elevators, sitting in conference rooms writing notes, or in the cafeteria (Stern 1998b).

I also discovered that this construct of the hidden curriculum provided a solution to the problem of why graduating medical students and residents do not appear to adopt all the professional behaviors that we expect. An example of a value that is both expected and taught in the hidden curriculum is the value of responsibility. Assuming personal responsibility for the care of patients is a core principle of medicine found in nearly every code written for the profession (Stern 1996). In the setting of clinical medical education, responsibility is taught nearly constantly. Every morning, a team rounds on "their" patients. Each team member has been assigned responsibility for one or more patients. All medical students know that they are to have the complete history, examination, laboratory tests, and latest vital signs on every patient. The medical students are responsible for reporting this information to the residents, and the residents to the attendings. Attending physicians are responsible for the final outcome of care, along with the myriad performance metrics of the hospital. There are no formal lectures about responsibility—it is taught in this hidden curriculum and remains consistent with our professional norms.

In contrast, there are some values that we intend to teach, and are taught (through the hidden curriculum) as the opposite. The hidden curriculum is far more powerful than any written code or any formal lecture about professional expectations. Take teamwork and interprofessional respect, for example. Like responsibility, these are generally considered goals of medicine and even play a key role in the most recent comprehensive accreditation standards for all residency training programs in the United States. But in the real-world setting of the hospital, interprofessional *dis*-respect is far more commonly taught in the hidden curriculum than interprofessional respect. (Note that this specific observation was made in the late 1990s, and I am open to the possibility that it has changed over time. I have not yet seen any contradictory data, however, and personal experience in the past decade has found this unprofessional value to be as pervasive as ever.) Take, for example, the following disparaging remark from an internal medicine resident in morning report about surgeons: "Well, you know what they say about surgeons: if they've done one before, then they've clearly seen it happen, if they've done two they have a lot of experience with it, and if they've done three then they've got an *extensive series*" (Stern 1996, 62). The idea that the work of surgeons is not evidence based, and they rely on their wits more than knowledge or science, comes through with sarcasm.

With the hidden curriculum identified as the intermediary factor between our expectations for education and the observed outcomes, the next logical question is how we might intervene to alter, interfere, or adapt this hidden curriculum to ensure the intended outcomes of professional behavior. The hidden curriculum, by the nature of being hidden, resists formal intrusion. Add a lecture to counteract its force, and students and residents simply go back to the hospital and continue to behave in the normative fashion that works well for the entire world around them (including their attendings, the nurses, other residents, other specialties, and so on). The hidden curriculum is in many ways the result of myriad noncurricular influences including personal beliefs, cultural norms, and organizational structure.

The Pedagogy of the Hidden

A key to understanding how one might influence change in the hidden curriculum is to understand how professional behaviors are naturally taught in the hidden curriculum. Though there may be many more pedagogical forms, two have stood out in my research in this arena: (1) parables, and (2) the physical and organizational structure of the learning environment.

Parables are a common pedagogical mode in the hidden curriculum. Parables are stories with a moral purpose. In popular literature, parables often are signified by their opening statement (for example, "Once upon a time"). In the context of medical training, we are always telling stories, but mostly we perceive these stories as simple medical histories with a formulaic narrative ("A forty-five-year-old male came to clinic with chest pain"). However, if observed carefully, there are other narratives that appear at first to be about patient care, but contain within them a moral purpose. In the context of medicine, these narratives also have a clear opening statement that signifies to the listener that this is a parable, not just a medical history. These parables often start with "I had this *great* case," or "When I was an intern . . ." Consider the following interaction overheard in attending rounds when a student asked the attending about the rate of nephrectomy after kidney biopsy:

In my whole career, I've been a nephrologist for 25 years. Uh, I've lost one kidney doing biopsies every year. And there was this schizophrenic patient who we biopsied, I did not allow the fellow to do the biopsy because I knew it was going to be a difficult one. I did it myself because I know I'm fast. And the patient screamed at the moment I was in the kidney, meaning that the kidney moved at the time that I was in there holding the outside and there was a tear in the kidney. We tried to do angiography to stop the bleeding. The kidney was finally removed, this patient lost the kidney. This was one of the most dramatic situations I've ever had, and it's actually quite rare to have a significant complication, to have a nephrectomy, it's one in one thousand. (Stern 1996, 79)

Of course the attending in this case could have just provided the answer: one in one thousand. But instead, he told a story, a parable that was intended to impart some of the principles of being a physician. I never asked this attending physician his intentions, but one can clearly see some values that might be learned by a student listener: responsibility, accountability, hierarchy. Although there are faculty development programs to enhance teachers' use of narratives to relate patient stories to assist them in managing their own emotional responses, and to engage with patients in a more personal fashion (Charon 2004), I am unaware of any programs that help educators use parables in a conscious and deliberate fashion to infiltrate the hidden curriculum.

The second pedagogical method in the hidden curriculum is the physical and organizational structure built into the learning environment. I believe that this pedagogical "method" is far more efficient and effective than any means relying on the individual behavior of teachers. The environment teaches in a hidden, but pervasive fashion. The first example I found of this was the teaching of confidentiality in clinical settings. Forty years ago, many hospitals kept charts on a clipboard hanging from the footboard of each patient bed, available for anyone walking past to peruse. Today, all medical records are electronic, kept on highly secure servers, and available only with password entry, often after the requisite warning that all patient information must be kept confidential. The structure of the educational environment enforces the behavior of confidentiality far better than do hours of lecture or even cautionary tales of senior faculty dismissed for improper access to a celebrity's chart.

From the annals of elementary school education, we know that cooperative or team learning started and stuck when schools stopped constructing classrooms with desks bolted to the floor facing the teacher's podium and allowed chairs to be moved into circles for group learning (Cuban 1997). When the physical fitness movement of the 1940s found its way into our schools, gymnasiums and football fields became a permanent structure of the educational landscape, encouraging all children to participate in a variety of sports, and resisting (by its sheer physical presence) any efforts to eliminate sports from the curriculum of secondary education in America.

So how might one harness the physical organizational elements of the learning environment in medical education to influence the hidden curriculum? I will provide one example here, but I expect there are many others playing out in hospitals and medical schools around the world. For the past decade at Mount Sinai Hospital, because of a need for efficiency and rapid bed turnover, patients admitted to the medical service were admitted to the first open bed, regardless of the team to which the patient was assigned. The resulting effect was that a teaching team could have patients spread across four to six separate units. In 2011, a group of faculty and residents convinced the hospital leadership that ward-based teams would allow for greater accountability for the metrics of care, and could influence a variety of metrics that the administration holds dear (including length of stay, readmission rate, and patient satisfaction). Though it was not designed to influence professional behaviors, we proposed that such an organizational change might well improve interprofessional relationships, enhance patient centeredness, and through these social mediators, lead to changes in patient satisfaction, pain scores, and more. With today's ward-based medical teams, a patient is admitted to a unit that is covered by a single team of attending, residents, medical students, nurses, social workers, and case managers.

Imagine the following scenario. In the past, a patient requested a pain medication by pressing the nurse call button. The nurse arrived, evaluated the patient, and looked to see if a medication was already prescribed. If not, the nurse had to find the physician. (Here's where the fun began.) The nurse looked up the doctor on call. As often as not, this was not the right physician, so another call had to be made to the covering physician. That physician was unlikely to be on the unit at the time, so he or she had to get to the unit when other activities calmed down. At that point, the doctor went in to see the patient, completed the evaluation, wrote the order, and tried to find the correct nurse to administer the medication.

With ward-based medical teams, the patient calls the nurse, who can easily find the physician assigned to the ward unit. The nurse knows who this person is because this team is on the ward all day long and works only on this unit for a month-long period. A quick conversation, evaluation, and order in the chart follows. The consequences of ward-based teams are as follows: (1) improved clinical care (less pain for patients, greater patient satisfaction, and improved patient outcomes); (2) improved interprofessional relationships (convenient communication between nurse and physician); and (3) enhanced teamwork (all members of the multidisciplinary team are aware of all other members caring for these patients).

Concluding Thoughts

In 2006 Maxine Papadakis and I wrote a review of how to teach professionalism in medical education (Stern and Papadakis 2006). We divided these methods into three categories: expectations (codes, oaths), experiences (both explicit and hidden), and evaluation (measuring professionalism). Although codes and oaths are essential, I believe that editing them or adding components has little effect on behavior. I also believe that measuring professional behavior is essential to the education of physicians. New metrics and accountability have helped us identify and dismiss those who are in the very small minority of unprofessional physicians who should not be allowed to practice. But new methods of measurement have little effect on the majority of students and physicians who behave professionally in most contexts most of the time.

Very few physicians are so morally bereft that they must be expelled from practice; very few physicians are so morally sound that they behave admirably in the worst of situations. I believe that only changes in the hidden curriculum can shift the behaviors of the vast majority of students and physicians who are likely to be influenced by context. I have outlined a few potential methods by which educators as individuals could effect change in the hidden curriculum, yet I believe that future research will demonstrate that organizational and structural change in the learning environment is the most potent and durable method for instilling professional behavior.

The organizational and physical structure of a hospital can potentially teach in the hidden. While research is ongoing to provide evidence to support this assertion, it is worthwhile for educators to consider the changes that could be made to create a learning environment that teaches professional values. Alert to opportunities like the ones I have just described, medical educators stand a chance to use the hidden curriculum to instill the values to which we aspire.

2: A Systems Approach to the Multilayered Hidden Curriculum

EDWARD M. HUNDERT

The invitation to write this chapter has been a wonderful opportunity for reflection. In the early to mid-1990s, as a student affairs dean, I saw every day how the hidden curriculum was adversely affecting the lives of our medical students. Action was clearly needed. Specifically, we needed both to prevent the hidden curriculum's damaging effects on our students' professional development and to harness its power to reinforce the positive values that continue to bring young people to the profession of medicine. A generous grant from the Charles E. Culpeper Foundation funded an empirical study of the hidden curriculum that I remember presenting as one of the three keynotes at the 1995 Association of American Medical Colleges (AAMC) conference, "Ethical and Professional Development of Medical Students and Residents" (Hundert, Hafferty, and Christakis 1996). We were finally focusing the profession's attention on these issues (Hundert, Douglas-Steele, and Bickel 1996; Wear 1997, 1998; Cruess and Cruess 1997a; Hafferty 1998; Stern 1998a). We were going to change the world—or at least the culture within which students and residents learn and work!

Fate sometimes has quite a sense of humor. In the late 1990s, I began a decade away from student affairs and research on student development, serving in leadership roles first as dean of a medical school and then as president of a research university. During those years, I was privileged to interact with people, processes, and organizations that can really make a difference. Whenever possible, I would try to exert a positive influence on the hidden curriculum issues I had studied. One of my fondest memories was of the time when I was moved to send out a university-wide email on election night 2004 as I watched the returns come in, expressing solidarity with our gay and lesbian faculty, students, and staff when the state where I worked overwhelmingly passed a referendum prohibiting access to benefits for same-sex couples. Over the weeks that followed, I was overwhelmed by literally thousands of emails—from all over the world—filled with gratitude and excitement at this expression of moral support. Leadership can make a difference, and I remember being glad, as those email responses poured in, that I had been part of the original group that tried to bring hidden curriculum issues to the attention of the leaders of medicine and medical education.

Even so, when I left the crush of those administrative leadership roles and returned several years ago to my first love of medical student teaching and learning, I was saddened to find that little had improved over the ensuing decade in these areas that I had previously studied. Although some of the worst kinds of sexism and gross faculty misbehavior were being weeded out of academic medicine during the 1970s and 1980s, any impact from our "hidden curriculum movement" of the 1990s was hard to discern. Both the mixed messages about what gets rewarded and the power structures that inhibit students from speaking up about it appear to be as ubiquitous today as they were fifteen years ago (even as there is more handwringing than ever about "professionalism"). What is definitely different now is the way I understand these matters as a result of my experience of the past two decades. Perhaps the best way to explain this change in perspective is with a "case."

As brief background, it is important to consider what we psychiatrists are fond of referring to as "framework issues" in the establishment of professional relationships. I remember as a resident going to my clinical supervisor for advice about a new patient who had presented to my clinic. During my intake interview, the patient had asked if I might be willing to fudge the insurance forms in such a way that she could get covered to come in more frequently for the treatment she both needed and wanted. Though some utilitarian calculation might have supported my conspiring with her to agree to this request, there were two larger problems my supervisor and I discussed. First, as a legal matter, one should never engage in insurance fraud, which is what such action would have constituted. But second, as an ethical and clinical matter, my wise teacher asked me to ponder the therapeutic future of a patient-doctor relationship established through an agreement to lie and break the rules. Why, if I agreed to lie along with her in establishing our "contract," would either the patient or I feel confident that *anything* said within that relationship should be assumed to have integrity and veracity?

Interestingly, a few years later, I was interviewing a candidate for a much-needed administrative assistant for my office. This candidate was the most "highly rated" person sent down from human resources, yet she asked me during the interview whether I might be willing to fudge one piece of information on the personnel form if I hired her, because doing so would entitle her to significantly better benefits more quickly, which would "help her out enormously." I had a "Yoda moment," recalling my clinical supervisor during my residency. Until that moment, this candidate had seemed like just the right person for the job. But why would I assume that her work would always embody the highest standards of professionalism if the very framework within which I hired her was itself breaking the established rules of hiring professionals?

As you may have already guessed, the case I would like to analyze here is a paradigmatic hidden curriculum issue: the lived experience of fourth-year medical students as they go through the mating ritual known as the "Match." The rules of the National Resident Matching Program (NRMP) are clear. These rules create a set of conditions that, if followed by all parties, brilliantly optimize the outcomes for the placement of students in the hospitals students want most and in the residency programs that most want those students in return. This "economic efficiency" of the Match algorithm is, however, entirely dependent on everyone's following the rules. The most salient of these rules expressly forbids either the programs or the applicants from making their rankings conditional on what the other party promises to do with its rankings. The rules are clear: a program is not to rank an applicant higher or lower on the hospital's list because of any promises from that applicant about where, on his or her own rank list, that applicant will rank the program. Specifically, the rules prohibit programs from even asking whether a student intends to rank the program number one (or anywhere else) on his or her list.

During the closing weeks of the process each year, when programs are finalizing their Match lists, fourth-year students spend a shocking amount of time in student affairs offices around the country asking for advice about how to respond to the many programs that break this rule by asking, directly or indirectly, for a promise that the student will rank the program number one. This rule-breaking behavior is worse in some specialties than in others, and in some programs and hospitals than in others (Jena et al. 2012). Some program directors organize the ritual to give themselves "plausible deniability," so that it is a faculty member not directly involved with running the residency who has the conversation with the applicant about his or her intentions; or, more commonly, who mentions to the applicant that "if you want to match here, it would be a good idea to send the chief a letter saying this is your number one." So each winter, in conversations with their trusted advisors on the faculty, close friends and family members, and student affairs deans, fourth-year students wrestle with the age-old dilemma of trying to be ethical when caught inside an unethical framework. The students are torn, and wonder: "If they are breaking the rules, don't they deserve to be lied to in return?" "If they are putting me in this situation 'illegally,' maybe I should just tell them I'm ranking them number one even if I'm not." And these students may have even read the empirical literature, which shows that, in some cases, such lying does in fact help students' Match results (Miller et al. 2003).

This case is important, because *the NRMP is the process by which every medical student in the United States gets his or her first job as a physician.* In legalistic terms, the NRMP literally establishes the contract for how new doctors enter their first professional role to care for patients in this country. In terms of professionalism, the NRMP process thereby establishes the moral framework for how physicians in America should be expected to exhibit professional conduct and practice medicine with integrity. When our students' lived reality of the very framework that establishes their first job as a physician is an experience involving strategic miscommunications, deception, and breaking of well-articulated rules, why are we surprised that concerns about professionalism are ubiquitous?

How are we to understand this unfortunate picture? Back in my days in student affairs, I was convinced that the program directors were to blame. There was no excuse for putting our students in this impossible situation; residency directors knew the rules as well as we did. I was part of a group of wonderful student affairs colleagues around the country, and we were not going to sit idly by while this misbehavior continued. We telephoned program directors to challenge them—but would of course do so only after Match day, so as not to potentially hurt our applicants who might be difficult to keep anonymous in these conversations. On my calls, I tried to explain the framework issue mentioned earlier: I challenged these program directors to *look inward* if they found that their residents were not living up to the highest standards of professional behavior! Why should they expect professionalism from their residents when, as training directors and role models, they had flaunted the rules governing the very process by which they hired these wonderful young people?

With so many student affairs colleagues busy making untold numbers of these same telephone calls to program directors, we never stopped to notice that all of our do-gooder efforts to "protect" our medical students were having little to no effect. Year after year we made our calls. Year after year the problem persisted, and it still persists today. The simple reason for this failure is that our efforts were *not directed at the actual source of the problem.*

The perspectives I gleaned in my subsequent administrative leadership roles suggest a more complicated picture than "program directors need to stop breaking the rules." Faculty members—even senior faculty members—have their own hidden curriculum of course, and, just like our students, we are all continually responding to the mixed signals and perverse incentives in our own work environments. I remember my first Match day as medical school dean, when all of the clinical department chairs reported jointly to me and the hospital CEO. When the CEO and I met with all of the chairs to learn about their results at the end of the day, they all proudly shared how successful their matches had been by detailing how far down their list they had gone to fill their program. "We had our best year ever—amazingly, we only went down to number fourteen on our list to fill all twelve slots!" one chair exclaimed. She must have seen the look of horror on my face, and it was all I could do in that moment to ask her to share instead with all the other chairs some of the attributes of the twelve people who had Matched—what medical schools they had attended, what accomplishments they had achieved, their diversity as a group—to get us excited about their joining us as trainees at our medical center.

After the meeting, I asked the hospital CEO (one of my favorite people) about the metric of "how far down the list we went" as a measure of success in the Match. He explained that this is the information the chairs request from their program directors, because it is the information filtered up to him for his annual report on the success of the Match to the hospital's board of trustees. I tried to explain not only why that metric is irrelevant, but worse, that it creates the incentive for our faculty to pressure students with conditional offers ("We'll rank you in one of our top twelve 'guaranteed' slots only if you promise to rank us first"), which is against the NRMP rules. I tried to explain how the Match algorithm ensures that if no one engaged in this behavior, we would get pretty much the same interns and residents, but we might go down to number twenty to fill those twelve slots. I told the CEO that I wanted to lead a campaign to start telling the chairs, program directors, and trustees that we never again want to hear about how far down the list they went—we only want to hear about the wonderful qualities of the new interns and residents they have attracted.

This case illustrates a *systems perspective* on the hidden curriculum because of the parallels that exist at every level in the hierarchy. Hospital CEOs have to navigate their own hidden curriculum. This CEO asked me what I thought the trustees' reaction would be when the new do-gooder dean informed them that we would—for the first time, and in contrast to the data received by their friends who are trustees at other teaching hospitals—no longer be informing the trustees how far down the lists we went to fill our programs. Would they not assume our Match must have gone worse than usual this year? And at the upcoming board of trustees meeting where I wanted to roll out this new plan, the CEO asked suggestively, "Didn't the two of us have some other tough things to discuss with the trustees in some other areas where things actually weren't going as well as we'd like, when the Match was in fact a big success?"

In an era when trickle-down theories have a highly charged connotation, such a systems-eye view of this Match-rules-breaking case suggests what I would call a *trickle-up* systems theory of the hidden curriculum, and I am not alone (Haidet 2008; Lucey and Souba 2010; Hafferty and Levinson 2008; Smith et al. 2007; Castellani and Hafferty 2006). The Match is just one example, and I could elaborate on many others, thanks to the large supply of case studies that are presented to me on regularly by third-year students at Harvard Medical School. Besides directing our sixteen-week required Medical Ethics and Professionalism course in the first-year curriculum, I have the joy and challenge of meeting every few weeks with third-year students who bring in "ethical issues from the wards" to discuss together in small, confidential groups. Although some of their cases are classic bioethics issues (end-of-life decision making and the like), the majority are classic hidden curriculum issues (Gaufberg et al. 2010). As the students describe with great emotion the behavior of some resident or attending physician that the students find unprofessional or otherwise problematic, I encourage them to ask themselves whether they think this person is a bad apple or just responding rationally to the incentives of his or her own lived environment. Very often, the incentives discerned by the students turn out to be some insurance-based formula driving clinical reimbursement rates, or a hospital policy that may have been designed with good intentions to solve some other problem, but is now having the unintended consequence of driving the behavior that the students see as inappropriate. There are, of course, some bad apples, but the majority of cases turn out to be systems issues of one sort or another.

Liao, Thomas, and Bell (2013) have recently pointed out the parallel here with the patient safety movement. As long as attention was focused on individual clinicians and their errors, it was impossible to begin to improve patient safety. It is only by taking a systems approach to safety that we can change the professional environment within which each person is trying to do his or her best. Here, I propose that exactly the same dynamic is at work for most hidden curriculum issues, and our attention needs to shift to multilayered systems if we are finally going to improve in these areas as well. Too many of our efforts to improve the hidden curriculum resemble the proverbial drunk looking for his car keys under the street lamp not because that is where he lost them, but because that is where the light is. We need to shift our attention to the root causes of these problems and stop treating symptoms. It turns out that most of the residency program directors getting those haughty calls from student affairs deans would themselves rather be following the NRMP rules; they do not want to be reporting their Match results in that irrelevant way either.

Two caveats are in order. First, in the spirit of looking inward, it is important that the conclusion of this chapter *not* be that we stop working at the student and faculty level to improve the professional milieu of medical education and focus instead entirely on how hospital boards evaluate their CEOs or on insurance reform to change reimbursement formulas. Indeed, even in the case example presented here, medical schools themselves frequently used to "advertise" what percentage of their students got their first or second choices in the Match, when this statistic should be equally irrelevant (and in fact, almost all schools have the same high first/second-choice percent fill rate, given the NRMP algorithm). I recall from my days as a student affairs dean one wonderful student who was torturing himself over his rank list because he knew his true first-choice program was such a reach, and he did not want to let the school down by hurting our statistics on what percentage of students land their first choice! We can still do a lot better just by focusing on our own behavior. (In a true systems solution to that particular subproblem, the NRMP has since stopped reporting to schools what percentage of their student body match to their first, second, third, and so on, choices to remove the temptation for this misleading advertising.)

My Delphic look-inward reminder is especially important during the current wave of curriculum reform at medical schools across the country, virtually all of which include a goal to improve the environment for the development of professionalism in the students who will go through the "new curriculum." Because previous waves of curriculum reforms have included a similar aspiration, I urge better attention to this systems perspective so that the next wave of curricula can be more successful in achieving this laudable goal. My main advice to these schools, by the way, is to focus more on the alignment of assessments, because experience shows that even the best-designed course or clerkship can stoke students' feelings of cynicism and bitterness when the stated and the lived assessment criteria are divergent.

The idea of building "professionalism training" into the formal curriculum has been around since the hidden curriculum movement emerged. In the late 1990s, approximately 90 percent of medical schools reported "teaching professionalism" in their curriculum (Swick et al. 1999). But if the systems issues at the root of many of our challenges remain unaddressed, it is even possible that teaching students an idealized view of professional values will set them up for even more cynicism and bitterness when they encounter the realities of the modern clinical world (D'Eon et al. 2007). My latest effort to address this in my own teaching has been to capture the hidden curriculum stories of our third-year students and, with their permission, use these as the cases in our first-year curriculum! In small groups at the end of the first year, we spend two hours discussing "ethical issues of doctors in training" using actual cases from the students just a couple of years ahead. The first-year students write short papers on strategies they can use to maintain their values in the face of such systems challenges, and we discuss these strategies together. Having started this a few years ago, we are already seeing some benefits for the third-year students, who, having discussed these issues in advance, report feeling more prepared (if not "fully immunized") for the realities that the clinical clerkships bring in this regard.

The second important caveat is that everything written here has been said before in one way or another (Bloom 1989; Hafferty 1998), so the question remains: Why do we think, "*This* time we really mean it that we're going to save the world—or at least the culture within which students and residents learn and work"? One lesson learned from my experiences away, in various leadership roles, is humility regarding the likelihood of achieving culture change even when you have the "commitment from leadership" that everyone knows is one necessary condition for such change (Souba 2010). All too often, misaligned governance structures induce the very behaviors in their organizations that people in those governance structures thrive on criticizing.

I am encouraged that today's leaders in academic medicine would sincerely like to do better on these issues. Indeed, I recall early discussions with Fred Hafferty and others about the pros and cons of popularizing the term *hidden curriculum* for these social forces. In talking with students and faculty, one can sometimes have a sense that these forces are hidden from the people in charge—the deans, hospital CEOs, and presidents—but in truth, these phenomena are discussed just as regularly and as passionately by the leaders. They are not hidden from anyone! I am not proposing that we change the term, but rather that "hidden" should be celebrated for its *irony* in this usage—something like a family secret that is known by absolutely everyone in the family but remains undiscussed so that all can pretend it is a secret. We have to be humble about how quickly large social forces can be redirected, and in the meantime we have to celebrate the ongoing efforts of outstanding role models, educators, and leaders at every level to continually validate and bolster the positive values of our students and residents.

Perhaps the most important lesson, therefore, is to never forget the positive aspects of the hidden curriculum (Tsang 2011). In those original 1990s empirical studies of student and resident professional development (Hundert, Douglas-Steele, and Bickel 1996; Douglas-Steele and Hundert, 1996; Hundert, Hafferty, and Christakis 1996), we found countless examples of true heroism among the residents, attendings, nurses, and others from whom our students learn about what it means to be a professional. The hidden curriculum literature tends to focus on the negative aspects of these social forces, but I like to remind everyone that if those parts of the brain that underlie professional values remain elastic enough at the age of our medical students and residents to be influenced negatively, we should take this as proof positive that we can equally powerfully reinforce the positive values that continue to bring young people to medicine. Professional development occurs within a multilayered, complex system, and we have to attack every level with positive energy if we are going to solve these problems. I encourage everyone to pick the level where they can have the most influence and get to work!

3: Education Reform and the Hidden Curriculum

The Canadian Journey

BRIAN DAVID HODGES AND AYELET KUPER

The Hidden Curriculum Emerges in Canada: From Midcentury Murmurs to a National Report

In 2009, the Association of Faculties of Medicine of Canada (AFMC) published a report titled "The Future of Medical Education in Canada (FMEC): A Collective Vision for MD Education." Produced through a process that combined empirical research with consensus building, this report articulated ten priority directions for medical education in Canada. The report was assembled as a synthesis of a variety of commissioned documents and reports, national working groups, expert panels, and consensus conferences, as well as an environmental scan. The environmental scan, in particular, was conducted over a period of two years (2007–9) by faculty members at the University of Toronto (including the authors of this chapter) and l'Université de Montréal, and consisted of three major elements: commissioned papers, national key informant interviews, and a process of thematic analysis (Hodges, Albert et al. 2011).

Most of the ten priority directions delineated within the FMEC report have been articulated in the past, often repeatedly (Whitehead 2011). Indeed, the historical record of twentieth-century North American medical education is replete with reiteration and repetition. A strikingly similar succession of articles and reports, published ten to fifteen years apart, liberally use a discourse of the "new" accompanied by rhetorically constructed urgencies, and call for attention to what are more or less the same problems (Whitehead, Hodges, and Austin 2013a). Such repetitive calls for medical education reform, followed by periods of forgetting and then rearticulations of the same imperatives, may serve to keep important issues at the forefront of discussion in medical education. On the other hand, they raise the concern that such repetition may, in fact, represent a distraction from actually changing anything (Whitehead, Hodges, and Austin 2013a) within conservative, change-resistant medical education (Bloom 1988). In either case, the repetitive nature of most medical education reports makes it all the more intriguing that two of the FMEC imperatives appear to be fairly novel, not having appeared in the plethora of past reports and documents (Whitehead 2011, 221).

The first of these novel FMEC imperatives, *interprofessionalism*, is beyond the scope of this chapter but has been taken up in detail elsewhere (Lingard 2012). This emerging discourse may reflect the fairly recent political and rhetorical construction of health professionals as members of teams, in contradistinction to the century-long image of the doctor as an autonomous individual whose competence was located only within himself or herself (Lingard 2009). Though it is too soon to say if the traditional individualist construction will actually be replaced, there is nevertheless an evolving discourse of collective, or team-based, competence. This change has already led to significant debate, both because it brings to light issues of power, hierarchy, and professional boundaries (Kuper and Whitehead 2012) and because it focuses on the cultures that socialize healthcare professionals in particular ways.

The second novel FMEC imperative is to *address the hidden curriculum*. The unprecedented appearance of a discourse about the hidden curriculum in this official context is quite interesting and challenges us to understand the historical antecedents of its emergence. Cribb and Bignold (1999) have argued that the lineage within medical education of the idea that later became known as the hidden curriculum can be traced to midcentury studies by sociologists of medical education Merton, Reader, and Kendal (1957); and Becker et al. (1961), who drew attention to "the central importance of the structural and cultural environment of the medical school to progress, educational experiences and the professional socialization of student doctors" (197). The emergence of this idea appears to represent a *moment* in medical education history, something that Michel Foucault called a *discontinuity* (Foucault 1972): a moment after which what had been taken for granted, what had seemed so normal, now appeared to be a *problem*.

These early sociologists did not, however, use the term *hidden curriculum*. That phrase was imported into medical education from the education literature (Jackson 1968; Snyder 1971) by sociologist Frederic Hafferty in the 1990s (Hafferty and Franks 1994; Hafferty 1998), concretizing the sociological notion into something that could be taken up by medical educators. Hafferty's efforts to bring medical education's attention to something heretofore invisible to it (except perhaps to sociologists toiling at its margins) have been repeated in the late twentieth century by other social scientists. For example, Janelle Taylor's (2003) paper, "Confronting 'Culture' in Medicine's 'Culture of No Culture'" (elaborated in this book), brought to light the ways in which medicine constructs *culture* as something external to itself, all the while acting as if medicine is not itself a highly specific and ritualized culture that varies across historical periods and geographic locations.

In summary, it seems that the notion of hidden curriculum was newly emergent in North American medical education at midcentury, and that it was concretized therein during the 1990s. We can also trace its subsequent dispersion and uptake in Canada as the twentieth century gave way to the twenty-first. During the decade following Hafferty's publications, the concept of the hidden curriculum was picked up in medical education by numerous writers, many of whom were sociologists or physicians with a social science orientation (Wear 1998; Woloschuk, Harasym, and Temple 2004; Lempp and Seale 2004; Haidet and Stein 2006). However, during the 2000s, the term was little used by medical education institutions, at least in Canada, suggesting that institutional medicine was not quite ready to deal with being confronted by social science–driven analyses of its culture and practices.

In Canada, a shift appears to have occurred with the publication of the aforementioned FMEC report and its ten priority directions. In retrospect, FMEC's environmental scan process (Hodges, Albert et al. 2011) was likely quite important in propelling the notion of the hidden curriculum to national prominence, where it survived the subsequent consensus-building phase of the project. Though the specific term *hidden curriculum* was not cited as often or as directly as some of the other emergent themes that made it to the final ten, it was clear during the research process that the essence of what the literature had more explicitly labeled as the hidden curriculum was nevertheless threaded throughout the project sources (Kuper et al. n.d.). Ultimately, the notion of a hidden curriculum, and a sense of an imperative to do something about it, appeared in the final Association of Faculties of Medicine of Canada report (n.d.). The section addressing hidden curriculum is reproduced in box 3-1.

It is interesting that the theme of hidden curriculum survived the national consensus process, which was heavily laden with institutional and organizational actors (Hodges, Albert et al. 2011). There were indeed some modifications to the associated directions for change, and reference to the

---

BOX 3-1

From the Future of Medical Education in Canada,
Association of Faculties of Medicine of Canada (n.d.)

Recommendation V: Address the Hidden Curriculum

The hidden curriculum is a "set of influences that function at the level of organizational structure and culture," affecting the nature of learning, professional interactions, and clinical practice. Faculties of Medicine must therefore ensure that the hidden curriculum is regularly identified and addressed by students, educators, and faculty throughout all stages of learning.

Rationale

The hidden curriculum encompasses what students learn outside the formal curriculum. It is pervasive and complex and can be deeply instilled in institutional cultures. In health education, the hidden curriculum cuts across disciplines within and outside medicine.

There are elements of the hidden curriculum that are positive in nature; however, many others have been identified as having a counterproductive effect on learning. The hidden curriculum often supports hierarchies of clinical domains or gives one group advantages over another. It sometimes reinforces the negative elements of existing reward and recognition systems and deters students from pursuing certain careers in medicine, such as family medicine. For these reasons, revealing and clarifying the hidden curriculum will be a challenging yet critical move forward for Canada's Faculties of Medicine.

Implementing this recommendation involves engaging both learners and teachers in identifying and acknowledging the hidden curriculum. This recommendation is made in the spirit of improving the socialization of physicians and ensuring that students and teachers acknowledge the hidden curriculum and its impact. It will encourage a process of self-reflection and self-analysis and will ultimately afford the opportunity to continually renew and reinvigorate the culture and value system of medical education. (23)

---

culture of medicine was dropped from the title. These changes can be understood as making more palatable recommendations that might have otherwise upset particular complacent certainties within medical education. Nevertheless, addressing the hidden curriculum did survive to take its place as Recommendation V. This speaks to the ongoing adoption of the idea of hidden curriculum into common parlance and to the recognition that it has now acquired a certain degree of legitimacy. Tina Martimianakis and Nancy McNaughton (chapter 8) explore the ways in which discourse helps us understand, describe, and address effects of the hidden curriculum in this book. Suffice it to say that in Canada in 2012, hidden curriculum had entered the everyday discourse of medical education.

Hidden Curriculum in Canada: From Emergent Discourse to Change in Practice?

It is, of course, important to articulate high-level directions for medical education, but as we have seen, these directions often remain unaddressed, with reports relegated to dusty shelves shortly after their publication. By contrast, some movements in medical education in Canada have had more enduring legacies. One of these is the well-known roles framework promoted by the Royal College of Physicians and Surgeons of Canada as CanMEDS (Frank and Danoff 2007). Widely cited and adopted in various forms by other health professionals and other countries around the world, the CanMEDS framework is an articulation of the seven roles that physicians must enact. In Canada, medical specialists originally only endorsed it, but the College of Family Medicine of Canada has since adopted its own version of CanMEDS. Though intended originally for postgraduate medical trainees, the framework has found its way into undergraduate curricula and continuing education programs of many health professions across Canada and abroad.

Much ink has been spilled about the advantages and disadvantages of dividing up competence into competencies (Rees 2004; Huddle and Heudebert 2007; Reeves, Fox, and Hodges 2009; Whitehead, Hodges, and Austin 2013b). However, for the purposes of this chapter, we will not describe the ongoing debates about the correctness or appropriateness of the CanMEDS framework. We will instead focus on the origin and the longevity of this work, through which CanMEDS has profoundly shaped medical education, assessment, and accreditation in Canada.

First, the origin: the CanMEDS framework was not invented by the Royal College of Physicians and Surgeons of Canada, but was instead adapted from an earlier framework produced by a project called Educating Future Physicians for Ontario (EFPO). Launched in Ontario, Canada's most populous province, after a highly publicized and unpopular provincial doctors' strike in 1987, the EFPO project sought to realign medical education with social responsibility (Neufeld et al. 1998). Following an extensive empirical study of the perceived needs and expectations of patients, families, public interest groups, and healthcare professionals, the EFPO framework proposed eight roles that Ontario society expected of its physicians. These roles are almost identical to the later CanMEDS roles, with the most prominent exception being the elimination of *physician as person* in the CanMEDS framework. The story of the EFPO project and the evolution of the roles concept into CanMEDS are told in a fascinating history by Cynthia Whitehead (2011).

Next, the longevity: the EFPO project conducted in Canada in 1987 was taken up as the basis of a competence framework that was widely operationalized throughout the following decades. Today, twenty-five years later, it is used in every aspect of physician education in Canada, and has been adopted in whole or in modified form in the education of many kinds of health professionals around the world. Clearly this work was not confined to a dusty shelf shortly after publication!

One might, therefore, ask, "What possibility is there that the FMEC report and, more specifically, the newfound legitimacy it both reflects and engenders for the notion of the hidden curriculum, will come to shape and change day-to-day practices in medical education?" If it is to be part of true medical education reform, then, like the CanMEDS framework, it will have to find its way into medical (and other health professions) training programs as well as into frontline healthcare practice settings. The latter is particularly important because "the hidden curriculum in medical education and the culture of medicine overlap because much of medical education happens in work (predominantly hospital) settings" (Cribb and Bignold 1999, 197). The hidden curriculum is also more about institutional culture than anything that can be located at an individual level: a true transformation will require a greater capacity for institutions such as medical schools and hospitals to "understand themselves" (195). Any meaningful uptake will thus be predicated on addressing culture and the hidden curriculum within institutional practices with respect both to medical education and to medicine more broadly, including learner assessment methods, teacher evaluations, promotion processes, and accreditation standards in educational institutions (for example, universities and colleges); or clinician assessment methods, reward structures, administrative organization, and accreditation standards in healthcare institutions (for example, hospitals and outpatient clinics).

A Possibility for Uptake into Practice?

In 2010 a charitable organization called Associated Medical Services (AMS), the same organization that funded and sponsored the EFPO project almost twenty-five years earlier, declared its interest in the hidden curriculum. Following a two-year environmental scan of the state of health professional practice and education, the board of AMS concluded that there was widespread support for a project that would invest in restoring the balance between technical competence and compassionate care (Associated Medical Services 2011a) through addressing the culture of medicine and nursing in Ontario and eventually Canada. After the publication of the FMEC report, AMS adopted some of that report's language and decided to focus on Recommendation V, "The Hidden Curriculum" (see Box 3-1). Today this AMS project, now called the Phoenix Project (www.theAMSPhoenix.ca), aims directly at understanding and addressing the hidden curriculum with a variety of initiatives, including the creation of fellowships and grants targeted at the phenomenon and activities to build a provincial and national discussion about compassionate care and the hidden curriculum.

Two province-wide summits were held in 2011 and were attended by leaders from medical schools, hospitals, government, and academia with expertise and interest in the hidden curriculum (including the authors of this chapter). One of these summits focused on medicine and the other on nursing, recognizing both the interest in addressing the topic from a multiprofessional perspective and the challenge of the observation that the term *hidden curriculum* itself, while now increasingly used in medical education, is almost unknown in nursing. There are, nevertheless, similarities between what is called the hidden curriculum in medicine and the construct of a "theory-practice gap" in nursing, both of which have deep resonance in nursing education and practice (Associated Medical Services 2011b). AMS hopes that its Phoenix Project will propel into practice new knowledge and strategies to understand the hidden curriculum and mitigate areas where those effects are negative, recognizing that there can also be positive dimensions to the hidden curriculum (2011b). To date, no other national education or healthcare organization has taken up FMEC's challenge to *address the hidden curriculum*, though clearly, a national effort is intended in the FMEC recommendations.

A True Shift or a Ride 'Round on a Carousel?

It remains to be seen whether the emergence of a discourse about the hidden curriculum in Canada will translate into substantively different practices, or whether, to borrow Whitehead's metaphor (Whitehead, Hodges, and Austin 2013a), it will simply end up being another ride around on the carousel. Certainly the adoption of the concept by a powerful national organization such as the Association of Faculties of Medicine of Canada appears to be meaningful. Attempts to concretize the notion and change practice (for example, the Phoenix Project) may represent a step along the way, much as the creation of the EFPO project turned what began as moral despair in the face of a doctors' strike into a set of curricular, assessment, and accreditation structures that could, at least in theory, reinforce the social advocacy functions of medicine. In this regard, it is worth noting that Whitehead (2011) provides a thoughtful critique of the degree to which the EFPO project was predicated on making medicine more socially responsive versus organized medicine's need to respond to a hostile environment in which public dissatisfaction threatened to reduce its autonomous powers of self-regulation.

There is, however, one worrying element in this unfolding hidden curriculum story. As noted, the FMEC report positions the "way forward" in a particular way wrought from national consensus (see box 3-2). These recommended directions do not acknowledge institutional responsibility to address the hidden curriculum. They instead locate this responsibility at the level of individual students ("choosing electives, engaging in research, getting involved in the community, and making career choices") and teachers (mentorship "to provide guidance for learners"), and rely on simplistic curricular interventions ("discussing the challenges of the hidden curriculum" and "sharing ways to address it"). This is most obviously problematic because "studies of the hidden curriculum cast doubt on the potential penetration and power of formal curriculum reform" (Cribb and Bignold 1999, 202).

BOX 3-2

Recommendations for change in medical education practice from the Future of Medical Education in Canada, Association of Faculties of Medicine of Canada (n.d.)

The Way Forward

Examples of strategies for addressing this recommendation include the following:

- Create culturally safe ways for students and faculty to make the hidden curriculum explicit and relevant to the formal curriculum.
- Encourage ongoing mentorship programs (student-student and faculty-student) to provide guidance for learners in such activities as choosing electives, engaging in research, getting involved in the community, and making career choices.
- Engage students and faculty from different schools in discussing the challenges of the hidden curriculum and in sharing ways to address it constructively.
- Expose students and faculty to the effects of the hidden curriculum on learners by using data and research. (23)

In addition, from the literature on culture change (for example, see Bloom 1988 on inertia to change), we know that the potent drivers of change in a cultural domain such as medical education are neither at the individual level nor primarily at the curriculum level but rather, necessarily, at the institutional and organizational level.

As Edward Hundert argues in this book (chapter 2), the hidden curriculum of microcultures must be linked to facilitative macrostructures. Continual movement upstream, from students to teachers to administrators and leaders, to the structures that govern them all, is necessary to understand the existence of and perpetuation of the hidden curriculum. To make meaningful change in hidden curriculum (and to get off the carousel) it will, therefore, be necessary to (1) make the hidden curriculum visible; (2) make the hidden curriculum "strange" by knowing our history and adopting a certain historical humility toward current practice; and (3) take responsibility for the hidden curriculum at an institutional and organizational level by engaging social scientists in our organizations and institutions, by informing decisions with evidence from a wide range of disciplinary perspectives (political, economic, sociological), and by opening the door to a discussion about what forms of knowledge actually underpin medical and health professional competence beyond the strictly scientific (Kuper, Whitehead, and Hodges 2013). Notably, this means that framing conduct and *professional behavior* as characteristics of individuals will have to give way, at least in part, to understanding how the choices made by individuals are shaped and constrained by *institutional* culture—which has important implications for assessment. Hafferty (1998) suggests a starting place, recommending that educators interested in locating the hidden curriculum examine institutional policies, evaluation practices, resource allocation, and institutional slang or nomenclature. In his words,

> The hidden curriculum highlights the importance and impact of structural factors on the learning process. Focusing on this level and type of influence draws our attention to . . . commonly held "understandings," customs, rituals and taken-for-granted aspects of what goes on in the life-space we call medical education. This concept also challenges medical educators to acknowledge their training institutions as both cultural entities and moral communities, intimately involved in constructing definitions about what is "good" and "bad" medicine. (Hafferty 1998, 404)

Acknowledgment

The authors are grateful to Elisa Hollenberg for editorial assistance.

PART II

THEORETICAL CONSIDERATIONS

This section opens with a chapter by Janelle Taylor and Claire Wendland that examines medicine's "culture of no culture" and also turns a rather critical lens on how work on the hidden curriculum has evolved over time. We place this chapter at the beginning of part 2 not because it seeks to summarize the theoretical landscape per se, but rather because it takes the status quo (in this case, how the hidden curriculum has come to be used within medical education) and adopts a contrarian viewpoint by asking, "What are we not seeing?" and "What *else* might be going on?" In these respects, this chapter operates very much in the spirit of the hidden curriculum by seeking to understand how work on the concept itself has taken on certain authoritative framings and thus itself participates in the paradox of making it possible for the hidden curriculum to remain hidden.

The Taylor and Wendland discussion is followed by chapters by Delese Wear, Joe Zarconi, and Rebecca Garden (chapter 5); and Heidi Lempp and Alan Cribb (chapter 6). Both Wear and Lempp were asked to participate because they had lead authored two of the most highly cited hidden curriculum articles to date (Lempp and Seale 2004; Wear 1998). Because of this status, they were invited to tackle any issues they desired using the hidden curriculum as a lens. Wear and her group discuss the role of implicit assumptions underlying two contemporary practices: (1) humanities as an appropriate and primary vehicle for delivering professionalism, and (2) what evaluation strategies come to be deemed appropriate and preferred to determine professional development. Their focus on the unseen and the unspoken is very much in keeping with core themes from Taylor and Wendland (chapter 4). Their story about the unintended consequences of outing the hidden curriculum should stand as a beacon for other attempts to address educational conundrums.

In chapter 6, Lempp and Cribb, in turn, continue this examination of the underlying logic of medical education with a focus on issues of prestige, status, stratification, and hierarchy both within medicine and between medicine and society. As in the preceding chapters, the authors ask how certain ways of knowing and doing are differentially embedded in both medical practice and medical education, and they continue with the theme of education as institutionalized structures of reproduction. The authors also examine how practices that have gained widespread visibility within medical education (including the hidden curriculum) remain muted or "effectively undermined or cancelled out (as vehicles of educational reform) through the governance of dominant, broadly technicist paradigms." Like Wear and colleagues, who look at professionalism, Lempp and Cribb provide us with a particular case study to illustrate their points—this time how "personalized medicine" and personalized (for example, patient-centered) healthcare may, via underlying assumptions and unexamined meanings, operate as countervailing forces driven by differing epistemologies.

4: The Hidden Curriculum in Medicine's "Culture of No Culture"

JANELLE S. TAYLOR AND CLAIRE WENDLAND

China Miéville's 2009 novel, *The City & The City*, is a noir murder mystery set in an imaginary, vaguely Eastern European setting where two entirely legally and socially separate cities, Besz and Ul Qoma, inhabit the same physical space. In the world of Miéville's novel, a frightening and very secretive agency called Breach polices the boundaries between the two cities and punishes those who trespass across those divisions. What separates Besz and Ul Qoma, however, far more than the actions of Breach, are the learned habits of "unseeing" that have been thoroughly internalized and are unthinkingly practiced by the citizens of the two cities. Although they walk the same sidewalks, drive the same streets, breathe the same air, and experience the same weather, inhabitants of each city have been rigorously schooled to *unsee* the people and the physical structures that belong to the other. As Miéville describes it, unseeing is a deeply ingrained habit of perception that must be instilled through a lengthy learning process.

We begin with Miéville's novel because it draws connections between group membership, socialization, institutional power, and habits of perception that we find provocative and usefully resonant with the topic of the hidden curriculum in medical education. Socialization—in medicine as in any other context—is as much about leaving old ways of thinking and acting as it is about taking on new ones. Unlearning is an important part of learning, and unseeing an important part of seeing. How does the "city" of medicine actively teach its inhabitants to *unsee* some things, processes, and people, through the same means and at the same time that it teaches them to *see* many others? How is unseeing enforced and policed? And how does seeing and unseeing relate to the hidden curriculum?

Learning to Unsee in Medical Education

At the bedside, in the clinic, and in the hospital hallways, much of medical learning is about what to notice (whether by seeing, hearing, feeling, or smelling) and what to ignore. Anyone who has learned to auscultate cardiac murmurs knows this process. When first a student's stethoscope lands on someone's chest, she hears a confusing array of sounds: her patient's inhalations and exhalations, the crackle of her stethoscope against his skin, the pulsing of her own blood in her ears, the valves of his heart closing, perhaps the voice of her instructor making suggestions. Learning to hear murmurs is as much about tuning out those distracting sounds—learning to distinguish field from background—as it is about hearing the subtler sounds of an aberrant flow of blood. Learning to see or to feel tissue planes in surgery is a similar process, and so is learning to make quick decisions in an emergency—in part by recognizing which actions are critical to maintaining life and which can be deferred, in part by relegating one's own panic to the background where it can be disregarded until after the fact. Unseeing, unhearing, unrecognizing, and unfeeling are essential skills of the effective clinician.

Ethnographies and memoirs of medical training show that case presentations are crucial to learning the unseeing that the city of medicine demands of its inhabitants (Anspach 1988). As medical training progresses, students learn to summarize medical histories and physical exams in shorter and shorter forms, even as the complaints and medical histories of the patients they see become more and more complicated. Punishments for breaching— for seeing and reporting what is construed as irrelevant to the clinical task at hand—may take the explicit form of a lowered grade. Unofficial censure by senior members of the medical team may be as subtle as inattention or as overt as comments like "We haven't got all day, *doctor*," or "Stop—just tell me what I need to know." Sometimes students' grades come to depend quite explicitly on their abilities to separate the important from the unimportant—to distinguish correctly what should be seen from what should be unseen (Good 2003).

We do not wish to claim that unseeing is a bad thing to be stamped out. It is a critical part of what makes medicine and other forms of specialized knowledge powerful. At the same time, unseeing has sociopolitical consequences. In medicine, norms of seeing and unseeing keep the focus on the individual patient's body. As trainees become part of medicine's professional community, they gradually learn to recognize bodily pathologies in their patients and to unsee (as irrelevant) the social pathologies and institutional structures that are powerful predictors of health and disease. They also learn also to unsee their own privilege and social position and the actions that maintain their professional prestige and in-group/out-group distinctions (Beagan 2000, 2003).

Ironically, but perhaps inevitably, blindness to social and institutional structures is not limited to medical *students*. It also is apparent in the discourse of those charged with teaching students, even in discussions of medical education reform and the hidden curriculum.

Unseeing the Hidden Curriculum

Fifteen years have passed since Frederic Hafferty published "Beyond Curriculum Reform: Confronting Medicine's Hidden Curriculum" (1998). The article has been enormously influential, as every chapter in this collection details, as indeed the very fact of this book's appearance attests. At the time of this writing, a literature-cited search in the Web of Science research database for published articles referencing Hafferty's 1998 article turns up no less than 320 publications (up from 319 a few days ago—and most certainly more, by the time you read these words).

One pattern that we, as cultural anthropologists, find striking within this literature is how frequently these articles describe or propose addressing the hidden curriculum through efforts targeted at *individuals*, whether faculty members or students. Individual faculty role models are urged, for example, to scrutinize their activities outside the classroom for what values they may be communicating to students. There is nothing wrong, of course, with encouraging people to engage in critical self-reflection; this is all to the good. The instrumental edge to much of this literature, however, gives us pause: faculty are to change their out-of-class behavior in order to "maximize the positive impact of the hidden curriculum" (Chuang et al. 2010, 316.e5) by "using the hidden curriculum to teach professionalism" (Rogers et al. 2012, 423). The hidden curriculum itself, far from being a problematic product of institutional structure and culture, is somehow reconceptualized as a tool to be manipulated by individuals toward desirable ends.

Others acknowledge the hidden curriculum as indeed a troubling presence, but propose that its influence can be counteracted by specific measures targeted at the level of individual students: "Exposure to . . . negative role modeling, may increase the likelihood of becoming cynical and adopting negative professional attitudes and behaviors. Reflective writing and feedback may mitigate this risk" (Karnieli-Miller et al. 2011, 369). Without changing much of anything else, in other words, educators are informed that they can inoculate students against the negative effects of the hidden curriculum by *adding* to the formal curriculum specific kinds of exercises designed to neutralize it.

The hidden curriculum, it would seem, often is conceptualized as being hidden within the aspects of individuals' lives that have traditionally lain outside the reach of the formal curriculum: their subconscious, their private thoughts, their extracurricular lives. One danger is that the hidden curriculum will be treated simply as a newly revealed territory not yet thoroughly colonized by the formal curriculum, and ripe for the claiming. (*Look!* Yet *more* time and activity to be carefully planned, scrutinized, documented, and assessed!) Armed with a limited and skewed understanding of the concept of the hidden curriculum, some now take it as a license to *extend* the formal curriculum: to plan not only what goes on in the classroom, but also what goes on "in the elevator, the corridor, the lounge, the cafeteria, or the on-call room" (Hafferty 1998, 404). Once every student and every faculty member has internalized and consistently demonstrates the appropriate attitudes, the hidden curriculum will disappear and medicine will be cured of its ills.

We see a second danger in this individualizing vision. Expansionist distortions of the idea of the hidden curriculum ignore Hafferty's clear admonition, "Any remedial effort that limits its focus to curriculum change does not challenge educators to examine the full range of influences . . . that compose the milieu of our medical programs" (Hafferty 1998, 407). If the hidden curriculum is grounded in the social organization of medicine, then no amount of fine-tuning the curriculum alone will address it; more fundamental changes will be required. Any approach that individualizes the hidden curriculum thus also systematically evades recognition of the structural constraints under which individuals act. It disregards Hafferty's insistence that the hidden curriculum is "a set of influences that function at the level of organizational *structure and culture*" (404; emphasis added).

This should perhaps not surprise us, however. The particular ways that the idea of the hidden curriculum has been taken up within medical education both reflect and tend to reproduce the *patterns of unseeing* characteristic of medicine's "culture of no culture."

Seeing the Hidden Curriculum in Medicine's Culture of No Culture

Let us consider the proposition that the hidden curriculum is situated not so much within individuals' private thoughts or lives as within the broader milieu, the "organizational structure and culture" of medical school. This presents us with a puzzle: If the hidden curriculum is situated in the social world that we inhabit, right there and observable everywhere around us, then in what sense (and from whom) is it actually *hidden*? To pose the same question in terms borrowed from Miéville, how have people learned to *unsee* certain aspects of the social and cultural structures all around them?

On one level, of course, this question is hardly unique to medicine. It is a version of the perennial Marxist question: Why don't the workers revolt? Why do people act in ways that are manifestly contrary to their own objective self-interest? Why don't they *see*? Not coincidentally, the concept of the hidden curriculum emerges out of broadly Marxist perspectives on education, which consider education as an institution that serves the function of socializing individuals to assume the ideas, values, assumptions, and expectations suited to the class position into which it helps slot them. Working-class kids get socialized into working-class jobs (Willis 1981), children of the elites learn to embody their privilege (Khan 2011), and those for whom education actually opens paths toward upward class mobility work mightily, quite apart from their studies, to acquire the tastes, habits, accents, and other forms of vital "cultural capital" that they did not inherit at birth (Bourdieu 1984). At the same time, however, Marxist perspectives on education also see education as holding the potential to become a radical force, by facilitating critical reflection and creating conditions for the emergence of class consciousness (Gramsci 2000; Freire 2000). Institutions of education systematically teach people to *unsee* their social world in ways that contribute to the maintenance of existing relations of class and power—but education *could* teach people to *see* their world clearly, and support their capacity to transform it.

When the idea of the hidden curriculum is invoked in medical education circles, these Marxist origins and questions rarely come up for discussion. This happens not necessarily because medical faculty or students are politically opposed to left-wing social movements—indeed, many consider themselves to be politically liberal or progressive. The simplest explanation is that most of those working in the field of medical education who use the term are simply not aware of its history. The writings of Karl Marx, Paolo Freire, Antonio Gramsci, Paul Willis, Pierre Bourdieu, and other critical scholars of education do not show up in medical school curricula, nor on the syllabi of courses generally required for admission to medical school, nor does one need to be familiar with them in order to perform well on the MCAT exams. Fred Hafferty, who of course *did* read such works in the course of his training as a sociologist, introduced the idea of the hidden curriculum into the literature on medical education, explaining it in an admirably clear and compelling fashion in an article published in a premier journal of medical education. Hafferty's article serves as the originary source for most in the field who engage with the idea of the hidden curriculum; few appear to have explored the idea beyond journals of medicine and medical education. Like experts in many other fields, medical experts tend to be quite thoroughly "disciplined" in their reading habits and citation practices.

We as social scientists, however, cannot be satisfied with an explanation pitched only at the level of individuals when those individuals think and act in patterned ways. When a group of people share a set of distinctive patterns of thought and social interaction, we may say that they share a culture. The word *culture* is very often invoked to explain the ideas and practices of other people. It is much more difficult to see one's own culture because it appears to be not cultural at all, but rather just the way things are: common sense, human nature, truth. When people in medical schools and hospitals—as well as courts, armies, and other modern institutions—label some spaces, people, and practices as "cultural," they simultaneously imply that their own spaces, people, and practices are somehow *outside of* culture and thus culture free. This way of thinking fits well with the conviction, shared by people within medical institutions, that medical knowledge is *real* (and therefore not "merely cultural") (Wendland, Taylor, and Hafferty 2013; Gershon and Taylor 2008). In this sense, medicine is arguably a culture of no culture, that is, a community defined by the shared cultural conviction that its shared convictions are *not* in the least cultural, but rather are timeless, universal truths (Taylor 2003).

We also might think of medicine as a "structure of no structure," a structure in which the patterned socioeconomic arrangements that direct power, opportunity, and comfort toward some and away from others are rendered invisible. Students, residents, fellows, and faculty in academic medical centers are keenly attuned to the hierarchies of power and prestige within the subsection of the medical world that belongs to doctors, it is true. They are insulated, however, from recognition of the sharper inequalities between those seeking (and paying for) medical care and those providing (and profiting from) it. Few doctors are directly involved in turning away patients who have the wrong (or no) insurance; few are directly involved in sending debt collectors after their patients. Few students know that the "standardized patients" on whom they learn to take (invented) social and medical histories do not earn health benefits for this work, and that for some this simulacrum of medical care *is* the only medical care to which they have ready access (Taylor 2011).

The curricula of medicine—formal, informal, and hidden—rigorously school practitioners in individualism as a habit of thought and practice, in ways that discourage, or even disable, social and cultural analysis. Medicine addresses itself to illnesses and injuries of bodies, using high-tech tools and the methods of laboratory science to identify a single cause and a targeted specific cure for each disease, focusing always on the individual's body, especially its interior. Questions concerning social and cultural worlds and their political ordering seem to lie beyond the bounds of what medical education can or should engage. Medicine is, of course, always taught, learned, invented, practiced, regulated, funded, and sought by *people*—and for that reason, is always irreducibly social, cultural, and political. But learning to *see* individual bodies in the ways that contemporary American medicine requires also entails learning to *unsee* whatever does not fit within a relentlessly individualistic framing—whether the social or cultural background of an individual patient, the political-economic sources of a disease, or the social hierarchies and cultural values of a medical institution.

Here, then, is the answer to our puzzle—though it is a puzzling answer: the hidden curriculum in medical education, although it is right there in plain sight, remains effectively hidden because of the patterns of unseeing characteristic of medical education. In other words, the hidden curriculum helps create the blind spots in which it then hides.

Unlearning to Unsee in Medical Education

Theoretical models have power. In the 1960s epidemiologists proposed the *web of causation* as a way to understand the complex and multifactorial nature of many substantial public health concerns such as cancers, coronary artery disease, common mental disorders, and so on. As Nancy Krieger pointed out thirty years later, the web of causation quickly became accepted as an unproblematic depiction of epidemiologic reality—and not as what it actually is, a theoretical model with certain specific implications. The web model plays into biomedical individualism by allowing (even encouraging) physicians to focus on "lifestyle" and "risk factors" closest to the individual and therefore presumed to be remediable. It levels distinctions among causative factors, fails to distinguish between determinants of disease in individuals and in populations, and—because it excludes history—cannot address why population patterns of health and disease change over time. Krieger (1994) proposed rethinking the web of causation by asking, "Has anyone seen the spider?"

The hidden curriculum too is a theoretical model with specific implications. The term *hidden*, though apt in many respects, may lead medical educators to think that simple exposure will resolve the problematic effects of the hidden curriculum. (Similar assumptions are involved in prescribing disclosure of financial conflicts of interest to strengthen medical research integrity.) Following Krieger's lead, we might ask who hid the hidden curriculum, where is it hidden, and why is any part of the curriculum hidden anyway? These questions reveal the power of the original formulation: taken as directed, the model of the hidden curriculum requires attention to structure and culture *within* medical institutions, and thus makes it impossible to think of medicine as either acultural or nonstructuring. In this regard, *hegemonic* might be a more apt adjective than *hidden*. The debt to Marx, Gramsci, and Freire becomes more obvious, and the path forward more difficult to redirect from revolutionary change to individual efforts at improved "professionalism." Attention to the hidden curriculum helps medical educators to re-see what has been systematically unseen.

The formal curriculum, prescribed by the Association of American Medical Colleges (AAMC) and presented in the textbooks, teaches an ideal medicine intended to diagnose and treat the disordered physiologies of individual human bodies. But actual human bodies (of doctors, patients, and medical students) live in human social and cultural worlds. The hidden curriculum hides in the gap between the ideal and the real practice of medicine, and it provides the lessons that students and educators need for the everyday work of medicine. The hidden and informal curricula, not the formal curriculum, teach American trainees how to guard against lawsuits or to bill office visits most effectively. The hidden and informal curricula teach Malawian trainees how to improvise diagnosis and treatment when "standard" measures are unavailable, or how to confront government officials when supply chains are broken or hospital budgets are insufficient to function (Wendland 2010)—and when it might be wiser not to. Everywhere medicine is practiced, these and related lessons of the hidden curriculum teach trainee doctors (students, interns, residents, registrars, and junior doctors) how to function in their particular medical milieu.

If we consider the hidden curriculum as instruction for actual medical practice, two interesting implications follow. First, the *content* of the hidden curriculum can be anticipated to be variable, probably much more variable than the content of the formal curriculum (Fins and del Pozo 2011). Unlike the formal curriculum, the hidden and informal curricula are not collectively prescribed by the AAMC and enforced by national certification examinations. Even more important, variability should arise because the actual conditions of practice vary substantially from place to place, era to era, payment structure to payment structure, and community to community. Second, understanding the problematic effects of the hidden curriculum will require understanding the problematic aspects of actual medical practice more broadly—and although exposing the hidden curriculum will not neutralize its effects, this may be an excellent first step toward that understanding.

Medicine is practiced by and on people. It is practiced over a huge portion of the globe. Even within any given nation, medical care happens in socially and culturally diverse contexts. In the United States, these contexts include rural clinics serving primarily Indigenous people and staffed by solo family practitioners, and teeming urban academic medicine complexes. At many of these places, students learn their work. We anticipate that careful attention to the hidden curriculum in a range of places will show far more variability than expected, and that some of this variability might illuminate the social and cultural structures that institutional medicine so often teaches its practitioners to unsee. Gibson-Graham (2006) famously proposed that "the end of capitalism" was actually around us everywhere, in alternative community economies and noncapitalist practices that were so small-scale that social theorists simply did not see them—had *learned* not to see them, in fact, by steeping in a language and worldview in which "economies" were large-scale systems. Perhaps our own habits of perception have rendered us unable to see the living grass cracking through the pavement of institutional medicine, and perhaps there already exist hidden curricula in which understanding individual bodies and their pathologies does not require unseeing their social, political, and economic contexts. Frantz Fanon, Rudolf Virchow, and Salvador Allende were, after all, physicians. Perhaps other possible curricula are waiting, hiding in plain sight, on the streets of the city of medicine.

5: Disorderly Conduct

Calling Out the Hidden Curriculum(s) of Professionalism

DELESE WEAR, JOE ZARCONI, AND REBECCA GARDEN

To be thoughtful about what we are doing is to be conscious of ourselves struggling to make meanings, to make critical sense of what authoritative others are offering as objectively "real."
—MAXINE GREENE (2005, 380)

To *assume*: to take for granted or without proof. In an educational environment obsessed with evidence, it seems odd that so many practices in medical education remain firmly in place without a shred of evidence that they are relevant, "true," or even effective. These assumptions operate within Hafferty's definition of the hidden curriculum—"among other things, the commonly held 'understandings,' customs, rituals, and taken-for-granted aspects of what goes on in the life-space we call medical education" (1998, 404). Every day in this life-space, we move through what Joanne Trautmann Banks refers to as "unseen worlds" (Trautmann 1982, 24), or perhaps more aptly, *unspoken* worlds.

In this chapter, we focus on current assumptions about professionalism and two factors in its expression in the undergraduate medical curriculum: (1) the medical humanities, designated by many as a primary vehicle for the "delivery" of the professionalism curriculum; and (2) various evaluative strategies—most notably competencies, benchmarks, and assessable outcomes—used to determine the professional development of students. Our focus on the medical humanities and our penchant for assessment in professionalism education arise from implicit assumptions underlying the nature and goals of each, assumptions that often work *against* what they claim to support—the ongoing professional development of physicians. Here we examine *assumptions as hidden curriculum*. We argue that such assumptions deflect serious investigation of the everyday practices surrounding professionalism education that have comfortably settled into the medical education environment and that impede our progress toward inspiring students about professionalism.

Professionalism: Contested Meanings

It has been long known and clearly documented that medical students become more cynical as they progress through the curriculum. A vast literature exists about this phenomenon, some of it theoretical, most of it descriptive, all with remarkably similar language (Becker et al. 1961; Christakis and Feudtner 1993; Newton et al. 2008). We know that such cynicism erupts when students experience mistreatment and powerlessness or witness physician behaviors that contradict what they have been taught about professionalism. As educators, our own cynicism about whether we can change the clinical culture of medicine may be justified, or it may be a self-fulfilling prophesy. Either way, we're not even embarrassed. Like the usual response to an ill-mannered eccentric relative acting out at a family dinner, we dismiss such behaviors and say, "Oh that's just the way he is . . . ignore him." We turn away from these culprits in the medical environment and focus our instructional efforts solely on their victims, the students. Our ignoring these behaviors, in turn, offers powerful lessons to students about how things really are in medicine, about what professionalism is, and about what it isn't.

Meanwhile, the professionalism discourse focusing on interpersonal, communicative, ethical, or "humanistic" aspects of medical care at the trainee level goes something like this: if we create lists of attributes denoting professionalism, talk about professionalism enough (or at least use the word enough), assess it enough, and offer enough "remedial" measures for reported lapses in it (in students only), students will become "professional" or demonstrate professional "competence." Indeed, the major accrediting organizations subscribe vigorously to such professionalism mandates for trainees. And the Association of American Medical Colleges (AAMC), the American Board of Internal Medicine (ABIM), and numerous other specialty organizations all address this elusive concept, defined by even more abstract concepts including virtues such as duty, respect, altruism, empathy, and truthfulness, among others. The term *professionalism* is used as though it were a common referent by us all, but in fact it is often merely a vaguely positive-sounding floating signifier that medical schools, accrediting bodies, medical school administrators, and faculty deploy to signal that they are serious about such virtues attached to it and thus are able to claim a moral high ground for medicine and medical education. It is at the local level where professionalism educational efforts are enacted, however, and it is there where the tension between abstractions denoting professionalism and the actual witnessed behaviors, practices, and attitudes of "professionals" arises.

Brainard and Brislen pose such problems most succinctly in their "view from the trenches" as medical students:

> The chief barrier to medical professionalism education is unprofessional conduct by medical educators, which is protected by an established hierarchy of academic authority. Students feel no such protection, and the current structure of professionalism education and evaluation does more to harm students' virtue, confidence, and ethics than is generally acknowledged . . . . Deficiencies in the learning environment, combined with the subjective nature of professionalism evaluation, can leave students feeling persecuted, unfairly judged, and genuinely and tragically confused. (2007, 1010)

Leo and Eagen (2008) write similarly about the flawed professionalism movement as they experienced its manifestations in their education, beginning with this statement: "Cringe . . . this is the reaction that many students have to the word *professionalism*" (508). The authors report that the "disdain, frustration, and hostility" are not because students believe themselves above discussions involving their professional identities, but because the lopsided focus on criticizing unprofessional behaviors in students "leads to an aura of negativity whenever the word *professionalism* is mentioned" (510). Given that students have so little authority in the educational setting, particularly in the clinic, they resent and resist being assigned sole responsibility for professional behavior while concomitantly being deprived of the power to critique its absence in their superiors.

Thus, the failure to address the "values being transmitted within the hidden and informal curriculum [that] are decidedly 'unprofessional' in nature" (Hafferty 2000a, 24) is a major cause of students' disdain of the "p-word" and is directly tied to the development of cynicism cited earlier. Yet, the drumbeats for assessing professionalism in *students* largely ignore these disturbing contradictions, and students notice the conspicuous absence of similar assessment efforts targeting the same behaviors in attendings (Leo and Eagen 2008). Instead, students face an environment of "excessive directives, lectures, rules, and moral pronouncements that they [find] repetitive and patronizing" (Goldstein et al. 2006, 873).

Unfortunately, and at the local medical school level, the term *professionalism* also frequently denotes a more pragmatic concentration on student behaviors, such as punctuality or appearance. In addition, medical educators designing curricula often turn to the field perceived as the humanizing counterpart to the potentially dehumanizing basic science curriculum and clinical training: the medical humanities. Such content is often deemed most appropriate for more intensive investigation (if not outright inculcation) of professionalism, particularly the virtues associated with it. Assumptions proliferate here as well, most of them unspoken, including how professional virtues can be "taught" directly, and where, and by whom. For many medical educators, the medical humanities—primarily ethics, literature, narrative inquiry, and writing—seem as good a place as any to address professionalism, if not to actually "teach" it.

Medical Humanities: The Foundation for Professionalism?

The assumption that professionalism issues are more at home in the content of the humanities than elsewhere in the formal curriculum is rife with misunderstandings and inaccuracies. Nonetheless, medical education has appropriated the humanities in several ways, particularly in the service of professionalism education. The Project to Rebalance and Integrate Medical Education (PRIME) is currently a major national movement insistently arguing that "the goals of medical ethics and humanities teaching should be clearly articulated and explicitly linked to consensus goals of professionalism and . . . to those aspects of professionalism that lend themselves to reliable evidence-based quantitative and qualitative assessment" (Doukas et al. 2012, 337).

To these and many other medical educators, it just makes sense that humanities inquiry leads to more compassionate, caring physicians. In fact, we often hear medical educators using the word *humanities* interchangeably with *humanism*, *humane*, and *humanist*. Likely reasons for these specious assumptions include equating humanities inquiry in medical education with a kind of liberal arts experience, however limited that experience might be relative to the entirety of medical education, and then proceeding with the belief that this modest dose of liberal arts equates with a robust liberal arts education. What is felt to be a rigorous academic course of liberal arts inquiry is most often actually a piecemeal, elective, and less complex and critical approach to humanities inquiry that is frequently seen as "stuck on" to the *real* medical education curriculum.

A long line of humanities scholars in medical education offer a phalanx of perspectives. K. Danner Clouser, prominent in the development of medical humanities over thirty years ago, argues that the most important benefit of the humanities in "technical-vocational training programs" such as medicine is *critical intelligence* (1986). Writing about literature in particular, Trautmann Banks points out that when we ask students to engage with literature during medical education, teaching them to read "in the fullest sense," we are training them *medically*: "To ask the medical student what is being said here—not at all an easy question when one must look at words in their personal and social contexts and when several things are being said at once—is to prepare him or her for the doctor-patient relationship" (Trautmann 1982, 26). Others contend that literary inquiry in medical education teaches students to "follow the narrative thread of complex and chaotic stories . . . to recognize the multiple, often contradictory meanings of events that befall human beings" (Hunter, Charon, and Coulehan 1995, 788). More recently, Catherine Belling has offered a meticulous description of the merits of all humanities study in medicine:

> The humanities resist the homogenization of social science metrics, for our focus is on the specific and particular, exactly those aspects of human texts that resist reduction. We value fine distinctions, even at the risk of defaulting to an n value of 1. This is precisely why the humanities are so valuable to medicine, for we offer a counterpart to the necessary reductions of the natural sciences. The unit of medicine is the particular patient, always irreducible. (2010, 940)

When students focus attention on complex but particular patient narratives, they also are coming to understand "contingency, context, and complex processes through which we construct meaning" (Gillis 2008, 11–12). And they come to understand how formulas and metrics and "evidence," however critical they are to understanding disease processes, have limited usefulness in understanding a particular patient. Such understandings involve "certain habits of mind, nuances to thinking, an appreciation for subtleties and ambiguities of argument," and may move students to "develop new kinds of doubts and anxieties, concerns and hesitations" (Brottman 2009). All these point to excellence in *clinical care*, not solely to professional virtues. To cede the medical humanities only to "virtue" building or "professionalism" is simply to get it all wrong.

Still, more assumptions remain that underlie a troubling lack of expertise that is ubiquitous in medical humanities teaching. Given that medical culture defines itself in part through a rigorous emphasis on areas of expertise and specialties involving serious regimens of study and practice, it is surprising that, when it comes to educating in the humanities (particularly when the humanities are being marshaled as a vehicle for professionalism education), there appears to be a nonchalant approach to even defining what the areas of study are, much less how they achieve anything of value for clinicians-in-training. Some argue that medical humanities approaches, such as the "study and creation of creative literature . . . encourage humanism and critical thinking and serve as a vehicle to improve care, commitment, and self-care," as well as teaching that "there are multiple perspectives, making suspect the privileging of any one perspective (e.g., the physician's versus that of the patient or family)" and inculcating skills in taking patient histories (Doukas et al. 2012, 337).

Yet, the educators making these claims do not provide any explanation of *how* studying literature or writing creatively teaches multiple perspectives, or how a student might avoid appropriating a patient's story or projecting her or his own experiences onto the patient, despite the fact that there is a formidable literature of critical arguments supporting and critiquing these assumptions and practices (Diedrich 2005; Garden 2007, 2010; Peterkin and Prettyman 2009; Squier 2007; Wear and Aultman 2005). Medical humanities scholars and educators draw on literary and disability studies' complex critiques of assumptions and practices regarding empathy and humanitarian issues in culture in order to develop pedagogical approaches that deconstruct, rather than reify, physician power in the clinic. Thus, medical educators who devise professionalism courses or programs by ostensibly founding them on the humanities disciplines should be careful to consult the deep literature, if not the deep bench of medical humanities experts themselves, in order to make persuasive claims and provide real outcomes for them regarding the humanities as a vehicle for training in ethical, compassionate, and professional conduct.

The problem of reducing professionalism training to a checklist of "competencies" recurs with the question of expertise. Emphasizing education in professionalism competencies by devising checklists of objectives and measurements that are easily packaged and reproduced (Doukas et al. 2010) makes it easier for non-experts—anyone, really—to teach the subject. Although administrators may trust that their students are engaging with complex sociocultural and ethical issues and getting the perspectives of the patient—through study in the medical humanities—students are more likely to receive yet another fragmented PowerPoint approach to a subject. Medical humanities scholars and educators with serious training and credentials do for students what specialists do for patients who need them: they bring a deep knowledge of the research, including the latest findings, to bear on experience and expertise in practice. Above all, they bring a nuanced approach to the assumptions too often made about the powers of the medical humanities.

Assessment and Professionalism: "Taking Apart the Art"

One of the most wildly enthusiastic movements in academic medicine over the past quarter century is the implementation of the competencies concept to denote students' knowledge, skills, and attitudes. The assumptions surrounding competencies include that some kind of *standard* exists that reflects a level students should achieve before moving on, and that there are ways to evaluate whether students meet these standards, ways that accurately capture whatever characteristic is under scrutiny. This may be easy enough for knowledge-based phenomena or for clinical skills, although Huddle and Heudebert's (2007) incisive article on the topic problematizes competencies even in those domains as overly reductionistic. However, turning assessment of professionalism into a series of benchmarks and rubrics is deeply flawed. Indeed, benchmarking professionalism lends a deceptive impression of exactness—of "real" measurement—to a phenomenon that is fluid and contingent, variably enacted by variable human beings. Judith Grant argues this point eloquently, that the totality of what physicians do is "far greater than any of the parts that can be described in competence terms." In fact, "they are making judgments, managing cases in the absence of definitive information, taking a multiplicity of factors into account . . . almost never replicating precisely the same approach because every case is never exactly like any other" (1999, 273).

Current critiques of the assumptions fueling the use of benchmarks, competencies, or other outcomes-based assessments of professionalism are beginning to appear with increasing frequency (Lingard 2009; Hodges

2006; Wear 2009). All are quick to state that such a critique does not attempt to replace competencies, or that learners should never be appraised regarding how they enact empathic and respectful caregiving to patients. Nonetheless, all point out serious problems with such assessment that uses empty benchmarking or competency-driven strategies, or with other forms of assessment that are actually coercive.

Coerciveness, for example, can occur during the "evaluation" of portfolios or reflective writing assignments using rubrics that purport to tell us where students are in terms of their professional development, a kind of surveillance that deems students professionally appropriate, or at least growing in that direction. When this is the case—when students' interpretive efforts in both oral and written language are subjected to various kinds of measurement that encourage adherence to prescribed, almost scripted conventional positions regarding professional attitudes—the "easier path (for students) is likely . . . to stay with the familiar and to avoid trouble which may arise from questioning established ways of thinking and acting" (Peterson et al. 2008, 3). Students learn (via a parallel hidden curriculum) that critique of medical culture, including any questioning of all that is taken for granted about the pedagogy of medical education, is not welcomed either by faculty or by a medical education marked by "the constant pressure to 'perform' according to imposed and often reductive standards" (Apple 2005, 15).

Where to Go from Here?

We have discussed some of the assumptions underlying the professionalism discourse and two factors in its expression: the medical humanities as a vehicle for professional development, and competency-based approaches to measure the professional development of students, often marked by excessive reductionism. We have argued that these assumptions often work *against* what they claim to support. Questions remain, most notably, what now?

Perhaps one place to begin is to move away from the term *professionalism* itself. It is fractured, used uncritically, and evoked punitively far too often; it is imbued with assumptions so variable that in any given educational location it slips away from a common referent. Jarvis-Selinger, Pratt, and Regehr offer what may be the most compelling argument for moving away from the "excessive reductionism . . . in discussions of professionalism" toward an exploration of the "interrelated *identities* that form the basis of what it means to be a physician" (2012, 1; italics added). By including the roles and responsibilities that emerge as students are learning the "practice" of medicine, a thoughtful "focus on *being* rather than exclusively a focus on *doing*" can begin to take place (1). Moreover, the coauthors argue that supplementing the work in developing measurable competencies with a consideration of professional identity formation may ameliorate two problems inherent in competency-based training: first, the tendency to atomize and fix what is essentially a dynamic and evolutionary process of becoming a physician; and second, the tendency to focus on minimally acceptable levels of "competence" as an indication of readiness to practice. Medical education could begin to reorient itself not only to thinking about making medical students and residents perform competently, but also to considering how their professional identities as physicians are evolving (Jarvis-Selinger et al. 2012, 5). Professional identity development requires far more than students' adherence to "rules"; to see-one, do-one, teach-one-type competencies; or to documentation of designated behavioral manifestations of abstract qualities such as altruism or compassion. Using an orientation toward professional identity development focused on *being* rather than *behaving* makes such reductionistic assessment of "being" increasingly problematic.

Students require a social environment that nurtures their individual identity development, which is no small order. Coulehan stated this succinctly over a decade ago when he argued that the first requirement "for a sea change in professionalism" is to "dramatically increase the number of role model physicians at every stage of medical education" (2006, 116). "This is a conscious, overt effort that includes full-time faculty members who exemplify professional virtue in their interactions with patients, staff, and trainees; who have a broad, humanistic perspective; and who are devoted to teaching. . . . [These] physicians are reflective, as opposed to non-reflective, in their professionalism [and] their presence would dilute and diminish the conflict between tacit and explicit values" (116). These are the role models who may engage students in the kind of ongoing reflective practice that acknowledges and supports their identity development at both the individual and collective level, "which involves a socialization of the person into appropriate roles and forms of participation in the community's work" (Jarvis-Selinger et al. 2012, 2).

And what of the humanities? We firmly resist assumptions that link humanities inquiry to professionalism any more than other disciplines or content are similarly bound. The humanities offer knowledge and skills that may move students toward becoming better *physicians*, in the same way courses on patient interviewing or population health or various clerkships do. In the end, the incorporation of the humanities into medical education can make a difference, if we cut through the decorative assumptions of their worth to what they can offer. But to make a difference, humanities inquiry must be ongoing and systematic in the regular curriculum, not relegated to an electives-only curriculum. The medium *is* the message, and curriculum time and course placement is one of the most powerful indices of what a medical school values, of who's in charge, of what knowledge is worth the most.

6: The Diversity and Unity of the Hidden Curriculum

Medical Knowledge in an Era of Personalized Healthcare

HEIDI LEMPP AND ALAN CRIBB

The hidden curriculum is a valuable lens revealing what sociologists routinely analyze as the reproduction of powerful biomedical discourses, because it highlights some of the concrete social processes through which the values of medicine are transmitted. The distinction between the official and the hidden curriculum not only makes explicit the ways in which some values, and value hierarchies, are effectively publicized while others operate below the radar, but also forces upon us the question of how these advertised and unadvertised elements are related. For example, the hidden curriculum is a useful focus for anyone interested, as we are in this chapter, in how the advertised "epistemic authority" of medicine relates to the less flaunted social and personal authority that doctors have over their students, junior colleagues, and other health professionals, not to mention patients or the public.

There is a risk, however, that talk of *the* hidden curriculum or *the* values of medicine itself rests upon and reinforces a concealed assumption that medicine is straightforwardly singular. In this chapter, we want to stand back from this assumption and reflect on the tensions between diversifying and unifying tendencies in medicine. Specifically, we want to contribute to the mapping of both the breadth and the depth of the hidden curriculum. In relation to breadth, for example, we shall indicate how medical cultures are constructed within and across different medical specialties (Hinze 1999) and how these constructions are mirrored in the existence of a status or prestige ranking system of medical specialties. In relation to depth, we shall suggest an analysis of the foundational and structuring effects of medical epistemology indicated, for example, by emphases on "closure" and authority. One of our aims is to review some of the potential tensions between aspects of breadth and depth, and we will conclude by briefly exploring competing constructions of the idea of personalized healthcare (Groves and Wagner 2005) as an illustration of these tensions.

The Breadth of the Hidden Curriculum

There is plenty of evidence within the broader spectrum of healthcare professional education literature of the multiple ways that the hidden curriculum remains a key factor shaping students' experiences. At the undergraduate level there is research evidence from dental education (Brainard and Brislen 2007; Wilson and Ayers 2004), medical education (Hafferty 1998; Lempp and Seale 2004; Mahood 2011; White et al. 2012), and nurse education (Bell 1984; Mayson and Hayward 1997; Partridge 1983), along with work on more thematic foci such as ethics (Hafferty and Franks 1994; Howard et al. 2012). For postgraduate education, the concept has been applied to anesthesia residency training (Gaiser 2009), the operating room (Lingard et al. 2002), radiology residency training (Anderson 1992), clinical orthopedics (Gofton and Regehr 2006), oncology (Buss et al. 2007), and internal medicine (Billings et al. 2011).

These publications highlight that what students learn is as important as what they are taught. Professional identity formation and socialization take place within strongly normative and hierarchical cultures, and students often discover what is valued in medicine and medical identities through subtle processes with potentially dramatic effects on, for example, loss of idealism (Billings et al. 2011), challenges to ethical integrity (Baldwin , Daugherty, and Rowley 1998; Mahood 2011), ritualized professional identity (Haas and Shaffir 1982; Spindler 1992), emotional neutralization (Hafferty 2000b; Hojat et al. 2009), tolerance of abuse (Frank et al. 2006; Paice and Firth-Cozens 2003; Wood 2006), conceptions of "good doctoring" or role modeling (Cruess, Cruess, and Steinert 2008; Wright et al. 1998), and acceptance of haphazard teaching (Lempp and Seale 2004).

It is also well recognized that the epistemological and social hierarchies and norms that separate medicine from "non-medicine" (whether manifest in lay or allied professional forms) have analogues *within* medicine. The loosely overlapping distinctions between "high-status" and "low-status" working contexts and agendas, between "hard" and "soft" forms of knowledge, and between specialist prestige and generalist respect—although continuously contested—are themselves reproduced through the hidden curriculum. In short, the "fact" that not all medical identities are equal is well known and learned, but it is not part of the official curriculum. Similarly, the existence of a prestige rank order of medical specialties (and of diseases) is well documented (Hinze 1999; Shortell 1974) but is not openly debated (Album and Westin 2008), although frequently discussed informally among medical students and healthcare professionals.

For example, with a focus on nine specialties, Furnham (1986) investigated the attitudes and beliefs of 449 preclinical and clinical medical students in three London University Medical Schools. Psychiatry was scored with the lowest status and was perceived as most unspecific, most imprecise as a body of knowledge, and an "unreal" area of expertise. Moreover, psychiatrists were seen as less stable people, who were keen to establish rapport with their patients. In contrast, surgery was viewed as a male-dominated "real" discipline, whose results were replicable, and with theories least removed from practice. Further, surgeons appeared most dogmatic, least interested in humanizing medicine, less concerned with treating the whole person, and least susceptible to the emotional demands of patients.

Similarly, Album and Westin (2008) conducted a cross-sectional survey of 805 senior physicians and 490 senior medical students in Norway, focusing on thirty-eight different diseases that require hospitalization across twenty-three medical specialties. Specialties associated with technologically sophisticated, immediate, and invasive procedures in vital organs located in the upper body were given high prestige scores (for example, myocardial infarction, leukemia, and brain tumor, usually found in younger patients, linked to neurosurgery; thoracic surgery; and cardiology medical specialties). In contrast, low prestige scores were assigned to diseases and specialties associated with chronic conditions located in the lower part of the body or without specific location (for example, fibromyalgia syndrome and anxiety); and with less invasive procedures and older patients, cared for by geriatricians, psychiatrists, or general physicians. The diseases with lower rankings are those often associated with the concept of stigma (Goffman 1963), and people's experiences of being stigmatized or discriminated against (Thornicroft, Rose, and Kassam 2007).

Hinze's interview study (1999) added a twist to these findings and uncovered a further silent and symbolic reality. Specifically, she highlighted a gendered hierarchy of medical specialties. Hinze's findings are that the prestige hierarchy of medical disciplines is not gender neutral, but shows a structure with men at the top and women on the bottom of the ranking ladder, symbolized by masculine (hands-on hard work and toughness) and feminine (passivity and softness) stereotypical connotations.

What these studies suggest is that medical specialization exists in a world of professional tribalism characterized by persistent gender stratification, the importance of professional status, and, in some cases, an emphasis on narrow specialist technical skills at the expense of softer, "less real" and "feminine" dispositions. The complex experience of being embedded within these different roles and settings no doubt diverges to some degree from these reported rankings and connotations, but these accounts, though involving simplifications, are not straightforwardly false. That is, students not only learn about medical hierarchies through the hidden curriculum but, insofar as they follow different patterns of training and select different kinds of specialist emphases, they are subject to different hidden *curricula*. Different clusters and configurations of values are subtly presented, stressed, and reproduced in different settings.

The Depth of the Hidden Curriculum

This story of relative diversity can also be seen with only a superficial implication of paradox as a story of unity. The boundaries between medicine and non-medicine are not particularly blurred—not least because the occupational and social positions of doctors are heavily governed, defined, and defended. Indeed, the glue that holds together the various domains of medicine within these boundaries is powerful. In this regard, medicine can be seen as a paradigm of the standard model within sociology of professions: the profession of medicine is a transaction between members of an occupational group and the broader society in which claims to distinctive forms of expertise and standards are traded for significant social status and authority.

Essentially, the same processes operate *within* medicine; that is, it is the claim to special professional knowledge that often underpins the relative social status and authority of doctors in their relationships with one another and with other health occupations. This can be seen quite clearly in microsociological studies where medical students often make discriminations about relative occupational prestige. They tend to do so by reference to the foundational role of "special" medical knowledge that is frequently linked to the hard-soft knowledge distinction as part of the formation of medical identity (Donetto 2010). The corollary of this logic is, of course, that forms of expertise that are less specific to medicine (or less specific within medicine) will tend to be of lower status, (for example, health promotion or medical ethics).

This broad equation between lower status and forms of expertise that are less medicine specific helps to explain the extraordinary resilience of some of the hierarchies in the hidden curriculum. No one is saying that caring dispositions or communication, and so on, are intrinsically unimportant. Indeed, many people, inside and outside medicine, stress the opposite and repeatedly seek to promote the importance of these qualities in the profession. However, a key element of the diversity and breadth of medical education reform is that more liberal, humanistic or sociocritical currents are differentially embedded in different areas of medical education. In the United Kingdom context, at least, many themes related to these currents (for example, person-centeredness) are well established across the official curriculum. But in practice, they have much greater hold in some areas of the hidden curriculum than in others. Areas of resistance, we are arguing, are not explained by anyone asserting that softer forms of knowledge are unimportant. Indeed, they are identified by medical students as positive qualities in medical role models (Lempp and Seale 2004). It is much more likely that these softer forms of knowledge are just less medicine specific, and therefore have less to contribute to the maintenance of the epistemic and social authority of doctors.

To recognize this underlying logic, that is, the foundational role that "special" medical knowledge plays in medical identify formation, does not depend on a critical reading of medicine. Students' induction into special and specialist clinical sciences is also central to those functionalist sociological readings of medicine that strongly affirm the profession. Doctors, individually and collectively, often are called on to provide socially definitive judgments on questions of huge personal and policy significance; and only the most anti-science skeptics would suggest that there is no legitimate place for highly specialist clinical expertise. Undertaking this socially important role involves closing in on scientifically better answers; closing down on open-ended questions of policy and professional action; and making practical, and sometimes technical, interventions (for example, the design and uses of reproductive technology options or health screening systems). Doctors are asked to take responsibility for these forms of closure and cannot be expected to do so from a position of epistemological agnosticism or relativism. However, the challenge, recognized by many inside and outside medicine, is how to keep this necessary emphasis on scientific and technical paradigms within its legitimate sphere, and how to ensure effective checks and balances from other forms of, and sources of, knowledge and social authority. In practice, this is where the hidden curriculum messages about relatively core and peripheral aspects of medical knowledge assert themselves again and again.

Sociological studies of medical students continue to suggest that the emphasis of medical education is for them to learn to perform competently, by acquiring "hard" knowledge, in a way that relatively sidelines caring behavior for example (Brosnan 2009). This reproduction of knowledge hierarchies is also reinforced through broader structural processes. For example, in the UK these hierarchies are deeply embedded in the ranking tables of the most successful medical schools. Those institutions that maintain a traditional science-oriented medical curriculum—for example, Oxford, Cambridge, and Edinburgh (Brosnan 2010)—achieve the highest standings and are able to attract the students with the top grades. In return, this helps to secure an elevated standing the following year and to gain further applications, funding, and prestige.

What are perhaps less well recognized than these institutional structures of reproduction are the metatheoretical structuring effects of medical epistemology. Here we are referring to the ways in which many relative departures from assumptions about either scientism or the social authority of doctors are both widely endorsed within medical education and the medicine profession, and yet, at the same time, are effectively undermined or cancelled out through the governance of dominant, broadly technicist paradigms. Those operating within alternative paradigms (for example, liberal or sociocritical perspectives) are often expected to explain and account for themselves through the foundational logics of "hard" knowledge and epistemic and practical closure. At a day-to-day level within medical schools, where these structuring effects are experienced viscerally, staff who are interested in "softer" areas are expected to justify themselves in ways that appeal to harder conceptions of knowledge (for example, through modeling, measurement, and experimental methodologies), whereas the reverse is very much rarer; that is, "hard clinical scientists" are much less likely to be asked to elucidate and defend the necessarily complex and contested values and purposes underpinning their own work.

Thus far, we have sought to provide a summary of what we mean by the breadth and the depth of the hidden curriculum and thereby give an indication of the potential tensions between them. Breadth, both in the sense of variations across curricula and in enriched and epistemologically diverse curricula, sometimes exists uneasily with depth, given the organizing power of the foundational and core logic of what is "special" about medical knowledge. To conclude, we want to suggest why these potential strains pose a crucial challenge not only to medical educators but also to the future of medical professionalism.

Personalized Medicine and Personalized Care

It frequently is suggested that professional education needs to evolve to reflect broader sociodemographic, cultural, and epidemiological changes (Album and Westin 2008; Frenk et al. 2010). One underlying concern is that medicine's professional ethos is outdated and has not kept pace with multiple present challenges to medical practice including, for example, the increase in long-term conditions and disability that are often complex and difficult to treat. There are, for instance, 15.4 million people in England (from a population of just over 53 million) living with one or more long-term conditions. These are defined as illnesses that cannot currently be cured, but can be controlled by medication and other therapies (Department of Health 2008a). It has been argued (Cribb 2000) that what these transitions require are more open-ended, diffuse, and complex healthcare approaches, which "imply the need for partnership rather than circumscribed technical interventions," or specifically working "with" people and not just "on" them (Cribb 2000, 917). These shifts are accompanied, in the UK health policy and elsewhere, by constant calls for reforms of healthcare that (1) view clinical conditions in the context of people's personal circumstances and biographies, and (2) are responsive to the values and preferences of individuals about the lives they want to be enabled to lead (Entwistle et al. 2012). Labels, such as person-centered or personalized care, are often used to capture these more diffuse and responsive agendas. It follows that medical students need to be educationally prepared for this different approach to healthcare; one that is broader than, and in some respects at odds with, the traditional scientific emphasis of medicine and its curricula.

However, against the background of this more "diffused" health agenda (Cribb 2000), there has been the rise of personalization in another, equally interesting but much narrower sense. Specifically, there has been a steady embrace of genomic and personalized medicine to guide medical decision making (Ginsburg and Willard 2009). In essence, this new area of medicine (and its further specialization) takes each person's unique clinical, genetic, genomic, and environmental information into account when assessing individual risks for developing a disease with the aim of prescribing individualized treatment plans. The guiding, arguably somewhat simplistic, principle for this emerging approach is "the right drug, at the right dose at the right time" (Hamburg and Collins 2010, 301). This new paradigm shift seems, at least in part, to be driven by the pharmacological industry and biomedical scientists, underpinned by commercial motivation.

The success of this shift will depend on accurate diagnostic tests (for example, as already applied in breast cancer and cardiovascular disease), translational science, and regulatory policies to protect patients (Hamburg and Collins 2010). Some authors have questioned whether this approach will provide satisfactory solutions to common diseases in the near future or contribute to better health and quality of life for the population (Baird 2001). Specifically, the complex interplay between environment and health; the link between human disease, lifestyle, and circumstances (for example, smoking, alcohol consumption, physical inactivity, and poor nutrition or sanitation); and human behavior with regard to medicine concordance have been suggested as challenges to this conception of personalized medicine.

This conception of personalized medicine is in striking contrast to the notion of personalized care planning recommended and endorsed by the UK government (Department of Health 2008b). The government's aims are to provide people with long-term conditions more control over which treatment and services they can receive, to meet their complex needs and offer support to self-care. In this vision of long-term care, patients appear to be more in the driving seat, and their participation plays an integral and important role in their continuing management pathway. Whereas *personalized care* emphasizes responsiveness to patient perspectives and agency, *personalized medicine* seems to emphasize a supply-side model in which scientists deliver inventions to clinicians (Perkins et al. 2007) who, in turn, deliver treatments to patients. Such thinking shows little commitment to how best to integrate the view of service users and public participation in healthcare (Thornicroft, Lempp, and Tansella 2011).

Conclusion

Personalized medicine shows the continuing power and utility of clinical science forms of expertise, and illustrates and reasserts the depth of the hidden curriculum and the foundational logic of "special" medical knowledge. However, personalized care shows the importance of broader epistemologies and conceptions of healthcare professionalism. It would be a mistake to dismiss the importance of either of these emphases. However, we argue, there is a danger: the way in which medical students are still enculturated in contexts that structurally valorize and privilege narrower rather than broader conceptions of expertise and professionalism.

PART III
METHODOLOGICAL AND ASSESSMENT APPROACHES

This section is a cornerstone of this book, due not only to the diversity and excellence of its contributors, but also to the current dearth of specifics about how one might go about examining the hidden curriculum. Because of his own groundbreaking work on measuring the hidden curriculum (for example, the C3 scale; see Haidet et al. 2005), we asked Paul Haidet (joined here by Cayla Teal) to provide a fresh look into how he might biopsy the hidden curriculum today. This is one of the many chapters in this book that could have been three times its length and still not be complete. Haidet and Teal chose to highlight one approach, the LOGIC Model, but the field is ripe for other vehicles. Following Haidet and Teal, we provide three additional windows into the hidden curriculum, including discourse analysis (Tina Martimianakis and Nancy McNaughton, chapter 8), narrative analysis (Pooja Rutberg and Elizabeth Gaufberg, chapter 9), and survey analysis (Dorene Balmer and Boyd Richards, chapter 10).

Once again, these are not the only tools one might use, but all four chapters provide us with distinctly different approaches for how we might gather information on the context and content of health professions education. These four chapters notwithstanding, tools for examining the subterranean domains of educational practices—and that do so relative to its more surface topography—remain one of the more underexplored elements in the overall body of work on the hidden curriculum. Readers also should note that there is a subsequent chapter (Kelly Edwards, chapter 20) on the culture of research training, but this chapter is framed more as a thematic case study (for example, how one might apply the hidden curriculum to research training) than as a specific methodological approach.

7: Organizing Chaos

A Conceptual Framework for Assessing Hidden Curricula in Medical Education

PAUL HAIDET AND CAYLA R. TEAL

Defined as the "the set of influences that function at the level of organizational structure and culture" (Hafferty and Franks 1994, 770), the hidden curriculum includes the behaviors of, and interactions among, learners, educators, and institutional leaders who significantly influence the intended messages of the formal curriculum. Although a hidden curriculum theoretically can influence learners and faculty in positive or negative ways, the medical education community most commonly has focused on students' adoption of behaviors or attitudes that appear to counter intentional educational efforts. For instance, student attitudes and behaviors may be influenced by the clinician who takes shortcuts in physical exams because "the detailed way students are taught is unnecessary in the real world"; by the educator who suggests that students should worry more about basic science than communication skills because "talking is easy"; or by the leader who financially supports young researchers, but not educators, because "researchers need protected time to develop." Persistent attitudes and behaviors such as these significantly impact learner development to the point that many educators and accrediting bodies in recent years have developed a strong interest in systematically identifying and measuring the hidden curriculum and, subsequently, intervening to improve the learning environment. Hidden curricula can exist in a variety of health education settings, but this chapter will focus on assessment specifically within the medical school context. Our purpose is to provide a conceptual framework to guide efforts to assess one's local hidden curriculum.

Assessing a Hidden Curriculum: Context Specific, Context Dependent

Although many educators can observe and articulate the overall effects of the hidden curriculum, what usually is not apparent is the constellation of

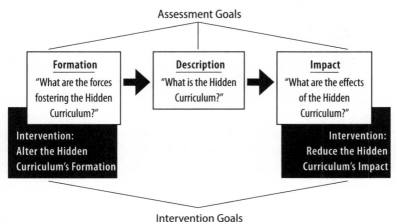

Figure 7.1

countervailing microforces, related to both formal and hidden curricula, that lead to these effects. Individuals, such as students, who experience this array of forces are left to try to pull meaning out of this seeming chaos. From the viewpoint of an assessor, some preparation is needed to hone the direction that will guide assessment activities.

Realizing that organizational cultures and hidden curricula tend to be in constant flux and to evolve over time, we propose a simplified schematic in figure 7-1 to organize one's initial focus in approaching assessment. As shown, one can assess the formation, description, or impact of a hidden curriculum, or some combination of the three. Most often, educators focus on the middle box, asking the question, "What *is* the hidden curriculum here at our institution, in our department, and so on?" However, interventions to address the hidden curriculum or its effects must necessarily be aimed at one of the other two foci, either through altering ongoing formation and reformation of the hidden curriculum itself (Cottingham et al. 2008) or by reducing its impact (Thompson et al. 2010). From an assessment standpoint, questions about formation or impact necessitate a broader scope than just understanding and describing. Description is an important first step for hidden curricula that are not well understood, but this first step should be coupled with an assessment of either formation or impact in order to adequately plan and evaluate an intervention strategy. In this chapter, we will focus on description and impact, because the current literature offers strong examples of these areas. However, information about where and how a hidden curriculum originated often is inherent in describing it.

Although writers and speakers often refer to "the" hidden curriculum, we assert that "a" hidden curriculum is a more accurate term. Empirical evidence suggests that the hidden curriculum is not one all-encompassing culture that affects every person and process across multiple institutions, but rather that there exist multiple local organizational cultures within individual medical schools and their affiliated clinical institutions (Haidet et al. 2006). This point is important, because when focusing on assessment, one first needs to define the "field of view" with respect to which hidden curriculum one intends to biopsy. The field of view can be defined by considering three questions: (1) "About what?" (2) "In what context?" (3) "As experienced by whom?"

As shown in table 7-1, the first consideration ("About what?") focuses on the *content* of the hidden curriculum. Hidden curricula in medical education have been discussed in relationship to behavioral and social sciences (Adler, Hughes, and Scott 2006), professionalism (Karnieli-Miller et al. 2011; Rogers et al. 2012), patient-centered care (Al-Bawardy et al. 2009), communication (Bell et al. 2010), evidence-based practice (Agrawal et al. 2008), and quality and safety (Bradley et al. 2011), among other topics.

The second consideration ("In what context?") focuses on the *context* of the hidden curriculum. Context can come in several different forms. Most important, hidden curricula usually are specific to the *entity* within which they occur—educational institutions, training hospitals, and so on. There also may be *administrative units* within which hidden curricula exist—departments, centers, divisions, hospital wards, and so on. Next, hidden curricula may occur within specific *structural or curricular units*—courses, particular educational teams, clerkships, and so on. Finally, there may be key *message bearers* whose interactions carry particular influence in disseminating the content of hidden curricula.

The third consideration ("As experienced by whom?") is the *lens*, or vantage point, through which a hidden curriculum is being experienced. Much of the literature focuses on students' and trainees' experiences, but faculty, nurses, institutional leaders, and others also can be affected by the hidden curriculum. The choice of the proper lens should be driven by one's goal or purpose in assessing a hidden curriculum.

Consider the two scenarios in table 7-1. The first explores a hidden curriculum influencing student beliefs about behavioral sciences training within preclinical medical education at a specific medical school. What are the contextual elements within which this hidden curriculum might exist?

TABLE 7.1

Examples of a Hidden Curriculum's Content, Context, and Lens

CONTENT (about what?)	(in what) CONTEXT?				LENS (as experienced by whom?)
	Entity (setting)	Administrative Unit (departments, divisions)	Structural Unit (curricular element)	Message Bearers	
The value of the behavioral sciences in preclinical medical education	A specific medical college	Pre-clerkship curriculum	A particular block of courses	Senior students; Course directors; Clinical faculty	Students
The feasibility of patient-centered care	A teaching hospital	Department of medicine	Medicine clerkship	Hospital administrators; Departmental leadership	Clinician educators

In the scenario, if one is interested in how students decide on which courses to prioritize in studying for exams, the structural unit becomes a particular block of courses including traditional basic science courses and a behavioral science course. Suppose that, after talking with preclinical students, one were to find that even though all the block courses are weighted equally in terms of course hours or credits, students are prioritizing material in the basic sciences based on the notion that "only those going into psychiatry will ever use the behavioral science material."

In this instance, one might target a combination of senior students and faculty as important message bearers. In this scenario, the senior students may be very influential, based on their observing the rarity of integration of behavioral science concepts among clinical faculty not working in psychiatry. Further, a well-respected course director might be overheard suggesting to students that the basic science courses require mastering of specific jargon and more work than the "commonsense" concepts in behavioral science. Identifying and understanding this hidden curriculum would require an assessor to identify these contextually specific behaviors and beliefs. In similar fashion, the second scenario describes the content, context, and lenses that one might choose in a scenario where clinical educators are role modeling less than patient-centered behaviors because clinical quotas regarding the numbers of patients seen are creating difficulties for actually engaging in patient-centered care.

In summary, before planning an assessment of a hidden curriculum, one must first be clear about what aspects of a hidden curriculum (formation, description, impact) one will focus on. If the ultimate goal is to intervene, the focus should include more than just description. Second, one needs to define the field of view with respect to content and context and select the appropriate lens(es) through which to view the hidden curriculum. Once these elements are appropriately defined, assessment is ready to begin.

A Conceptual Model for Organizing Efforts to Assess Hidden Curricula

In this section, we adopt the Logic Model (W. K. Kellogg Foundation 2004) as a framework for organizing efforts to measure hidden curricula. The Logic Model was specifically designed to organize program development activities and to tie outcomes to programs. As such, it has proven to be a useful tool in guiding program evaluation. Although previous use of the model has focused mainly on *planned* programs, we posit that it also has utility for organizing efforts to assess *unplanned* programs, such as hidden curricula. The Logic Model, depicted in figure 7-2, directs attention to five aspects of a hidden curriculum; two of these aspects focus on the description, and three focus on the impact. As shown in the figure, the five aspects consist of *inputs* or resources, *activities*, *outputs* or immediate products, *outcomes* or intermediate results, and *impact* or longer-term effects of a hidden curriculum. In the following paragraphs, we examine each aspect.

The first aspect is the *inputs* of a particular hidden curriculum. In a formal curriculum, inputs consist of those things that are invested to support the curriculum—basic content, individuals who teach, time set aside for teaching, and so on. Similarly, in hidden curricula, the inputs are the underlying premises and messages that comprise and sustain a particular hidden curriculum. Most often, the premises of a particular hidden curriculum establish expectations of how members of the educational community (teachers, students, and so on) should think or act. For example, in a study of messages that faculty encountered in their institution (Haidet and Stein 2006,

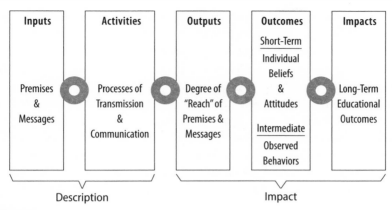

Figure 7.2

S17), the following statements were listed as representative of the kinds of things they had heard or talked about:

- There is always ONE right answer to any problem.
- Doctors never admit to not knowing something.
- Solving social and personal problems is not a primary goal of medicine.

These three statements all relate to an underlying premise, namely, that "uncertainty or complexity are to be avoided." This premise, though not always explicitly stated, supports and sustains the actual statements that *are* made by teachers, students, and others, and guides their behaviors as well. This underlying premise, then, is an important input of the particular hidden curriculum that those faculty experienced. Efforts aimed at assessing the inputs of a hidden curriculum have most frequently been conducted as qualitative inquiry. For example, qualitative approaches have been used to examine premises about integrative medicine (Adler et al. 2006), value of knowledge versus skill in medicine (Eva et al. 2011; Bernabeo et al. 2011), organizational perspectives on medical education about Indigenous peoples (Ewen et al. 2012), value of palliative care education (Fernandes et al. 2008), paternalistic attitudes toward patients (Lamiani et al. 2011), gender roles in clinical care (Lempp and Seale 2006), selection and presentation of clinical cases (Turbes, Krebs, and Axtell 2002), and cultural competency education (Wachtler and Troein 2003). Qualitative methods in the form of interviews, focus groups, ethnographic methods, and various observational techniques are specifically useful for exploring hidden curriculum inputs. On the other hand, if the premises already are well understood and the point of assessment is to examine to what extent competing premises are held by influential members of the community, then attitudinal survey methods might be an appropriate alternative.

The second aspect in the Logic Model is *activities*. The activities of hidden curricula are analogous to the structures (courses, and so on) of and methods (pedagogy, and so on) used in formal curricula. However, unlike formal curricula, the activities of hidden curricula are informal, unplanned, often spontaneous, and likely nonlinear as well. Examples could include casual conversations in workrooms and offices, observed hierarchical relationships in the context of medical care teams, and patterns of interaction among healthcare personnel. These activities serve to transmit and communicate the premises of the hidden curriculum. In the literature, qualitative methods have been used to identify modes of premise transmission. Examples of these include how attitudes about professional behavior were transmitted to students (Adkoli et al. 2011) and how persistent beliefs about working with selected patients were maintained in an organization (Ewen et al. 2012). A variety of new techniques may be useful for assessing activities of the hidden curriculum. Social network analysis may be helpful for identifying common paths by which premises are transmitted, that is, from whom to whom? Quantitative survey-based methods may be particularly useful if the survey instruments are based on advance qualitative work. For example, survey methods have been used to explore student perceptions about end-of-life care and the educational modalities through which they gained those perceptions (Billings et al. 2010). Data from surveys also might be useful in path analysis for determining the relative importance of various modes of transmission and types of message bearers.

As shown in figure 7-1, assessments directed at identifying inputs and activities are answering the descriptive question, "What is the hidden curriculum?" If the activities responsible for transmitting or communicating the premises result in their adoption, then the premises might start guiding the behaviors of those who pass through a particular hidden curriculum. The Logic Model suggests that evidence of adoption would exist in outputs, outcomes, and impact. Assessment of these would focus on answering the overarching question, "What is the impact of the hidden curriculum?"

In a generic Logic Model, *outputs* are considered service delivery units, such as numbers of courses or students taught. Even though hidden curricula are not planned, there are still outputs in the form of the numbers of people that are reached by the premises of the hidden curriculum. Short-term and intermediate outcomes, then, result from the delivery of the premises, and impact consists of the long-term effects. All of these elements are straightforward in a formal curriculum. For example, the outputs of a traditional curriculum might consist of the number of courses, sessions, clinical experiences, and so on. The *outcomes* are learner knowledge and skill, while the *impact* consists of learners' success as residents and eventually as physicians. Because of the informal nature of hidden curricula, these three concepts shift, particularly with respect to outputs.

As a result, an assessment strategy needs to focus not on service delivery units, but rather on the reach or extent to which learners come in contact with the premises or the agents (teachers, role models, administrators, and so on) who will foster adoption of premises. Measurement in this realm could consist of a combination of qualitative and quantitative methods. Of all the elements in our Logic Model, outputs have been studied the least with respect to the hidden curriculum. However, one intriguing study used survey methods to explore student attitudes about professionalism (the outcome) and how this outcome linked to students' reported degree of exposure (the output) to faculty unprofessional behavior (the activity) (Johnston et al. 2011). Studies such as this provide some insight into the importance of measuring outputs by suggesting that frequent or powerful communication activities can significantly perpetuate the hidden curriculum's premises.

The fourth aspect of the Logic Model focuses on *outcomes* of the hidden curriculum. We suggest that short-term outcomes consist of individuals' beliefs and attitudes, and that intermediate outcomes consist of their observed behaviors. Assessment techniques to measure outcomes can include either qualitative methods (for example, field observations of behavioral, coded video or audio recordings) or quantitative methods (for example, surveys), though the proliferation of attitudinal surveys as well as surveys assessing self-report or observed behavior make quantitative methods more likely. Further, both types of outcomes (attitudinal and behavioral) can be explored in tandem. For example, outcomes of hidden curricula with respect to patient-centeredness have been explored in medical education (Haidet et al. 2006; Al-Bawardy et al. 2009; Krupat et al. 2009) using the Patient Practitioner Orientation Scale (Krupat et al. 1999), which measures patient-centered attitudes, and the C3 instrument (Haidet, Kelly, and Chou 2005), which measures student recollection of observed behaviors among both students and faculty. Other survey studies have explored students' attitudes and behavior resulting from hidden curricula about professionalism (Johnston et al. 2011), preparedness for providing end-of-life care (Billings et al. 2010), patient safety (Madigosky et al. 2006), and career choice (Hunt et al. 1996).

The last, and perhaps the most commonly measured, aspect of hidden curricula is their *impact*. The focus of measurement here is usually on the long-term outcomes (attitudes or behaviors) that are presumed to be a result of time spent and experiences encountered within a particular hidden curriculum. Such measurements are typically quantitative and have included surveys, objective structured clinical exams, attitudinal measures, 360-degree evaluations, and evaluation of particular choices (such as specialty choice). Unfortunately, longitudinal impacts, especially on learners who encounter hidden curricula early in their training, are not commonly studied, and very little literature exists to date on the subject.

The Logic Model in Action

In this final section, we present a hypothetical example using concepts from this chapter. Our intent is to demonstrate the use of the Logic Model to develop a comprehensive, focused plan for assessing a hidden curriculum. Before we begin, we raise two issues for consideration. First, when identifying premises as part of assessing inputs, it may not be necessary or feasible to try to follow *all* of the premises encountered. Rather, it might be more efficient to identify one or a few premises that seem particularly powerful and then focus predominantly on those. Second, although the Logic Model implies a linear, causal relationship between elements such as outputs, outcomes, and impacts, the reality might not be strictly linear or causal. For example, attitudes and behaviors may be forming simultaneously, creating the opportunity to measure both in a single survey.

Example: Assessing the impact of a comprehensive and demanding anatomy course on students' patient-centered attitudes in the pre-clerkship curriculum.

Imagine that students at Anywhere Medical School start their medical education with a ten-week immersion course in anatomy that consists of lectures, gross anatomy lab dissections, radiograph interpretation, and histology. Imagine that this course starts during the second week of medical school, meets every day in some fashion, and runs concurrently with a two-sessions-per-week introductory course in physical examination and patient-physician communication. Anatomy faculty are highly engaged in teaching their courses, and have passionately defended the need for students to learn the subject comprehensively and early as a "foundation for subsequent medical problem solving and decision making." The dean of the pre-clerkship curriculum at Anywhere Medical School is interested in the extent to which students gain or lose patient-centered attitudes based on their experiences in anatomy, given its large and early footprint in their educational experiences. Rather than just measure students' attitudes before and after the anatomy course (which might show a difference but might also be secondary to a variety of other influences beyond the anatomy course), you decide to assess the hidden curriculum with respect to patient-centered care as it pertains to the anatomy course.

Using the Logic Model, you first focus on the anatomy course-specific inputs, or the premises and messages, with respect to patient-centered care. You start by reviewing the literature and brainstorming a list of areas that seem to reside at the intersection of anatomy and patient-centered care, such as studying, patients, the human body, cadavers, death and dying, and others. You then use a combination of field observations (sitting in on lectures; observing gross anatomy lab) and interviews to explore what messages and premises exist about these issues. Let's assume that you find and decide to focus on two particular premises with respect to anatomy and patients-as-human-beings (a core tenet of patient-centered care): (1) an informal premise that anatomy should take precedence over all other concurrent courses, and (2) a point of view that tends to systematically deconstruct the human body into component parts, obscuring one's personhood.

In order to determine whether these two messages are systematically influencing students in a way that erodes patient-centered attitudes, you would need to measure the activities, outputs, outcomes, and impacts of the anatomy course, focusing on these messages and their effects on patient-centered attitudes among students. For the activities and outputs, you might design a mixed-methods study aimed at uncovering modes of transmission of the premises and determining the extent to which such modes are reaching students in the first-year class. Such processes might include overt teacher comments during lectures and labs, the influence of teaching assistants during laboratories, advice from upper-level students assigned to first-year students in mentoring or big brother–big sister programs, advice from faculty mentors or advisors, and others. Measuring the extent and reach of such processes could be done with a survey of the first-year medical students.

If your survey of activities and outputs suggests that the premises achieve a large reach among first-year students, you might then decide to measure short-term and intermediate outcomes. Two important short-term attitudinal outcomes related to the premises might be (1) beliefs about the value of prioritizing studying anatomy over preparing for the physical diagnosis and medical communication course, and (2) views about the relative importance of fixing underlying biomechanical derangements as opposed to addressing the social or psychological needs of patients. Again, this might be done in a survey of the first-year class using items designed specifically to address these issues or previously validated instruments that measure these or closely related constructs. The behaviorally based outcome measures that you might tie to these beliefs could consist of time spent studying anatomy relative to preparing for other classes, and perhaps students' focus in communicating with patients in simulations and patient encounters during the concurrent physical exam and communication course.

Finally, the impact might be measured with a survey of student attitudes toward patient-centered care before and after the anatomy class. As mentioned at the beginning of this example, one could have pursued only this last step. However, without measuring the other aspects directed by the Logic Model, it would have been difficult to develop specific connections to the anatomy course, or to determine the power and extent of any hidden curriculum that existed within and around the course. Such data would be important to examine before intervening in the anatomy course or elsewhere.

Data Collection

This chapter focuses mainly on primary data collection; that is, data collected expressly for the purpose of measuring a hidden curriculum. However, as in other areas of research and assessment, it may be quicker and more convenient to conduct a secondary analysis of already existing data that may have been collected for some other purpose. In the case of assessing hidden curricula, secondary data has the same characteristic problems as it typically does for any evaluation or research project: the data must be useful given the research question, must be available and accessible, and must be of high quality. Because hidden curricula are highly dependent on context, meeting these three criteria may be even more challenging than for other research or assessment tasks. If the secondary data was collected to answer broad questions, it may lack the focus necessary to fully understand a hidden curriculum. On the other hand, secondary data from too specific a question may not have the relevance needed to explore a hidden curriculum. For example, many schools recently have been collecting data about student burnout that may point to the existence of disconnects and schisms in the learning environment. Although this may suggest the possibility of a hidden curriculum, it may not lend itself to exploring fully or pinpointing causal elements in that hidden curriculum.

Conclusion

We advocate for a focused and comprehensive approach to assessing hidden curricula that exist in medical schools and teaching hospitals. Such an approach would include advance work to answer these questions: "About what?" "In what context?" "As experienced by whom?" This advance work would be followed by a plan that uses a variety of methods to explore the inputs, activities, outputs, outcomes, and impacts of a particular hidden curriculum. We believe that this approach will provide useful information about the nature of the hidden curriculum, potential targets for intervention, and elements to monitor in assessing progress toward improving the learning environment for students and faculty.

8: Discourse, Governmentality, Biopower, and the Hidden Curriculum

Maria Athina (Tina) Martimianakis and
Nancy McNaughton

We know that culture, structures, and institutions impact learning (Freidson 1986; Good 2003; Muzzin 2001); that professional identity is formed and negotiated in everyday activity (Becker et al. 1961; Beagan 2000); and that educational practice includes struggles over what counts as knowledge with material implications including access to resources, equipment, and decision making (Bourdieau and Wacquant 1992; Gieryn 1983). What we know less about is what happens when we label aspects of the curriculum "hidden" and create the imperative for addressing the effects of learning that are not explicitly controlled by learners or teachers.

Foucauldian discourse analysis provides the opportunity to address the importance of the hidden curriculum as an active social practice. Such an approach allows the researcher to make visible the gaps between espoused, formal, and enacted expectations, as well as to examine how a focus on the hidden curriculum is productive inside and outside medical training contexts. Operationalizing a Foucauldian approach can take on multiple forms, all of which recognize criticality and the material effects inherent in intersecting discourses and what they make possible in practice. A number of resources exist that guide the researcher into the intricacies of this type of exploration (Kuper, Whitehead, and Hodges 2013).

In this chapter, we draw on Foucault's concepts of discourse, governmentality, and biopower to explore how the hidden curriculum, as an object for medical education intervention and management, relates to medicine's professional project (Foucault 1994; Lemke 2001; Skelton 1997).

Discourse Enacted: An OSCE Professionalism Case

A medical resident walks into an exam room where she sees a sixty-year-old man seated on the exam table in a gown. The resident has read on the candidate instructions that the man has come into the clinic today because his left knee has been bothering him so much that he can no longer comfortably walk a reasonable distance or crouch down. The resident asks the man for the location of the pain as well as its history. As she moves to examine the man's knee, she notices that the patient has become restless and that his breathing is shallow and faster than at the beginning of the encounter. She is about to ask if the patient is comfortable when the man collapses to the floor.

An examiner observing the interaction is filling out a checklist and at this point in the encounter is waiting to see how the resident responds to this sudden turn of events. Will the resident take the time to adjust the patient's gown so that when he regains consciousness he will not be embarrassed to find himself naked? Will the resident maintain a professional vocabulary that respects the patient as a person, even if the man is not apparently awake to hear her?

This is an Objective Structured Clinical Examinations (OSCE) station, in which the resident is being assessed across a number of professionalism criteria that are understood to be an essential part of a clinician's critical thinking, decision making and professional demeanor. It has been designed to make visible the implicit expectations about professionalism that accompany the knowledge and procedural skills related to knee pain.

OSCEs are currently considered "state of the art" in health professional assessment for their effectiveness in measuring a range of behaviors, skills, knowledge, and attitudes in trainees. The OSCE format is made possible by two interrelated ideas: first, that "clinical performance has to be proven by testing, measurement and recording," and second, that "it also needs to be psychometrically acceptable and defensible" (Boursicot et al. 2011, 371). The act of teachers observing and grading trainees as they conduct history taking, physical examination procedures, diagnosis, and management of standardized patients is enacted as part of an explicit curriculum and educational enterprise that assumes trainees can be taught to align their performance of technical skills and expertise with espoused professional norms.

In our example, however, the correct values, beliefs, and attitudes (those that will increase the resident's score on the checklist) may well differ from those enacted by the trainee's teachers in the workplace. As such, this OSCE station is also an assessment of how well this candidate can manage the effects of the hidden curriculum. The construct of the hidden curriculum, as Frederic Hafferty describes, "highlights the importance and impact of structural factors on the learning process. Focusing on this level and type of influence draws our attention to . . . the commonly held 'understandings,' customs, rituals, and taken-for-granted aspects of what goes on in the life-space we call medical education" (Hafferty 1998, 404).

Although this OSCE station does not exist in its current form (to the authors' knowledge), it raises several issues that this chapter will explore related to the construct of the hidden curriculum and its uptake as a regulatory and disciplining technology in medical education. If the candidate fails this station, who else fails with her? The candidate will be denied the passing grade needed to move forward in her studies and receive the credentials necessary to practice. But what about the resident's teachers, or the medical school at which she studies, or the hospital where she works? What consequences will they face if this resident fails this station? Issues beyond the professionalism of this resident are also at stake in this exercise.

Discourse

Discourses are practices that systematically form the objects of which they speak (Foucault 1972, 49). Discourses can be understood as an "interrelated set of texts and the practices of their production, dissemination and reception that bring an object into being" (Phillips and Hardy 2002, 3). Discourses develop over time and are dynamic. They have the appearance of "truths" and are related to in unproblematized ways. According to Foucault, there is no natural progression from one discourse to another. Rather the emergence, reproduction, and dominance of a particular discourse are always contingent and relational.

Discourses represent dominant ideas and create particular material relationships between individuals and between individuals and institutions. Their constitutive properties can be witnessed through the performance and negotiation of professional identities. For example, "teacher as expert" versus "teacher as facilitator" are distinct subject positions supported by differing theories of what makes a "good" teacher. A co-constituting relationship exists among the teacher as expert, the learner as empty vessel, and curricula organized around foundational knowledge. Pedagogical approaches that support this notion of teacher as expert include didactic methodologies. In contrast, the teacher as facilitator starts from the premise that learning is about process. Although foundational knowledge is important, good teaching is not premised on how much the teacher knows, but rather on how well he or she can lead learners to the knowledge they seek. Various learner-centered teaching approaches, as well as faculty development programs, support this discourse of teaching. Parsing the discursive relations that support one or both forms of teaching in a given context would also provide unique insight into the hidden curriculum, for we might also expect that both the teacher and the student would have a different relationship to the hidden curriculum depending on which discourse of teaching or learning was dominant in the particular educational setting.

Such analysis could also focus on isolating and describing statements and practices that are shaped historically in institutional settings through social relations that impact learning implicitly. Returning to our case example, making sense of the situation through the concept of discourse might begin by troubling the taken-for-granted assumptions that as educators, we can create clinical examinations that are "objective" and "standardized" (Hodges 2009). We might also explore how learning is shaped by the idea that empathy and humanism can be taught and then measured. More broadly, such an approach might direct us to investigate how these ideas have become entrenched and taken for granted in our educational practices, and what other objects, relationships, and rules they make possible. We might study which aspects of the hidden curriculum are being evaluated in contexts where teachers are asked to assess student performance using global rating scores or 360-degree evaluations. Or we might even ask, what happens when educators or administrators commit to addressing the effects of the hidden curriculum using checklist approaches, as a way to account to external stakeholders? (Martimianakis 2008).

The relationship an organization or a community of educators will have with the hidden curriculum will depend on the discourses that dominate in their context. In North American medical schools, professionalism and the hidden curriculum are interwoven conversations: the hidden curriculum is evoked as a way to speak about our failure or success as educators in teaching espoused values such as professionalism. Further, it would be hard to argue against the idea that professionalism relates to notions of altruism. But in European settings, altruism and the practice of medicine are not necessarily linked. Understanding how and why professionalism and altruism have historically emerged as interrelated in North American contexts will expose not only how the hidden curriculum operates in the formation and reproduction of norms, but also how it contributes to the construction of readily identifiable, if not openly acknowledged, markers of professional identity that are historically and geographically specific (Hafler et al. 2011).

Foucault's work reminds us that various ideas about the hidden curriculum will engage differing discourses and thus should be taken to be both embodied and enacted. The goal, then, is to identify the strategies used to systematically maintain and reproduce the possibility of certain discourses in a given context and the ideas and possibilities that become obscured in the process (Foucault 1972). Such an approach can account for the ways in which certain forms of knowledge emerge as more relevant and useful than others at a given point in time, like physician ways of "knowing" the body, psychoanalyst ways of "knowing" the human psyche, and educator ways of "knowing" the curriculum. Those who are not trained in the proper knowledge are not trusted or sanctioned socially to heal the body, the soul, or the curriculum.

Foucauldian discourse analysis differs from other analytical approaches applied to the hidden curriculum in that it does not premise learning solely as an educational practice. As such, discourses can be investigated as forms of social action that create effects in the classroom but that also link activity in the classroom to activity outside the classroom. When professionalism is studied as a discourse, the ideas and statements linked to the term *professionalism* have meaning outside of explorations of occupational change and the professional projects of specific occupations. This linking of ideas across sectors makes visible the material implications of professionalism discourses inside and outside the classroom, and offers a pathway for studying how these discourses are used as a form of governance: "In many of the new occupational contexts . . . professionalism is being used to convince, cajole and persuade employees, practitioners and other workers to perform and behave in ways which the organization or the institution deem appropriate, effective and efficient" (Evetts 2003, 411).

Culturally, the discourse of professionalism is reproduced every time a behavior that strikes us as odd, out of place, rude, or worrisome is labeled unprofessional. Studying professionalism through a Foucauldian lens makes visible the contestable nature of its meaning (Hodges, Ginsberg et al. 2011; Martimianakis et al. 2009). Often, what is considered professional behavior for a trainee may be challenged once he or she is in the work setting where the "real" practice of medicine takes place.

Returning to our OSCE case, a Foucauldian analytic lens raises additional questions. How might the activities of educators who are trying to instil the espoused values of professionalism in trainees be undermined by management approaches that draw on different discourses of professionalism that rationalize the importance of efficiency and austerity? This gap between what is being espoused as professional and what is possible to enact in practice is the most often-cited example of the hidden curriculum and attributed generally to teachers who do not model what they teach (Jaye et al. 2006). A Foucauldian reading would explore discourses of role modeling and the expectations they place on teachers to "fix" (regulate) the hidden curriculum, of which they are part. Such an analysis would also challenge us to consider why medical schools are trying to construct trainee behavior to fit a discourse that operates according to different institutional demands than those encountered in the workplace. We might consider how OSCEs and other forms of assessment contribute to the socialization of trainees into the medical profession but also instill in them the importance of complying to the espoused values of future communities they want to belong to, or in Foucauldian terms, create the conditions for "docile bodies" that can be further worked and improved upon in contexts outside formal schooling (Foucault 1995, 136–38). This leads us to explore the Foucauldian construct of governmentality and its utility in making visible the ways in which medical education's interest in making the hidden curriculum visible relates to broader sociopolitical relations.

Governmentality and Biopower

Foucault introduced the notion of governmentality to explain how a de-centered process of governing emerged alongside a mentality of rule that oriented social, cultural, and political practices to the needs of the capitalist market and the neoliberal state (Foucault 2004). For Foucault, the term *government* had expansive meaning and included not only the exercise of power through formal instruments of ruling, but also the way in which individuals draw on particular discourses to authorize their day-to-day behavior. As Rose explains, "Government is achieved through educating citizens in their professional roles and in their personal lives—in the languages by which they interpret their experiences, the norms by which they should evaluate them, the techniques by which they should seek to improve them" (1998, 76).

Foucault introduced the notion of governmentality to explain how a de-centered process of governing emerged alongside a "mentality of rule" that oriented social, cultural, and political practices to the needs of the capitalist market and the neoliberal state (Foucault 2004). For Foucault, the term *government* had expansive meaning and included not only the exercise of power through formal instruments of ruling, but also the way in which individuals draw on particular discourses to authorize their day-to-day behavior. Government then, in the Foucauldian sense, refers to the "conduct of conduct" (Lemke 2001, 45). Foucault shifted the focus away from questions of the exercise of power *over* subjects by other subjects, groups, or institutions to discussions of *how* struggles of power constitute individuals as both subjects and objects of power (Tamboukou 2003, 8). More specifically, the act of making an individual subject is a form of power applied in the context of everyday activity, "which categorizes the individual and marks him by his own individuality, attaches him to his own identity, imposes a law of truth on him which he must recognize and which others have to recognize in him" (Foucault 1982, 212).

Central to this idea of subjectification is Foucault's notion of biopower used "to describe the government or management of populations" through systematized ways of knowing the body as a singularity or a collective (Jaye et al. 2006, 141). Biopower is linked to modern institutions including medicine, public health, and education. As Rabinow and Rose suggest, "Biopower . . . entails one or more truth discourses about the 'vital' character of living human beings; an array of authorities considered competent to speak that truth; strategies for intervention upon collective existence in the name of life and health; and modes of subjectification, in which individuals work on themselves in the name of the individual or collective life or health" (2006, 195).

According to Foucault, biopower captures the shift "towards the techniques of governance that both discipline and regulate social experiences" (Rich and Miah 2009, 166) and is often premised on preventative rationales. Consider the issue of teenage pregnancies and the various strategies that are currently used to prevent them, including sex education classes, abstinence campaigns, and the distribution of free condoms. Several subjectivities are created in the process: teens as "high risk" with respect to their sexual choices, and authorized knowers who have solutions to the problem. Although teenage reproduction was typical in years past, today it is considered "unwanted," "dangerous," and "risky."

> Babies born in the U.S. to teenage mothers are at risk for long-term problems in many major areas of life, including school failure, poverty,

and physical or mental illness. The teenage mothers themselves are also at risk for these problems. (American Academy of Child and Adolescent Psychiatry 2012, par. 1)

Applying a governmentality lens to thinking about teenage pregnancies, we might consider how these truths (risks associated with teenage pregnancies) are used to control and regulate "deviant populations," in this case, teenagers who have not yet finished their education and thus will have a hard time leading productive lives, thereby ending up dependent on the state. Or we might think about the physician and the field of medicine, and their role in creating the "knowing" for this type of governing; and consider how efforts to empower and prevent through patient education and family counseling contribute to the reproduction of neoliberal rationales including rational planning, individualism, economic efficiency, and standardization (Turunen and Rafferty 2013). We might consider the pedagogical techniques currently used to shape the communication between physicians and teens around topics related to sexual intercourse, sexual orientation, abortion, family planning, and so on; and we might ask how "commonly held" understanding, customs, rituals, and taken-for-granted aspects of what goes on in the life-space we call medical education interfere or support the construction of teen pregnancy as risky. In the process, we would be able to challenge "medical educators to acknowledge their training institutions as both cultural entities and moral communities intimately involved in constructing definitions about what is 'good' and 'bad' medicine" (Hafferty 1998, 404).

Biopower is linked to the medical gaze. In *The Birth of the Clinic*, Foucault described how the medical gaze became part of a broader apparatus of governing sociopolitical relationships. As the relationship of science and medicine became institutionalized, the physician became the vessel through which the knowledge of the body flowed, and his or her subjectivity was irrevocably linked to the ability to channel this knowledge. Through science, the physician was given the gift of the "gaze" and assumed the responsibilities as well as all the privileges of exercising the gaze (Foucault 1994, 55). The application of the medical gaze is a form of boundary work that is intimately linked to medicine's professionalization project. By identifying new medical objects to which to apply the medical gaze, medicine has "the ability to limitlessly expand its possibilities on a practical level, as each region of human action can potentially be an object of medical intervention and management" (Alexias 2008, 172). Indeed, in 2004 Hodges argued that the medical gaze has extended to the field of medical education, as physician-teachers work to "know student bodies," that is, to understand the mechanics of learning and being a trainee in order to be able to diagnose diseases of the curriculum. Hodges described a number of micropractices involving self-reflection, self-assessment, and self-regulation that encouraged docility in both teachers and trainees. Close to a decade later, the effects of the medical education gaze are much more pronounced and, more often than not, rationalized on a need to make visible the hidden curriculum.

Recently, the deanery of our school sent a letter to all faculty asking them to stop using teaching cases that began with a patient presenting with a condition to a specialist that had been misdiagnosed by a family practitioner. Apparently, such cases abound and were thought to stigmatize family practice and dissuade students from choosing family medicine as a future career. To make this point, an excerpt from a student reflection was cited, with the explicit permission of the student. Here, the medical education gaze is thus turned back onto teachers through the very techniques used to "discipline" students to the espoused ideals of the profession. It is within this space where pedagogy meets ethics that we come to consider what role the discourse of the hidden curriculum will have in shaping the future of medical practice.

In the end we are reminded that Foucault does not locate the micropractices of power "within conspiratorial group interests or the linear historical process of class, race or gender struggle" (Skelton 1997, 186). Indeed, because power circulates through discourse, there is always the possibility that individuals can strategically use prevailing rationales to resist institutional forces, a particularly relevant issue in relation to discussions of how to harness the positive potential of the hidden curriculum (Karnieli-Miller, Vu, et al. 2010; Sternod 2011).

Conclusion

In this chapter, we have examined several ways in which an analytic approach drawing on the Foucauldian concepts of discourse, governmentality, and biopower can make visible the political work that educators and trainees carry out. Whatever else we deem as an overarching mission for medical schools, their social contract in contemporary Western societies is to prepare trainees to assume social, economic, and civic responsibilities as physicians upon graduation.

Our goal in this chapter was to outline how schools, as socializing and normalizing environments, contribute to the management of populations and individuals (Rose 1998; Popkewitz and Brennan 1998). Through the micropractices of pedagogy, including classroom teaching, writing, grading, examinations, rewards, and punishments, schools operate to produce "docile bodies" that "may be subjected, used, transformed and improved" (Foucault 1995, 136–38). The idea that the body can be known and therefore molded to particular ideals without the use of brute force has made educational contexts, especially medical schools, coveted objects of regulation and a central tenet in contemporary forms of governing (Bragg 2007; Jaye at al. 2006). As we have shown in this chapter, these ideas are especially relevant to discussions of the hidden curriculum.

The use of a Foucauldian analytical approach allows us insight into how the hidden curriculum, like the discourses in which it participates, can be investigated as a form of social action that creates effects in the world. By interrogating how particular ideas dominate and sometimes thwart espoused professionalizing goals, we can begin to act to change practices, decisions, and formations with better insight into how our actions within medical school relate to other facets of our lives.

9: Medical Student Narratives and the Hidden Curriculum

Pooja C. Rutberg and Elizabeth H. Gaufberg

All new learning looks at first like chaos.
—ADRIENNE RICH

Storytelling reveals meaning without committing the error of defining it.
—HANNAH ARENDT

Medical students tell stories all the time—they create written narratives for the chart, condense patient information to fit the boxes in electronic medical records, share detailed patient histories in morning report and brief ones for sign-out, recount funny experiences in the cafeteria and painful ones in quiet moments. These and other narrative forms, when used in specific situations, may further a variety of important goals such as clinical efficiency, diagnostic accuracy, and emotional decompression. Similarly, narrative can serve a variety of educational purposes. When used thoughtfully and effectively, narrative assignments can harness the fundamental human instinct to tell stories as a way to make sense of the world and communicate our experiences with others. When we require students to write about their experiences with the explicit intention of helping them connect to their core values within cultures that do not always support those values, narrative can help shape healthy professional formation. In essence, narrative both reflects and shapes the hidden curriculum of our educational environments.

For the purposes of this chapter, we define *student narrative* as a student writing assignment that involves the telling of an event or experience. Narrative is distinct from other rhetorical modes such as exposition, argument, or description. Here, we explore the ways in which student narratives can serve as *windows* into the hidden curriculum and the cultural contexts in which students work and learn. We describe how student narratives can act as *mirrors*, allowing reflection on experience and a glimpse into our own deeply held values as students, faculty, and citizens. We also discuss how narratives can become *bridges*—creating linkages between an individual's core values and experiences, as well as connecting with members of a larger community of learners. Finally, we review various ways educators are using student narratives in medical education, and we touch on practical issues including confidentiality and approaches to assessment.

Narrative as a Window into the Hidden Curriculum

Student narratives have the potential to show us what is going on in our learning environments by allowing us to explore and begin to understand the intrinsic influences and implicit codes that shape medical training. Accurately elucidating these factors can be challenging for medical educators who are socialized by the hidden curriculum and, as such, are often unable to fully auscultate its heartbeat. Medical students are ideal participant-observer anthropologists, bringing fresh eyes and unacculturated minds into medicine. Once immersed in the culture and subcultures of the medical world that they have long desired and worked hard to join, students tend to absorb the assumptions, behaviors, and values that surround them. They absorb and are absorbed. Writing enables students to pause, reflect, and sustain awareness and curiosity about this new world; at the same time, it provides educators with rich information about that world, which includes its hidden curriculum.

Researchers can aggregate and analyze narratives using grounded theory and other qualitative methods to illuminate common themes in the hidden curriculum (Gaufberg et al. 2010). Student narratives have helped educators understand the positive and negative experiences that shape students' moral, ethical, and professional development (Karnieli-Miller, Vu, et al. 2010); their engagement with the hierarchy of medical culture; the impact of poorly defined and regulated evaluation criteria (Gaufberg et al. 2010; Brainard and Brislen 2007); and the differing, and sometimes conflicting, implicit assumptions and messages in different clinical settings (Bernard et al. 2011). In this manner, narratives anchor the discussion of the hidden curriculum in students' lived experience.

Similar to looking through a window, there will always be things just outside our view when using narrative to access the hidden curriculum. Even when students seem to write openly, there will be influences either hidden from the students themselves or so taboo that students do not feel comfortable writing about them. Analyses of student narratives have noted these voids, with examples including the paucity in the narratives of explicit emotional responses to events (Karnieli-Miller, Vu, et al. 2010), reflections on competition with peers, or the role of nurses and other health professions colleagues in patient care (Gaufberg et al. 2010). By listening carefully for these silences and omissions, educators can bring the *hidden* hidden curriculum into view.

Narrative as a Mirror

The value of narratives in medical education extends beyond helping us see what surrounds us; it also helps us see ourselves more clearly. Narrative can help students and educators answer the questions of who we are and what we bring to our work. As with a mirror, a narrative reflection may provide an accurate image, but one that is subject to interpretation. What we see in the mirror depends on how we feel and what prior knowledge and biases we bring—reflection cannot be divorced from emotion, cognition, and imagination.

Understanding ourselves and our work through reflective practices has been variously described as the thoughtful consideration and exploration of experiences and knowledge (Wald et al. 2012); a "habit of the mind" that allows for attentiveness, curiosity, and self-awareness (Epstein and Hundert 2002); or, alternatively, an "active interior state" that uses cognitive, affective, imaginative, and creative means to understand experiences (Charon and Hermann 2012, 6). Through the process of writing and reflection, hidden curricular messages come into awareness, allowing the opportunity to make choices about what to integrate into or reject from a developing professional identity. The ability to use narrative for self-reflection, self-awareness, and self-growth, however, is not necessarily an innate skill (Mann, Gordon, and MacLeod 2009). Educators have adopted various methods, described later in this chapter, to nurture and develop reflective practice in their students.

The importance of reflective practice has been elegantly described by Biggs, who suggests that the mirror analogy is more useful in an expanded form: "A reflection in a mirror is an exact replica of what is in front of it. Reflection in professional practice, however, gives back not what is, but what might be, an improvement on the original" (1999, 6).

Narrative as a Bridge

Within a constructivist understanding of how people learn, students experience a complex learning environment firsthand, and then create meaning from their raw experience through developing and testing constructs. The process of creating a narrative allows the medical student to make linkages between concepts that he or she may have learned in the preclinical years (professionalism, altruism, integrity, respect, service) or those that come from personal life (kindness, love, fairness, forgiveness, courage) to those from actual clinical experiences (Epstein 1999; Bolton 2009). All too often, a student's lived experience is at odds with the values that he or she has been taught are of paramount importance to the profession. Disparities between core personal and professional values and actual experience can be explored and sometimes reconciled within a narrative (Gaufberg et al. 2010; Brainard and Brislen 2007). By bringing these connections into awareness, narratives have been shown to help students develop their professional identity (Quaintance, Arnold, and Thompson 2010).

When used within a framework of meaning making or "discovery," sharing stories can help learners remember and sustain the core values that brought them to medicine in the first place (Rabow et al. 2010). By acting as a bridge in this manner, reflection can serve to prevent and reverse the development of burnout, a dire consequence of dissonance between one's core values and actions, characterized by cynicism, alienation, dissatisfaction, and emotional exhaustion (Benson and Magraith 2005).

As narratives are discussed in community—in the form of peer-group reflection sessions, online discussion boards, medical school publications, town-hall style meetings—a broader group understanding of the meaning of experiences can evolve. In the sharing of stories, there is also the possibility of building bridges between individuals who come to the practice of medicine from differing backgrounds and experience, and of developing a shared morality among learners. This is one way that students join the long, proud lineage of physicians (Rabow et al. 2010). By creating opportunities to reflect on the meaning of our work with others in the context of explicitly shared values, narrative also builds a bridge between the formal and hidden curriculum and, in the process, transforms both self and community.

Practical Applications

Following are some examples of how educators use narrative to support student learning and professional development. Some narrative assignments are more intentionally analytic, using rubrics that aim to build cognitive and critical thinking skills; others seek transformation at a deeper emotional level.

- Aronson et al. (2011) at the University of California–San Francisco School of Medicine have developed and studied a guide for critical reflection called Learning from your Experiences as a Professional (LEaP). Based on the SOAP note format, the guide pushes students beyond merely reporting experiences (subjective) to considering their experiences from multiple perspectives (objective), synthesizing their learning (assessment), and finally making a plan to address future similar situations (plan). This guide has been shown to increase reflection scores of third-year students.
- At the Warren Alpert Medical School of Brown University, Wald et al. (2010) have developed a preclinical narrative medicine curriculum in which students discuss responses to structured questions. Faculty provide feedback using the "Brown Educational Guide to Analysis of Narrative (BEGAN)" that involves careful reading, identifying salient quotes to extract themes and lessons learned, using reflection-inviting questions, and providing concrete recommendations. This framework is intended to cultivate students' reflective capacity and highlight their insights to promote self-awareness and self-confidence. There is an accompanying rubric (REFLECT) to assess student reflective capacity, which is discussed later in this chapter (Wald et al. 2012).
- Charon and Hermann (2012) at Columbia University have described a model of *writing as discovery*, where reflective skills are taught from writing itself. Students receive training to equip them with skills to represent and recognize the complexities they encounter in their medical training as stories. The narratives are read aloud in collaborative workshops where teachers, trained in the art of close reading, highlight narrative features to help the students recognize hidden content in their writings. This reciprocal process nurtures both writing skills and the reflection that arises from the act of writing.

- Harvard Medical School Cambridge Integrated Clerkship (CIC) students are using narrative as a means to explore and build a common understanding of the system issues they encounter in their clinical work. The students have self-organized regular CIC Systems Rounds, which occur in the evening at student homes. Students come prepared to respond to this group-generated prompt: "Tell us a story about something you experienced that reflects a 'blindspot' in the system. . . . It can be anything that made you angry, frustrated, sad, grateful or curious about our health care system that affected a patient's health care: a frailty, a gap, an act of kindness when no one else was looking." The students are gathering their stories in a "scrapbook," have begun to engage in qualitative thematic analysis of the narratives, and are contemplating how best to use them for personal, community, and system growth (Ellison-Barnes et al. 2012).

- At George Washington University School of Medicine and Health Sciences, Chretien, Goldman, and Faselis (2008) have integrated web-based technology and reflective practice through the use of reflective writing class blogs. During a four-week rotation, students add reflective posts to a class website. Students are encouraged to comment on classmates' posts, and a faculty facilitator provides feedback on every post. This innovative curriculum has been described to facilitate interactions between peers and the instructor to promote deeper reflection, provide near real-time support for distressing events, and efficiently allow many students to benefit from a single faculty role model.

- Branch (2005) at Emory University has described the use of critical incident reports as a way to explore ethics and professional values in medical education. In these reports, learners are asked to describe professional incidents that they judge to be personally important. The value and efficacy of using these reports is attributed to the focus on learner-chosen transformative experiences as a starting point for group reflection.

A Note of Caution: The Hidden Curriculum of Student Narrative Assignments

As with any formal curricular assignment, faculty are well advised to consider their own assumptions and motivations in assigning students to write narratives, as well as the hidden curricular messages that might be hitchhiking along with the assignment. We send messages to students about *what we value* by where in the curriculum assignments are placed, whether they are required or elective, how they are framed, what prompts we choose, whether faculty engage in the same activities as students, as well as whether and how we assess them. When integrating narrative into a curriculum, faculty must think deliberately about all of these areas because these messages are among many that students are prioritizing at any given moment.

- Place in the overall curriculum: Are narrative assignments "carved out" in a patient-doctor or reflective practice course, or are they assigned as part of a core clinical rotation? Are they relegated to the preclinical years when there is often more available curricular time, or prioritized as a means to process actual clinical experiences? When we assign narratives at multiple points in the curriculum, including during clinical experiences, we give students the valuable message that writing and telling stories is something integral to effective and ethical practice.
- Role modeling: Students are quick to pick up on any disparity between what we ask them to do and what we do ourselves. What do students see (if anything) in the clinical setting that they can call "narrative" or "reflection"? Conversely, what things are clinicians currently doing that might be termed "reflective," reframed as "storytelling," or reinterpreted as "narrative"? When physicians on the faculty write, share, or publish narratives themselves, students get the message that narratives are of central importance to what we do as physicians, that storytelling and making meaning is an iterative process that is important over the life span of the physician.
- Goals of narrative: Are faculty clear (with students and themselves) regarding the goals of assigning narratives? Beyond the general hope that writing will be "good for students" or "build professionalism," we must be intentional about our anticipated outcomes of the assignment and communicate this clearly to our learners. Are we asking them to write in order to foster self-awareness, hone reflective capabilities, explore ethical dilemmas, make meaning, support professional identity formation, process the emotional experience of doctoring, engage in culture change or advocacy efforts, or provide data for research purposes?

Clearly communicating our intention is especially important when we collect narratives for research purposes, because students can end up feeling either like guinea pigs or spies unless we properly frame our inquiry. For what purpose are we asking them to make themselves vulnerable and take the time to write? How is the relationship of faculty to students and their stories affected if those stories become "data"? Do we protect the students against reprisal if we publish their narratives as part of research or quality improvement efforts?

- Prompts: How do we select prompts or reflective triggers? Students' narratives are typically framed and confined by the assignment, making it crucial to intentionally select a prompt that reflects the educational or research goals of the narrative. Do we use prompts, some of which may focus students' attention on challenges and problems, or do we use appreciative inquiry, which can access and engage the positive aspects of a learning community (Suchman et al. 2004)?

- Privacy: What messages do we as faculty convey about the private-versus-public nature of narratives? Are students protected from sharing narratives with other students—that is, do they submit to a faculty member, or are they encouraged or even required to share with others? What is the right balance between privacy and safety and the stance that storytelling and reflection are something we must encourage and require students to do in the community as professionals?

- Assessment: Do we assess or evaluate student narratives? Is the assessment formative (to be fed back into a student's learning, growth, and development), or is a summative or evaluative grade given? What messages are conveyed with each? This is discussed later in the chapter.

- Context and confidentiality: Does our educational community value narrative? The successful incorporation of narrative assignments requires a community that values and legitimizes reflection and prioritizes it in an overfull curriculum. In addition, students need a safe environment, mentorship, peer support, and protected time to be able to develop their reflective capacity (Mann, Gordon, and MacLeod 2009). Reflective practice requires adopting a different learning framework from the one many students know—a framework free from censure, in which there are no experts and no "right answers." Rabow, Wrubel, and Remen (2007) describe the concept of *interactional safety*, where students learn the technique of "generous listening" and participate in establishing in-group ground rules such as the confidentiality of peers' revelations.

Successful groups can do much to protect and nurture fellow members, but educators must still be clear with students about the limits of confidentiality with respect to harm to self or others, or significant student maltreatment. If a concerning passage or shared reflection is encountered, direct engagement with the student is usually sufficient to clarify risk and resolve the issue. In nine years of a reflective practice group at the Harvard Medical School CIC, the authors of this chapter have always been able to work through issues with students and have never felt the need to violate student confidentiality.

The relationship between narrative and the hidden curriculum is complex and paradoxical. On the one hand, narrative and reflective writing are wonderful tools for exposing and exploring the hidden curriculum. On the other hand, reflective writing is subject to its own hidden curriculum. Fortunately, the very process of writing and sharing gives us an opportunity to explore, hold, and sometimes resolve such tensions.

Student Narratives, Feedback, and Evaluation

There is a healthy debate among medical educators about whether to assess or evaluate narrative writing. Good educational practice links assessment to the goals and objectives at hand. Decisions about whether and how to give feedback, assess, or evaluate any aspect of student performance must be made in light of educational goals.

Wald and coauthors (2012) recently published their experiences developing REFLECT (Reflection Evaluation for Learners' Enhanced Competencies Tool), which is applied by faculty to medical student narratives as a means to evaluate and give feedback on levels of reflection—from habitual action to critical reflection. The coauthors use the tool to provide formative rather than summative assessment, to avoid stimulating a formulaic approach to narrative construction in the interest of getting a good grade. In a commentary on the Wald piece, Coulehan and Granek (2012) agree that the rubric is a useful guide, primarily because "the content, context and style of accurate reflective feedback are so different from most teaching in the clinical setting that even experienced clinical faculty are apt to flounder" (9). Charon and Hermann (2012), cautious of assessment, suggest different methods of faculty-student interaction around narrative that corresponds to a somewhat different view on the role of writing in medical education. Rather than use writing "to measure the attainment of the skill of reflection after that skill has somehow been attained elsewhere . . . writing is used to attain the state of reflection" (6). Writing is a way to access inner experience, thoughts, and emotions through a process of discovery.

For better or for worse, students learn about what is important to us in large part by what we assess. External forces such as accreditation requirements have a major impact on assessment, but to our knowledge, such mandates have not deeply penetrated the world of storytelling. Faculty must consider what messages we give our students when we do or do not evaluate their narratives. We must consider if and how the process of assessment will affect the process of writing, and whether it might support or undermine our goals. One educator on a medical education listserv shared her fear that rating scales "will be the death of real writing" (Charon 2009). No doubt, a polished narrative containing all the elements on a reflective practice checklist can be produced by most medical students without anything truly transformational taking place. This underscores the importance of finding ways to promote intrinsic motivation to write and share stories in the interest of examining and learning from experience. We are struck by Coulehan and Granek's (2012) observation that faculty may see the process of teaching and giving feedback on reflective writing as very different from teaching and giving feedback in the clinical domain. We are compelled to ask, why is this? What might teaching and feedback look like if our faculty truly viewed storytelling and reflection as habits integral to good medical practice?

Student Narratives and Culture Change

From the very first day of medical school, we become responsible for the cultures in which we work and learn. Narratives have the potential to help us shape and change these cultures as we undergo individual and communal transformations. Our students share their own values and experiences in what can be thought of as "stories of self." Discussion in groups in which core professional values and collective wisdom can emerge builds a "story of us." Public narrative can extend those conversations to the "story of now," engaging entire communities in transformational action (Ganz 2008).

Conclusions

Narratives have the power to call attention to everyday experiences and to connect experiences to deeply held personal and professional values. Individual students, small groups, and large communities can uncover and explore these explicit and implicit values, allowing positive elements to be emphasized and negative ones to be reformed. Sharing stories will always be something we do as human beings. Perhaps someday the practice of reflection will be woven into the fabric of medical culture and may be less needed as a formal curricular offering. For now, each student narrative is a treasure chest with much to offer. Our work as educators is to help reveal their value to the student and his or her community.

10: Bounded and Open

A Personally Transformative Empirical Journey into Curricula, Objectives, and Student Learning

DORENE BALMER AND BOYD F. RICHARDS

Encouraged to move beyond the editorial boundaries of writing for an academic journal, we (Boyd and Dorene) use the openness of dialogue to tell a story about an interview study set in the context of curriculum reform and the underlying discovery process that drove the reform. The results of our interview study reveal the variability of student learning, which occurs in the interplay across curricular boundaries, including the hidden curriculum, in a learning environment that is unavoidably open.

Prologue

BOYD: Even though I have worked as a medical educator for nearly thirty years, my thinking about medical school curricula recently was transformed by the findings of an interview study with fourth-year medical students conducted in the spring of 2011. Consistent with our roles as educational consultants, Dorene Balmer and I sought data about students' lived experiences relative to recently adopted schoolwide learning objectives to inform ongoing governance discussions among curriculum leaders. Our goal was to help leaders plan curricular revisions designed to ensure that students had sufficient opportunity prior to graduation to achieve every objective.

In our interview study, we asked students to retrospectively identify, via a task of assigning points, where in Columbia's curricula they had acquired the knowledge, skills, and attitudes associated with the new schoolwide objectives. We also asked them to estimate the amount of time dedicated to each objective. Using this framework, students tended to identify that much more learning took place outside of the formal curriculum than I had expected. I share pie charts for three objectives, each illustrative of other objectives with similar patterns.

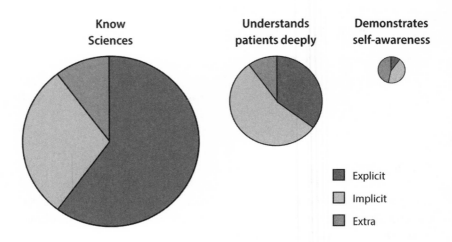

Figure 10.1. Pie charts for three of ten learning objectives, each representing students' assigned points for (1) where learning related to objective occurred (sections of pie: explicit-, implicit-, or extra-curriculum) and (2) relative amount of focus on objective during four years of education (size of pie).

Having read much of the emergent literature about the hidden curriculum over the years, I realized that students learn a lot of important things about being a doctor outside of the formal classroom. Nevertheless, my mental model of curriculum at the time simplistically assumed that learning experiences occurred in the formal, explicit curriculum, and that these experiences occasionally were overshadowed by competing, and almost always negative, learning experiences in the hidden curriculum. Based on the results shown in the figures, my mental model of curriculum now assumes a complex interplay of experiences, which, at best, are guided by elements of the formal curriculum, but often occur elsewhere.

DORENE: Coming into medical education through the "back door" of clinical practice, I was intrigued by the idea of exploring students' lived experience relative to the new schoolwide objectives. After fifteen years of clinical experience at a large children's hospital—years spent working alongside attending physicians, fellows, residents, and other health professionals as they cared for children and their families—I knew that profound learning occurred in the clinical classroom, and I came to appreciate the power of the implicit curriculum. I avoided using the term *hidden curriculum* because the learning I saw and heard about often converged with the explicit curriculum, even though it lacked the structure, organization, and predictability of the explicit curriculum (Balmer et al. 2009). For me, the interview study reinforced my mental model of curriculum. The chance to go beyond merely describing the implicit curriculum and potentially make it "legitimate," by showing how it contributed to medical students' achievement of schoolwide objectives, was appealing. As a qualitative researcher, I envisioned collecting data through in-depth interviews. What I wasn't prepared for was the value of giving form, via quantification, to students' relatively illusive and formless experience.

Conception

BOYD: When I arrived at Columbia in the summer of 2007, curriculum reform was well under way. Most faculty and students seemed engaged and excited about the proposed structural revisions to the four-year curriculum focused on reducing the preclinical curriculum to eighteen months in order to make time for students to differentiate themselves with a required scholarly project and electives after a twelve-month major clinical year. I felt privileged to participate in frequent discussions needed to work out the details of these changes as they cascaded down through the levels of organization that comprise a curriculum—from courses to sections and on to lectures, or from learning activities to formative assessments and on to summative evaluations.

After several months as a participant observer, I began to notice how little we made reference to existing curricular objectives. It appeared to me that everyone's attention was simply consumed by the pragmatics of the mandated structural changes. Not long after Dorene joined me in the Center for Education Research and Evaluation, we recognized a tremendous commitment to quality in terms of both process and outcome in the faculty with whom we were engaged. A culture of excellence prevailed in which many long-standing values were assumed to be present without being explicitly articulated or discussed.

As educators, Dorene and I came to believe that one of the best contributions we could make to the reform initiative would be to use our skills in group facilitation to lead a discussion about the quality of fit between planned curriculum changes and the existing curricular objectives. In a rapid succession of meetings, we discovered that we needed to set aside the existing stated objectives and initiate a deeper discovery process to uncover the implicit objectives and values upon which faculty had been basing their curricular decisions.

The first step in this discovery process was to identify the content, or the "what," of these implicit objectives. We accomplished this through Dorene's careful inductive coding of more than twenty-three curriculum documents, followed by a series of working sessions with students and faculty to translate the codes into value statements that became our objectives. The second step was to gain a sense of the "how," that is, how these objectives were manifest in the lived experiences of students. This second step was the motivation for our interview study.

DORENE: Like Boyd, I noticed that the existing curricular objectives were not part of the everyday language of Columbia faculty and students. However, this is not to say that guiding principles were nonexistent. Faculty and students readily expressed values and beliefs about the medical education Columbia could and did provide. Boyd and I, along with a group of willing partners, were commissioned by the vice dean for education to champion new schoolwide objectives. Thus we began a journey toward creating a new framework of objectives that was not only compatible with core competencies, such as those embraced by the Accreditation Council for Graduate Medical Education (ACGME), but also reflected the mission, priorities, and unique qualities of the institution (Balmer, Richards, and Drusin 2010).

With the vice dean's support, Boyd and I organized a group of twenty faculty members and students, and encouraged them to cluster concepts from curricular documents into categories that represented the knowledge, skills, and attitudes of a Columbia physician. Then, we worked with two smaller groups of faculty members and students that met weekly over the course of four weeks to refine the categories and ultimately construct objective-type statements. Both groups favored a less reductionist approach, so we ended up with ten expansive statements of aspiration. Moreover, both large-group and small-group activities provided a venue for faculty and students, collectively, to reflect on what Columbia meant to them and to articulate their dreams for what students would take with them after graduation. Thus, our schoolwide objectives were not a comprehensive, itemized list of what students should be able to do, but aspirations for who they were expected to become.

One year after the creation of our schoolwide objectives, Boyd and I facilitated another group of faculty members and students. Our purpose was to operationalize our decidedly aspirational objectives to align with the Liaison Committee on Medical Education (LCME) mandates to govern by objectives. Again, we observed a resistance to a reductionist approach. Faculty members and students saw the achievement of schoolwide objectives as, in their words, "a sense of accumulated accomplishment" rather than a detailed checklist. We left the meeting with a greater realization that, for the most part, faculty members and students preferred objectives that were more about "being a doctor" than "doing the work of a doctor" (Jarvis-Sellinger, Pratt, and Regehr 2012).

Having identified the "what" of our schoolwide objectives, Boyd and I were ideally positioned to understand the "how." We conducted this interview study to help us understand how the objectives actually played out in students' lived experience as they traversed the explicit, implicit, and extra-curriculum at our institution.

The Interview Study

BOYD: The basic design for the interview study emerged from one of the regular meetings I had with Dorene: we would give students 100 points for each objective, and ask them to think aloud while assigning the points to different categories of curricula to represent the portion of learning they would attribute to each. We reasoned that the recorded think-aloud transcripts would help reveal students' rationale for their point assignments, and that the point assignments would provide data that we could easily average and compare across students and across objectives—and not exceed my limited abilities as a statistician.

Our biggest challenge in building on this basic study design was how to define the categories of curricula for students to use to classify their learning experiences. After several conversations and false starts, we created six categories based conceptually on a 2 x 3 matrix: curriculum phase (preclinical versus clinical) and type of curriculum based on its relationship to the "formal curriculum" (explicit, implicit, and extra). According to the definitions we shared with students at the commencement of each interview, the *explicit curriculum* included learning activities that are specified within the formal curriculum such as course syllabi. The *implicit curriculum* included learning activities (that is, the "hidden" or "informal" curriculum) that occur in the context of the formal curriculum, but are implicit, such as the modeling of behaviors of residents. The *extracurriculum* included learning activities that occur outside the formal curriculum, such as participation in clubs, volunteering in New York City, and so on. In the decision to use the terms *implicit* and *explicit*, we drew upon the work of Eliott Eisner, who distinguishes explicit as curriculum the school "advertises" (for example, printed course materials) and implicit as what is taught through institutional culture and organization as well as through interpersonal interactions with instructors (1985).

In the spring of 2011, Dorene and I invited eighteen students who had completed their major clinical year and whose schedules made it convenient to participate in the study (for example, they were in town on electives or taking time off to do research). These students comprised about 12 percent of the student body and represented diverse clinical interests. They also were among the last to journey through the old curricula and served as a baseline for eventual comparison to students from the new curriculum.

We did the first couple of interviews together to work out the interview protocol; then Dorene conducted most of the others. The interviews ranged from 30 to 150 minutes, mostly depending on the pace at which students were able to make their point assignments and talk at the same time. We audiotaped and transcribed verbatim every interview. The protocol went as follows:

- We gave students a worksheet with the curriculum definitions at the top and the schoolwide objectives listed alphabetically as rows in a matrix. The columns were the six curricular categories.
- Students read and verbalized their understanding of each curricular objective.
- Students used the worksheet to one-by-one assign their 100 points for the objective. Occasionally, we would interrupt the students and ask follow-up questions to solicit their level of confidence.
- When they had assigned points to all ten objectives, students then assigned another 100 points across all ten objectives, again thinking aloud, to reflect the relative quantity of learning that occurred for each objective.

DORENE: Although the quantitative data helped us represent something that Boyd and I could walk around and examine—an architectural framework, so to speak—the more nuanced qualitative data helped us inspect its unusual arches, its unexpected buttresses. Students' comments shed light on why they assigned their learning experiences to one of three curricula: the explicit, the implicit, and the extracurriculum. The interviews yielded a collection of narratives that helped us appreciate how students made sense of the myriad events and interactions they encountered outside the explicit curriculum, and how they adapted new understandings stemming from experiences in the implicit or extracurriculum to what they had previously learned in class. Often, the narratives came in the form of stories, like this one:

> I'd seen a patient in the psych ER who had literally just attempted suicide two hours earlier. The attending was like, "Just go talk to her," but I was like, "I can't talk to her. I've never spoken to a patient who has just attempted suicide." He said, "Well, how would you imagine starting that conversation? You just have to do it." I was like, "What if I say the wrong thing? What am I going to do if I break down because this is, like, very emotional?" He said, "You just have to go talk to her. She is a regular person; she just has a lot of issues and problems." And that's how you learn it. You don't learn it from the attending telling you what to ask. You don't learn it from thinking about it and saying, "Maybe I shouldn't mention the word *suicide* because she just attempted suicide." You just go and you do. With every patient it's different, but that's how you learn.

As a qualitative researcher, I was accustomed to being able to identify relatively circumscribed, emergent themes within narratives. But in this interview study, the overriding theme was *variability*. Each student had diverse learning experiences and a distinct narrative. Students themselves talked about variability and the uniqueness of their idiosyncratic learning experiences, as they pertained to the schoolwide objectives, like this:

> I feel like it [my experiences] wouldn't be opposite and it wouldn't be extremely different, but I think it would be different . . . . For me, I struggled at times with the emotional part of school and I think because of that struggle, it made what I learned outside of school [about self-awareness and personal wellness] more important than what I learned through the school.

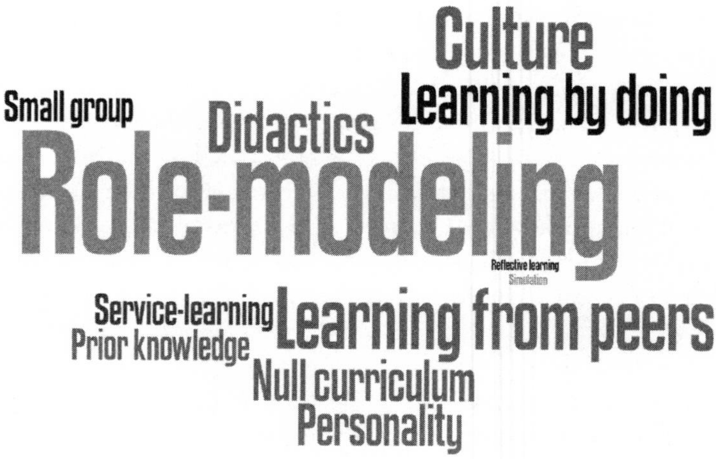

Culture
Learning by doing
Small group **Didactics**
Role-modeling
Reflective learning
Simulation
Service-learning **Learning from peers**
Prior knowledge
Null curriculum
Personality

Figure 10.2. A schematic representation of the process of socialization leading to identity formation including the major factors that influence the process.

Nonetheless, Boyd and I did identify a few general patterns in the data. First, we heard a lot about the prevalence and cogency of learning in the implicit curriculum. As displayed in figure 10-2, learning from role modeling, either positive or negative, was predominant. As seen in the figure, other words represented different ways of learning in the implicit curriculum (for example, what students picked up from peers, the culture, and by doing the work of a physician) and tended to surpass learning via didactics or small-group discussions in the explicit curriculum.

Second, Boyd and I noticed that students tended to understand learning in the preclinical phase of medical school differently than learning in the clinical phase. Learning in preclinical courses often was recognized as part of the explicit curriculum, with a focus on medical knowledge and the foundations of clinical practice. As shown in the pie charts in figure 10-1, students attributed much time acquiring medical knowledge to the explicit curriculum. In contrast, learning in the clinical years often was attributed to the implicit curriculum. Although this learning may have been more powerful, it consumed relatively less time. For example, one student talked about learning teamwork like this:

> In the explicit curriculum, they stress that you're an important member of the team. But in the implicit curriculum, you quickly realize that

you're not an important part of the team, that you can easily be skipped, and you learn that good residents don't do that.

Third, we came to realize that for some students, learning in the extracurriculum was pivotal to their sense of achieving several schoolwide objectives. In other words, the extracurriculum was much more than just student support services. This was most notable for objectives that pertained to personal well-being or to research and discovery. For example, one student said this:

> When you talk about new knowledge, I think of this as research. It's mostly extracurricular, although we certainly do some thinking about research in the clinical years. I was involved in research the summer between my first and second year, so I would say the majority of this for me came through my extracurriculars.

Impact

BOYD: Over the past few months, I have noticed repeatedly the impact of our findings on my work as a medical educator. Three recent events come to mind by way of illustration. Early in the spring of 2012, a colleague, who also was a member of the curriculum renewal team, remarked that he had just had a conversation with a fellow graduate from Columbia, in which he concluded that the school's "current curriculum is much different than the one they had experienced as students many years ago." In my mind, I immediately questioned what my colleague meant. Which curriculum was he referring to? Was he just thinking about the explicit curriculum in which we had recently made some very noticeable structural changes—for example, shortened preclinical curriculum to make room for a scholarly project requirement during the clinical curriculum and intersessions inserted between blocks of clinical clerkships? Was he identifying changes in the implicit curriculum as well—for example, quality of resident role models, increased emphasis on students teaching fellow students, and increased opportunities to build meaningful relationships with faculty? Or was he thinking about differences in the extracurriculum—for example, club activities, summer research, student-run clinics, and volunteer opportunities in the city? Prior to engaging in this research, I never would have thought so broadly about these alternative possible references to differences in curricula.

In the summer of 2012, the medical school held its first annual curriculum summit. Late one afternoon, seventy-five faculty and students gathered in Riverview Lounge, a large open area with windows facing the George Washington Bridge and the Hudson River. After short presentations showcasing the status of the Columbia curriculum three years after reform was initiated, faculty and students broke into working groups to consider the progress to date in integrating our schoolwide objectives into all facets of curriculum governance. In response to concerns expressed in these energetic discussions, the entire group resolved to create one-page structured narratives for each of the ten schoolwide objectives, as they applied to the pre-clinical and clinical phases of training. The goal would be to clarify and add depth of understanding about the competencies and milestones included within each objective statement in a manner that focused on the sum of the parts more than the individuals parts themselves. The results of our interview study had a powerful influence on our thinking about these narratives. They motivated us to be more thoughtful in referencing learning and feedback opportunities present in the implicit and extracurriculum, opportunities we may have overlooked prior to doing this research.

In the fall of 2012, during a brainstorming session in a weekly faculty meeting led by Dr. Rita Charon, I found myself smiling inwardly as the conversation turned toward the need to more explicitly cultivate students' teaching skills within our curriculum. There I sat, sensing the pleasure of seeing many of the conclusions that Dorene and I had reached in exploring the results of our research being championed by this group of enthusiastic and experienced educators. The group clearly recognized the powerful role peers and residents play in students' learning, especially in the implicit curriculum, and beautifully articulated the far-reaching benefit of preparing our graduates for their teaching roles. This discussion affirmed for me important institutional progress away from seeing the LCME standard of ensuring effective resident teaching as a burden, and toward embracing the value of enhancing resident teaching and role modeling because of its central role in student mastery of many schoolwide objectives in the implicit curriculum. I felt I had come one step closer to understanding how faculty responsible for governing the curriculum can fulfill their responsibility beyond just the explicit curriculum.

DORENE: As the interview study drew to a close, and the new curriculum became the status quo, I better understood the limits of what I could contribute as a researcher and education specialist. I could incite conversations about the legitimacy of learning outside the explicit curriculum, but I could not sustain these conversations in places that mattered most. Fortunately, it was evident to all who participated in the development and implementation of our schoolwide objectives that we, the Columbia community, needed a tool to capture—to give form to—students' lived experiences, across the explicit, implicit, and extracurriculum, so that they too could appreciate all the dimensions or facets of their learning. It was also clear that we were well positioned to create a tool that capitalized on Columbia's rich tradition of narrative medicine. In this tradition, reflection is in the act of writing, and every writer needs a reader, someone who, by witnessing, helps the writer understand what just happened (Charon 2006).

The tool we chose was an electronic portfolio, and our readers were faculty who, trained in the narrative medicine tradition, were comfortable with close reading. The overall goal of the portfolio has been to nurture students' reflective capacity as self-regulated learners and future physicians, and to help them document their level of achievement of schoolwide objectives prior to graduation. We believe the portfolio will aid in students' consolidation of learning in the explicit, implicit, and extracurriculum, and in the integration of learning opportunities as they engage in structured reflections about their ongoing achievement of schoolwide learning objectives and form their own professional identities.

To date, efforts to create a portfolio at Columbia have evolved, from a reflective writing group that artfully composed reflective prompts to each schoolwide learning objective, to a curricular subcommittee that drafted guiding principles for the portfolio, to a technology task force charged with constructing an e-portfolio in our course management system, to naming a faculty director who would help shepherd the portfolio into the curriculum, and to piloting the portfolio with a group of medical students who met monthly to write, read, and share their experience of both.

For me personally, this interview study, and the discovery process that surrounded it, has enhanced my commitment to doing research that has direct application. It has also taught me to trust the process of partnering with the consumers of research, in this case, the medical students and faculty who make Columbia what it is.

Coda

Now, two years after initiating our interview study, would we do it differently? Our answer is, "Probably not." Our findings have influenced us individually, and given us fodder for many provocative discussions. Although we have a greater appreciation for the synergy that can happen when quantitative and qualitative approaches to inquiry are used to explore phenomena in medical education, this interview study has brought to light new issues with which to grapple. For instance, how do we hold students' unique lived experience in one hand, while holding the need to provide an equitable educational experience for all students in the other? How do we support the belief among students and faculty members that competency is as much about *being* as it is about *doing*, and at the same time dutifully meet minimum standards put forth by accrediting bodies?

We would like to think, then, that our study has generated a meaningful ripple through the ranks of faculty members, students, and others involved in medical education at Columbia. The findings have helped us shift our thinking about the implicit curriculum as primarily a negative force to a mostly positive one, and encouraged us to learn from students' lived experiences even when we are surrounded by the drone of discussions related to the explicit curriculum. In sum, our journey has taught us that, despite our best efforts to guide learning via schoolwide objectives in the explicit curriculum, "learning happens."

> Learning cannot be designed. Ultimately, it belongs to the realm of experience and practice. It follows the negotiation of meaning; it moves on its own terms. It slips through the cracks; it creates its own cracks. Learning happens, design or no design. (Wenger 1998, 225)

PART IV

THE HIDDEN CURRICULUM AND HEALTH PROFESSIONS EDUCATION

This section forms the centerpiece of this book. It is intended to provide a big-picture, 50,000-foot overview of how the hidden curriculum has been, and might be, applied to four domains of health professions education: medicine (Michael Rabow, chapter 11), nursing (Lisa Day and Patricia Benner, chapter 12), allied health (Virginia Wright-Peterson and Claire Bender, chapter 13), and interprofessional education (IPE) (Jill Thistlethwaite, chapter 14). Each of these four educational domains has a different history. Medical education has generated the largest body of work on the hidden curriculum, followed by nursing—with relatively little presence of this concept within the fields of allied health and interprofessional education.

The relative abundance of materials in medicine forces Rabow, not unexpectedly, to organize and present a rather substantive body of literature. In turn, although nursing has made comparatively little formal use of this concept, nursing has long been concerned with the classroom-theory and clinic-practice disjunctures it has observed, and therefore has a long history of work on a parallel concept, the *theory-practice gap*. In turn, the relative absence of the hidden curriculum as an analytical tool within allied and interprofessional health education means that these chapters stake out new ground. Obviously, there are other health occupations not represented in this volume—pharmacy and dentistry being two of many. Although such broader representation would have enriched the book, this also would have made it considerably longer. Finally, and while we were writing this section, Jill Thistlethwaite was awarded a Fulbright scholarship to travel the globe further exploring issues facing IPE (and, she hopes, the hidden curriculum of IPE) at a time when all health professions schools struggle to teach and practice healthcare in a less hierarchical and more team-oriented manner.

11: Becoming a Doctor

Learning from the Hidden Curriculum in Medical Education

MICHAEL W. RABOW

In a narrow sense, physicians are defined by an academic degree and a professional license. Historically, these have been based on what physicians know and can do—using a specialized fund of knowledge, cognitive abilities, and procedural skills taught by a rigorous curriculum and training in science and technology. Although the professional development of physicians does involve the accumulation of a body of knowledge (learning from the formal curriculum), it also includes the powerful influences of interpersonal relationships and the social and education milieu of medical school (learning from the hidden curriculum). How medical students become physicians involves the hidden curriculum at its core. Physicians are defined partly by what they know, but also by who they are—the values they hold, and the commitments they make.

This chapter addresses the questions of how the hidden curriculum is taught and what medical students learn from it. Also reviewed is the evidence of discordance between the formal and hidden curricula, and how medical students respond to these conflicts. Finally, future directions in addressing the challenges and opportunities of the hidden curriculum in medical education are considered.

How the Hidden Curriculum is Taught

That there is a hidden curriculum in medical school is beyond question. The editors and chapter authors of this book, as well as many others, have identified clearly and analyzed creatively the hidden curriculum in medical education. The content of the hidden curriculum is efficiently transmitted early during training and continuously thereafter through a variety of mechanisms.

Interpersonal Interactions

Walking into the first day of medical school, students start learning from two key teachers of the hidden curriculum: role models and peers. In interpersonal interactions with faculty, near-peers, and peers, students learn from both their teaching experiences and their clinical experiences (Haidet and Stein 2006; Karnieli-Miller et al. 2011; Lempp and Seale 2004; Haidet et al. 2008).

ROLE MODELS

Faculty physicians teaching medical students in the first years of school serve as role models and begin to shape how a student construes what it means to be a physician. Once students start to participate in clinical care, they are exposed to influential role models across the hierarchy (attendings, house officers, and medical students). Students' observations of how supervisors spend their time, what they appear to value, and the advice they offer serve to communicate to students what doctors are supposed to do and not do.

Although formal mentoring is rare, and students are often left to deal with powerful experiences and emotions on their own, informal role-modeling relationships are both ubiquitous and haphazard (Ratanawongsa, Teherani, and Hauer 2005; Gaufberg et al. 2010). Role models generally do not receive training or salary support for this work, and students observe both positive and negative behaviors (Karnieli-Miller et al. 2011; Lempp and Seale 2004). The quality of role modeling is inconsistent (Baker, Wrubel, and Rabow 2011; Burack et al. 1999). However, these relationships are particularly important in what students learn and in their professional development (Haidet et al. 2008). Student relationships with faculty role models impact learning outcomes, including students' intrinsic motivation to learn (Haidet and Stein 2006). Moreover, student-faculty relationships may presage some aspects of the clinical relationship that students eventually will forge with patients.

PEERS

Peer relationships are core in the hidden curriculum, partly because fellow students help each other interpret the meaning and implications of the formal curricula. Peer influence helps establish a student's sense of the relative importance of didactic content ("Do we really have to study this?" "Are you going to that lecture?") and the desirability of various attitudes and values

("My resident is so strong he totally blocked that admission from the ED.").

Near-peers, slightly ahead in the process of training, let students know "what it's really like," interpreting the clinical services' unwritten codes and values (Hundert, Hafferty, and Christakis 1996; Fernandes et al. 2008). Medical school peer relationships are powerful, with some evidence suggesting that friendships actually impact learning and grades among medical students (Woolf et al. 2012).

Learning Environment

Interactions with role models and peers are also part of a larger source of hidden curriculum for medical students that can be described as the educational and social milieu of medical school, that is, the *learning environment*. The medical learning environment has both general profession-wide elements as well as local features (which show tremendous variation among different medical schools). The medical learning environment can be seen as a type of culture with its own vocabulary, customs, and values (Gaufberg et al. 2010). The learning environment is a complex system of influences, and includes the regulations and pronouncements of professional organizations, institutional policies and resource allocation decisions, the formal curriculum (including its structure and curricular content), medical school rituals, experiences of mistreatment, and learner assessment and evaluation.

INTERPRETATION OF POLICIES AND THE FORMAL CURRICULUM

Educational structure (for example, how much time is committed to a topic in the curriculum) and funding allocations create meaning for students. The regulatory bodies and institutions of the medical profession create a hidden curriculum for students. ACGME (Accreditation Council for Graduate Medical Education), AAMC (Association of American Medical Colleges), NBME (National Board of Medical Examiners), and LCME (Liaison Commission on Medical Education) determine what medical students must learn to satisfy the requirements for licensure. Through what hoops must students jump? How much time are students asked to devote to learning versus providing useful service during their clinical encounters, and are there protections in place to prevent overwork and mistreatment? The formal messages of a particular medical school also serve to deliver unofficial, but powerful messages. What do the formal curricular subjects offered, and the time allotted to them, say about the medical school's values?

RITUAL

Ritual events can communicate compelling messages to students. Students are outfitted in potent symbols (the white coat, the stethoscope), and the identity of a physician is molded by events with symbolic meaning (anatomy class, writing medication prescriptions, offering a prognosis). The white-coat ceremony, taking the Hippocratic oath, or memorial services in anatomy class each suggest meaning to students about the role and commitments they are to assume as physicians (Wear 1998; Rabow, Wrubel, and Remen 2007). Routine clinical experiences also can take on ritualistic significance for students—staying up all night on call, taking a history on sensitive topics, dealing with death and dying, or the social and existential boundaries crossed during physical examinations, deliveries of babies, or surgery.

STUDENT MISTREATMENT AND ABUSE

The mistreatment of medical students deserves special attention in the discussion of the sources of the hidden curriculum. "Teaching by humiliation" and "dehumanization" have been reported widely (Lempp and Seale 2004; Gaufberg et al. 2010) with more than one-quarter of residents in one study reporting having been required to do something "immoral, unethical, or personally unacceptable" (Baldwin, Daugherty, and Rowley 1998, 1198). How medical students themselves are treated, both officially and informally, delivers a message to medical students about how they can or should treat patients (Benbassat 2013). Are there official policies for self-care or days off? Are there explicit and implicit rules about sexual harassment and protections for gender, sexual orientation, and ethnicity? Medical students learn by official policies, but also by whether these are enforced and on whom.

EVALUATION AND FEEDBACK

Ultimately, assessment, evaluation, and feedback clarify for medical students what really matters to their teachers, school, and profession. What is on the test? What are the domains of evaluation? What are required competencies? What are the consequences of failure in each of the domains (content knowledge, doctor-patient relationship, professionalism, and so on)? Research demonstrates key deficiencies in evaluation and feedback. In one study, attendings were unlikely to respond even to "perceived disrespect, uncaring, or hostility toward patients by members of their medical team" (Burack et al. 1999, 46).

What the Hidden Curriculum Teaches

All the sources of hidden curriculum offer some sense to medical students about what they are expected to know, what attitudes they should hold, and how they are supposed to behave. The teachings of the hidden curriculum span the whole of medical education, influencing what scientific content is attended to, and how students think (what cognitive processes are valued), as well as highlighting attitudes and values that contribute to medical professionalism. Although preclinical coursework is important, clinical experiences appear to be much more influential in the development of student identities and attitudes.

Identity and Role

The hidden curriculum guides the professional formation of medical students, influencing their professional development and their growing identity as physicians. Hidden curricular influences help determine professional behavior and career choices. The hidden curriculum communicates to students what their appropriate professional role is, sometimes with the loss of important elements of personhood (Rabow, Evans, and Remen 2013). Although equality is espoused, gender roles continue to be communicated. In end-of-life (EOL) care training, clinical clerkship experiences "affected students' developing professional identities by affording opportunities to manage strong emotions, understand the challenges of transitioning to residency, and gain a sense of self-efficacy as future physicians providing EOL care" (Ratanawongsa, Teherani, and Hauer 2005, 641). The learning environment has an impact on medical students' choice of specialty and career interests. Students learn in a milieu where primary care (versus subspecialty) clinicians and careers are valued and reimbursed differently.

Relationship

Relationship dynamics influence identity, attitudes, and behaviors. The interpersonal relationships developed by medical students are influenced by the hidden curriculum and impact their relationships with other healthcare workers, physicians, and patients.

Interprofessional relationships: Students often learn about a traditional model of medicine that posits the physician as an independent, infallible hero. Fitted in this model is the tendency toward paternalism as well as medicine's slow uptake of interprofessional education. The model insists that physicians know what is right, are central, and ultimately are more important than other clinicians in the care of patients. Physicians are taught to be individuals, be in charge, not seek help, and be sufficient unto themselves (Benbassat 2012). In accordance with this model, medical students are taught primarily among themselves, by physicians. Senior residents on call overnight sometimes describe their situation as "being the only one in-house," despite the hospital being filled with other experienced health professionals. In this sense of role, trainees discount the expertise of nurses and professionals from other disciplines.

Intraprofessional relationships: The hierarchy of power in medicine (students at the bottom to attendings at the top) is buttressed by the hidden curriculum (Gaufberg et al. 2010). Humiliation and hierarchy remain core elements of medical education (Lempp and Seale 2004). Students often learn not to question superiors, and perhaps to treat those lower in the hierarchy as they themselves were treated. Functioning on clinical teams as an interchangeable Student A or Student B, students may learn that their contributions to care are based only on their knowledge or technical abilities, rather than on unique elements of their personhood.

Physician-patient relationship: Role modeling of the physician-patient relationship can be extremely negative, and students frequently observe professional lapses and patient mistreatment (Karnieli-Miller, Taylor et al. 2010). In one study, nearly three-quarters of residents reported observing the mistreatment of patients (Baldwin, Daugherty, and Rowley 1998). Research suggests that students become increasingly paternalistic and distanced from patients over the course of training, experiencing "disapproval, mistrust, and negative judgment toward laypersons" (Michalec 2012, 267). With such distance, and a hidden curricular focus on cognitive and technical aspects of care, comes the well-documented loss of a key clinical skill—empathy.

Attitudes and Values

Medical school hidden curriculum tends to value science over humanism. Students learn to manage information better than relationships. Although efforts are under way in some corners to reverse this, the hidden curriculum still tends to value interventional, high-technology clinical care, making teaching humanism difficult. Communication skills training is given limited time in the curriculum; humanism courses may not be valued or required. There is a declining interest in careers in primary care among medical students.

In addition to the loss of empathy already noted, the hidden curriculum appears at least partially responsible for recognized declines in medical students' patient-centeredness and attitude scores (Woloschuk, Harasym, and Temple 2004). Research has documented the growth of cynicism (Dyrbye, Thomas, and Shanafelt 2005) and the decline of idealism over the course of training. The hidden curriculum can support the prejudices with which students arrive, including against patients with mental illness (Benbassat 2012).

The hidden curriculum tends to value action, rather than reflection or observation. It appears to have little tolerance for uncertainty (Benbassat 2012). Through a focus on tests and procedures transmitted through near-peer supervision and attending feedback, students are taught to "do everything" in the face of uncertainty.

Moral Development

Although medical schools do routinely offer formal teaching in ethics, the hidden curriculum, over the course of classroom and clinical experiences, serves as a primary source of ethics training (Hafferty and Franks 1994). Student decisions in the face of difficult dilemmas are influenced by a desire to please superiors, implicit values in the learning environment, and evaluation pressures. Notably, research has documented a decline in moral reasoning over the course of medical training and has identified the hidden curriculum as one of the causes (Feudtner, Christakis, and Christakis 1994; Hren, Marušić, and Marušić 2011).

Medical Professionalism

Ultimately, the hidden curriculum teaches about what it means to be a physician (Haidet and Stein 2006). The hidden curriculum fundamentally impacts students' understanding of professionalism (Karnieli-Miller et al. 2011). In a surgery clerkship, three-quarters of students reported a change in their idea of professionalism, including "identifying specific behaviors that they planned to adopt or avoid as part of their own professional conduct" (Rogers et al. 2012, 424). Students learn from more advanced students about what physicians do and do not do, struggling with the complexities of physician emotion, empathy, and professional relationships (Fernandes et al. 2008).

The hidden curriculum teaches students about medical professionalism by directing their professional formation, sculpting their identities as physicians, and influencing their moral development. Critically, however, the teachings of the hidden curriculum are not always positive or in line with the ideals of traditional or official professionalism statements and oaths (Rabow, Wrubel, and Remen 2007).

Discordance Between the Hidden and Formal Curricula

Not all hidden curricular messages are concordant with each other, and the hidden curriculum can conflict with the explicit messages of the formal curriculum (Stern 1998b) or with a student's own personal beliefs or values (Phillips and Clarke 2012). Faculty can say something but actually believe and practice in a different way. Content can be offered with a nod to political correctness, but then care can still proceed with values wholly different from those officially promoted. This *curricular discordance* has been documented in end-of-life care as well as in ethics training, both in the United States and in Europe (Gaufberg et al. 2010; Phillips and Clarke 2012). For example, students are taught explicitly about the value of caring for patients with kindness and compassion, but students report countless examples of seeing patients be mistreated or talked about disrespectfully. Students must deal with the discordance of being mistreated themselves as compared to how they are being told to treat patients.

This widely identified curricular discordance has educational and personal consequences for medical students. Students may not learn well if teachings are not *consistent* (Stern 1998b). Personal growth may be hampered, rather than promoted, if the hidden and formal curricula are not aligned. Hidden curricular messages and clinical training experiences can overpower formal classroom messages to be ethical and treat patients with respect and compassion, resulting in an erosion of ethics, the stunting of student moral growth, a loss of empathy, and crises of conscience (Feudtner, Christakis, and Christakis 1994; Hren, Marušić, and Marušić 2011; Solomon et al. 1993; Hojat et al. 2009). Curricular discordance in end-of-life care training has been associated with poorer attitudes toward end-of-life care, less regard for institutional values, and educational dissatisfaction (Rabow, Gargani, and Cooke 2007). Dyrbye documented declines in student mental health (2005). Coulehan describes constriction of student focus to simple technical or intellectual competencies in the face of curricular discordance (Coulehan and Williams 2001).

Future Directions: Reflection and Discernment

The future of hidden curricular learning lies, first, in trying to make the messages as clear and consistent as possible; and second, and even more important, in empowering students with the lifelong skill of discernment in the face of discordance.

First, being clear and consistent about the intended learnings of medical school—more closely aligning hidden and formal curricular messages—can decrease student distress and help students understand what they are to learn. Efforts to incorporate training in professionalism into the hidden and formal curriculum are under way. Faculty development is key, as is improved evaluation and feedback (Steinert et al. 2007). The Healer's Art is an elective course for medical students now offered at seventy medical schools in the United States and internationally (Remen, O'Donnell, and Rabow 2008). Students have described how the course aligns its formal and informal curriculum, allowing students to place their personal mission in the context of a safe community of inquiry (Rabow, Wrubel, and Remen 2007). Notably, although the presence of even an elective course signifies some institutional commitment, this message is less strong than if the curriculum is required. At Indiana University School of Medicine (IUSM), making the formal and hidden curricula more consistent has been an active goal, supported from the top of the organization (Litzelman and Cottingham 2007). IUSM has used appreciative inquiry, faculty development, and organizational change to "create simultaneously an informal curriculum that models and supports the moral, professional, and humane values expressed in the formal curriculum" (410).

Second, despite well-intentioned efforts to minimize it, some amount of curricular discordance is *inevitable*, and students must learn how to manage these unavoidable conflicts. Not all role models are positive role models. Some of the messages out of the mouths of attendings in long white coats are wrong. The task for students is not just to learn everything taught in the formal and hidden curriculum, but also to discern among the often-conflicting messages what they ultimately believe. In this way, curricular discordance is a central element of professional formation and growth. Being exposed to new perspectives and values, including those in direct opposition to personal beliefs, requires students to negotiate dilemmas and offers an opportunity to challenge prejudices or reaffirm long-held beliefs. At the core of innovations at IUSM, as described in the Flexner Centenary issue of *Academic Medicine*, "the goal of professional formation is to tether or anchor students to their personal principles and the core values of the profession and help them navigate through the inevitable conflicts that arise in training and practice" (Rabow et al. 2010, 311).

In the face of discordant curricula and complex influences, student reflection, both individually and among his or her professional community, is essential to afford students the time and perspective to make the best choices in discerning among conflicting teachings. Building in support for both individual student and group reflection has been accomplished informally in attending ward rounds as well as formally with longitudinal electronic portfolios, reflection-focused courses in palliative care, online humanism curricula, peer discussion groups, critical incident processing, panel discussions, and sharing in a safe community of inquiry.

Ultimately, in more closely aligning the hidden and formal curricula, and in promoting the development of the critical skills of reflection and discernment among students, medical schools may better be able to have students actually learn what schools are hoping to teach.

12: The Hidden Curriculum in Nursing Education

Lisa Day and Patricia Benner

Academic nurse educators who intend to prepare new nurses for practice are becoming aware of a hidden curriculum—an unofficial program of learning that parallels the approved, explicit curriculum. Through the hidden curriculum, students learn values that teachers are not necessarily intending to teach. The hidden curriculum is found in the classroom, laboratory, and clinical learning environments, and can create confusion and less-than-optimal outcomes for students and faculty because hidden assumptions cannot be readily noticed, much less examined. Perhaps the most troubling aspect of the hidden curriculum in nursing is evident in hospitals and other practice settings where student nurses complete part of their education and training. Though all student nurses go to clinical sites for part of their learning, and academic nurse educators intend to prepare these students to take up clinical practice, there is a separation between academic schooling and practice-based learning that creates a discontinuity between formal education and practice—the so-called education-practice gap.

In recent years, the education-practice gap has widened greatly and most frequently reflects advances in practice that are not yet taught in schools. Healthcare settings have become more complex and multilayered with regulations and technologies that change rapidly. At the same time, nursing school curricula, teaching, assessment, and grading have emphasized theory and elevated decontextualized content over the practical, context-dependent know-how that allows nurses to navigate complex healthcare systems; knowledge acquisition is emphasized while situated knowledge use is all but ignored. For students learning a practice, abstract theories and decontextualized content are sometimes necessary, but never sufficient. Nurse educators know this, and nursing schools incorporate clinical learning into the official curriculum. However, the message students get from the hidden curriculum—that is, the implicit and unconscious devaluing of practice-based learning in context and the privileging of theory-based content knowledge—is different.

In this chapter, we will identify the structures and assumptions present in nursing education that support and sustain this hidden curriculum; discuss ways in which aspects of the hidden curriculum are detrimental to student nurses, nurse educators, and the nursing profession in general; and suggest changes in nursing education that will result in a redefinition of learning for professional practice that is relevant to nursing and all professional education.

Support for the Hidden Curriculum

Theory over Practice

Historically, the system of nursing education and schooling has built and sustained a structure that privileges theory over practice for knowledge development, and formal decision-making models over practical reasoning in real situations (Sullivan and Rosin 2008). This hidden curriculum is based on an unquestioned academic preference for formal, theory-based decision-making models and criterial reasoning over practical reasoning across time, through changes in the situation or changes in the clinician's understanding of the situation. As Bourdieu (1990) and Schwartz and Sharpe (2011) have pointed out, one's grasp of the nature of the particular situation is at the heart of practical reasoning. Empiricists' confidence that the right abstract theory or theories are necessary to organize practice in an elemental, bottom-up manner ignores the importance of perceptual grasp of the particular in real clinical situations that require nurses to understand what is at stake and what the situation demands as it unfolds over time. The privileging of generalizable theory as the primary source of knowledge over engaged practice in particular situations perpetuates and is perpetuated by the disconnection of practice-based learning in clinical environments from the teaching and learning of theory that takes place in classrooms.

The view that knowledge that is abstracted and separated from practice is more trustworthy and more useful because it is objective and can be generalized and applied in many different situations is firmly established in Western science. Evidence-based practice in nursing holds up as the gold standard the empirical evidence generated by randomized, controlled studies, while labeling knowledge that is embedded in and comes from practice as merely anecdotal. In this structure, knowledge that is based on formal features and criteria generated while disengaged from practice is more valuable than knowledge that is situated, that is based on family resemblances and holistic recognition, and that attends to the particular.

These empirical assumptions are further demonstrated and supported by a common notion among academic nurse educators that student nurses must be taken out of the practice setting in order to learn the concepts and theories associated with nursing in an abstract and decontextualized way before they can apply these concepts and theoretical knowledge in practice. Many nursing courses are structured to enact this truism: professors deliver abstract theory via classroom lectures and test students' knowledge of concepts and content before they move them to laboratory and clinical settings for application exercises. This model is further supported in nursing education by the appeal of theories that assume learning is a purely cognitive endeavor involving the acquisition and organization of content in the mind; knowledge is understood as formal cognitive mental representation that gains clarity and strength when it is separated from context. The higher importance of theoretical understanding over situated, practical know-how is further emphasized by evaluation strategies; although student nurses do spend time learning in practice settings, they are most often graded on written assignments and exam scores that mimic the multiple-choice questions found on the licensing exam for registered nurses (NCLEX-RN).

In studies of learning a practice, Benner and colleagues (Benner 1984; Benner, Tanner, and Chesla 1996; Benner, Hooper-Kyriakidis, and Stannard 2011), Eraut (1994, 2004), Lave (1988), and Lave and Wenger (1991) have called into question the wisdom of separating learning from context. Benner and coauthors (Benner 1984; Benner, Tanner, and Chesla 1996; Benner, Hooper-Kyriakidis, and Stannard 2011) have described the knowledge embedded in nursing practice and how practical knowledge is gained experientially. According to Lave and Wenger (1991), learning is always situated, and beginners learn practice through social engagement with a community of practice. These perspectives on situated learning locate learning in the understanding and use of knowledge in particular, meaningful contexts. This is in contrast to the "culture of acquisition" (Lave 1997, 17) common in many nursing schools where acquiring knowledge is the ultimate goal.

The view of learning as knowledge acquisition, theoretical understanding, and organization of decontextualized mental content can no longer be supported even in the most theoretical of disciplines. For example, Lave's (1988) study of how adults learn and use mathematics demonstrates the important part that engagement in a meaningful situation plays in human cognition, and shows that most often, the demands of the practical situation form the conditions of possibility for retrieving and using whatever formal theoretical knowledge they have access to. Adults who were placed in everyday practical settings where they understood the situation and where something of value was at stake for them were easily able to solve the same kind of mathematical problem that they were not able to solve in the abstract on a decontextualized, formal exam. This supports the idea that students learn to solve math problems not only through the decontextualized theoretical constructs of the formal math curriculum, but also as part of the contextualized but unplanned and unacknowledged learning that happens in everyday practice.

Like adults learning and using mathematics, nurses learn and use their knowledge in particular contexts that are filled with meaning and value. When a nurse is placed in a practical context that solicits a certain response, she or he is able not only to access and use theoretical knowledge, but also to construct new knowledge specific to the situation. The adults studied by Lave (1988) used many more methods to calculate the math problems they confronted in everyday situations than they had learned in formal math courses. Similarly, nurses and nursing students who are engaged in situated, practical reasoning across time in actual practice are engaged in a form of productive thinking that is guided by the demands, resources, and constraints of the situation. Instead of the metaphor of "applying" knowledge—which is mainly useful in relation to standardized procedure guidelines—the dominant metaphor becomes "using" and "generating" knowledge in open-ended, underdetermined clinical situations. The kind of knowledge use that nurses engage in their everyday practice is responsive to the particular and, as such, cannot be standardized and applied regardless of context. This practical know-how is best learned while engaged in a meaningful situation that solicits a response from the learner (Lave and Wenger 1991; Benner, Hooper-Kyriakidis, and Stannard 2011; Rosch 1975; Rosch and Mervis 1975).

Overlooking the Body and Skilled Embodied Know-How

The elevation of theory and the mental aspects of practice evident in nursing's hidden curriculum also ignore the role of the body in cognition and learning. Cognitive scientists and philosophers working in the area of embodied cognition describe the fundamental role of the body, and the experience of the world that comes to us through our bodies, in thinking and the development of what is commonly referred to as mental content. In contrast to the Cartesian view, where mental content resides in the disengaged mind of a subject who is isolated from a world of objects, proponents of embodied cognition understand cognition as arising from the integration of mind, body, and world (Gallagher 2009; Kelly 2000). In this view, the body is essential to thinking, and one's body shapes how one experiences and thinks about the world.

The unspoken assumption in the way education is structured in schools of nursing is that the body is not important to learning or thinking. This is particularly problematic in nursing, where embodied skilled know-how and perception play such an important role in the practice. The cognitivist understandings of thinking, learning, and knowledge that show up in nursing school curricula, teaching, and evaluation emphasize mental content primarily acquired through formal conceptual models and theory. This is evident in the way coursework and testing require nursing students to memorize sets of facts related to disease processes, medical and surgical treatments, and the steps of the nursing process including specific assessments and standard nursing diagnoses and interventions.

Much of the content knowledge needed for nursing practice—for example, normal vital-sign parameters, the mechanism of action of certain classes of medications, and the normal ranges of some laboratory values—is suited to a cognitivist approach. However, although nurses do need to memorize many key facts, much of nursing practice requires hands-on, embodied engagement with equipment and embodied, relational involvement with patients and clients. Despite the embodied nature of the practice, in many schools of nursing, even the psychomotor skills nursing students learn are taken up in a cognitivist way. In skills-lab exercises, students study sets of steps along with their theoretical rationales, and then apply these steps to equipment in a laboratory with relatively little time for practice. For example, one clinical nursing skills textbook (Perry and Potter 2006) lists twenty-one steps for the skill of assessing a radial pulse, each with a rationale. The assumption seems to be that if the student assimilates the steps of the task into her or his mental content, she or he will be able to accomplish the task physically. This representational view of the mind embedded in a decontextualized, disembodied approach to knowledge does not integrate the physically situated know-how that is vital to nursing practice (Gallagher 2009).

Detrimental Effects of the Hidden Curriculum

Nursing practice involves physical and mental engagement in situations that change over time, in which patient, client, family, or community well-being is at stake. Academic nurse educators intend to prepare new nurses for a dynamic practice environment in which they will be lifelong learners. Nursing education's hidden curriculum undermines this goal by giving students the idea that learning is a matter of assimilating static mental content that will then be applied in practice. Academia's elevation of theory and theory-based empirical knowledge overlooks practice as a legitimate source of knowledge. This separation of the school curriculum from actual nursing practice sets up students for a jarring shift from schooling to the practice environment and workplace learning (Lave 1988; Lave and Wenger 1991).

If student nurses have been taught to value theory over practice and that learning involves only acquiring mental content, they will be less prepared to recognize the learning that occurs in practice and less able to incorporate lifelong learning into their everyday practice as nurses. Thus, nurses' skills of clinical inquiry in actual practice situations will be virtually untutored and will remain hidden. The hidden curriculum also increases the risk that the practice-based knowledge nurses do acquire will be overlooked or lost.

Another damaging aspect of the hidden curriculum in nursing is that it creates and reinforces the separation of the academic nurse educators, who *teach* and know *what and why*, from the practicing nurses, who *do* and know *how and when*. Nurse educators come to academia from practice. Most often, these nurses have developed expert know-how in an area of clinical nursing practice before they earn an advanced degree and join the faculty of a school of nursing. The separation of theory and practice in academia forces academic nurse educators to teach theoretical concepts that are isolated from lived practice; this can alienate them from their own nursing practice and result in dissatisfaction with teaching. In these ways, the hidden curriculum in nursing education may be at least partly responsible for faculty shortages in schools of nursing, the difficult transition from school to work that many new nurses experience, the high turnover in the first year of clinical nursing practice, and the quality and safety crisis in healthcare.

Overcoming the Hidden Curriculum

In addition to being rooted in empiricist notions of knowledge, the hidden curriculum in nursing is also embedded in a rational-technical model of professional practice. In this view, becoming a professional requires only the acquisition of a discrete, specialized body of content knowledge; being a professional means being a keeper of this content (Parsons 1958). Solving the problem of the hidden curriculum in nursing education will require a new way of thinking about professionalism and about professional practice, and a recognition on the part of nursing school faculty of the knowledge and wisdom embedded in the practice.

A New Paradigm of Professionalism

William Sullivan, in his book *Work and Integrity* (2005), has provided an alternative to the rational-technical view of professional learning. In Sullivan's view, learning in a professional discipline such as clergy, engineering, law, medicine, or nursing involves work in three apprenticeships: (1) the cognitive apprenticeship, where students learn the theory and knowledge required to understand the nature and goals of the practice; (2) the skills-based apprenticeship, where students learn the skilled know-how required to engage in good practice; and (3) the apprenticeship of ethical comportment, where students learn the values of the practice and how to embody and enact the notions of good in their everyday actions. The best professional practice, and the best education for professional practice, integrates all three of these apprenticeships.

In his description of the three apprenticeships of professional education, Sullivan (2005) takes issue with the view of professionalism proposed by sociologist Talcott Parsons (1958) as merely ownership of a body of knowledge and control over who may enter the practice. Instead, Sullivan understands professional practice as also requiring socially embedded know-how and a commitment to a community of practitioners who share similar or the same notions of good (MacIntyre 1984). In this view, which is connected to Aristotle's idea of *phronesis* (Aristotle/Thomson 1956), practice is a way of knowing in its own right, and those engaged in practice are not simply applying theoretical knowledge, but are engaged in a larger, overarching instantiation of values through knowledge and skills use. What the integration of the three apprenticeships means essentially is the reconnection and integration of theory and practice. Nurses must learn a body of theoretical knowledge, but this knowledge will be useless unless it is connected to the lived, embodied practice of nursing and used to instantiate the values of that practice.

Sullivan (2005) broadens our understanding of professionalism by including values- and skills-based apprenticeships in addition to unique theoretical knowledge in his description of professional education. It may be difficult for nursing and medical school faculties to adopt this view of professional practice when so much of what nurses and physicians must learn involves abstract scientific knowledge. Medical and nursing educators are, however, beginning to understand the importance of a more holistic view of professional formation and are adopting teaching and learning methods that attend to values (Benner and Sutphen 2007; Rabow et al. 2010).

Acknowledging the Wisdom of Practice

Formal conceptual and scientific knowledge are essential for the practice of nursing and medicine. However, in order to be useful to nurses, knowledge must be situated in particular clinical situations. Nursing students, and students in other practice disciplines, must learn to use the knowledge they acquire from lectures and textbooks in an actual practice situation. Knowledge use of this kind is a form of productive thinking that goes beyond the mere application of decontextualized sets of rules, techniques, and algorithms. The rule-based algorithms and formal criteria that often are emphasized in nursing school classrooms are static snapshot forms of reasoning; knowing these rules may be necessary to nursing practice, but will never be adequate. Clinical reasoning in nursing is reasoning across time about the particular, through changes in the situation and changes in how the nurse understands the situation. Clinical reasoning across time, assessing patient responses, trends, and trajectories, should form the core of nursing education and should be the basis of student evaluation and grading.

A shift in attention from disengaged critical thinking to engaged clinical reasoning will require academic nurse educators to recontextualize their teaching. Instead of presenting taxonomies of facts outlined on slides and handouts, teachers will have to involve nursing students in real, practice-based problem solving and coach them to think and act (Benner et al. 2010; Benner, Hooper-Kyriakidis, and Stannard 2011; Schwartz and Sharpe 2011). Instead of loading students with theoretical content knowledge before they enter practice, nurse educators who are interested in overcoming the hidden curriculum will recognize the value of the teaching and learning that comes from engagement with the practice—contextualized learning that integrates the three apprenticeships of professional education.

There are many ways to reconnect theory and practice and classroom and clinical learning, including team-based and problem-based learning, narrative pedagogy, unfolding case studies, and simulation. In *Educating Nurses* (2010), Benner and colleagues provide examples of the kind of teaching that integrates clinical and classroom learning and equalizes the value of theory and practice. Using case studies and situated coaching to contextualize learning in classroom and lab settings, and bringing these learning environments closer to clinically based learning, the teachers described in this book demonstrate their commitment to practice as a source of knowledge. By assigning a final grade, or some percent of a final course grade, to students' clinical work, faculty can send the message that learning from practice is as valuable as learning theory and abstract concepts.

Conclusion

In the past thirty years, there has been a burgeoning interest in the nature of a practice discipline—that is, a socially organized body of knowledge with notions of good practice and good outcomes internal to the practice that is self-improving and develops over time (MacIntyre 1984; Schwartz and Sharpe 2011). Teaching and learning a practice requires practice-specific pedagogies that take into account the specific demands, resources, and constraints of that practice. For example, the signature pedagogy in law education is that of case law; in medicine, a discipline-specific pedagogy is using case studies and ward rounds to teach differential diagnostic reasoning and specific situated strategies for ruling in and ruling out diagnoses. The signature pedagogy in nursing is situated coaching, so that students learn to make qualitative distinctions and recognize trends and changes in the patient's responses to disease and illness.

Becoming a nurse requires much more than knowledge of theory, content, and abstract concepts. It requires situated coaching; embodied, situated thinking and action; experiential learning; clinical inquiry in actual clinical situations; clinical reasoning across time in particular cases; and the engaged embodied agency of the student-clinician as she or he takes up the knowledge and skills and forms the character necessary to become a good practitioner. Socialization is present and necessary, but not sufficient; the student must actively engage his or her own self-understanding, commitments, and agency in embodying the practice.

In sum, the pedagogical strategies needed for teaching a practice require integration of knowledge acquisition and knowledge use, and require teachers to understand situated use of knowledge as a form of productive thinking and not the mere application of well-learned formal techniques or principles. As long as knowledge acquisition eclipses knowledge use and practical reasoning, nursing and other healthcare students will continue to experience a hidden curriculum that ultimately impedes the best clinical knowledge development and sound use of scientific evidence.

13: Making the Invisible Visible

Uncovering the Hidden Curriculum in Allied Health Education

VIRGINIA WRIGHT-PETERSON AND CLAIRE E. BENDER

To date, much has been written about the hidden curriculum in the medical school curriculum. However, there is very little published literature regarding hidden curriculum being identified in allied health education. First, what is allied health education? Where does allied health education take place? As an example, take a look at a typical operating room in any academic health center where you might find the following personnel:

STAFF	STUDENT
Physician/surgeon	Chief resident, resident, medical student
Physician/anesthesiologist/ CRNA	Resident, student nurse anesthesiologist
First assistant	Student
Surgical technologist	Student
Central supply technologist	Student
Nurses (not considered allied health)	Students

Depending on the type of case, pharmacist, respiratory therapist, and cardiovascular invasive specialist staff and students could also be involved.

This scenario demonstrates the large and diverse number of learners of the healthcare team in this common place. Allied health education can involve all members of the healthcare team other than physicians and, in most cases, undergraduate nurses. In this environment, where team-based care is vitally important for highest quality patient care, the opportunity and necessity for multiple levels of team-based learning exists, and thus, the opportunity exists for the hidden curriculum to develop.

This chapter will pose the following questions in regard to allied health education and the hidden curriculum:

1. Does it exist?
2. If so, what are the similarities to the medical school curriculum?
3. Are there differences in comparison to medical education, and what are they?
4. What opportunities are there for allied health educators to recognize and teach the hidden curriculum?

First, we need to define what the hidden curriculum means as allied health educators. Hafferty (1998) has categorized medical education into at least three interrelated, overlapping spheres: (1) the formal curriculum; (2) the informal curriculum, which is unplanned, unscripted, but involves interpersonal forms of teaching and learning that take place between faculty and students; and (3) the hidden curriculum, which is defined as a "set of influences that function at the level of the organizational structure and culture." Hafferty also shares that the hidden curriculum "highlights the importance and impact of structural factors on the learning process" (1998, 404). The hidden curriculum may relate to the program and the institution's culture; its classrooms and buildings; its policies, processes, and procedures; the faculty; and institutional slang. It is about the unspoken, unwritten messages that are being sent to the students by their environment. Hafler and colleagues (2011) extend the influences of the hidden curriculum to faculty development in medical education.

We agree with Hafferty that much of what is taught *and learned* in allied health education takes place not within formal and informal program instruction, but within the invisible or hidden curriculum in allied health education.

Hidden Curriculum in Allied Health Education

1. Does the hidden curriculum *exist* in allied health education? Although there is very little formal reference to allied health education in the literature (Bradley et al. 2011; Tsai et al. 2012; Viggiano et al. 2007; Gofton and Regehr 2006), through our observations over the past three decades, we believe it does. Our formal medical literature search using keywords "allied health education and hidden curriculum" has revealed the references just listed. Specific examples are included in our examination of the similarities and differences with medical education noted in the following sections.

2. Let us begin with the *similarities* we have observed between allied health education and medical education (which include medical students as well as medical residents and fellows). In allied health education, the formal curriculum includes the typical classroom or didactic setting, online instruction, laboratory simulation, and clinical education, which is the hands-on learning in the real-world setting. It is a highly concentrated, intense period of study that is competency based and has the goal of passing the appropriate certification or board exam. The informal curriculum includes lessons learned from the interactions between faculty and student, the role modeling of faculty and instructors, the observed excitement of the faculty about teaching and the profession, and their passion and energy for providing the best care to their patients. The hidden curriculum is the unknown, yet fearful world of the organization, with all of the policies, procedures, and processes, and the dos and don'ts found in the student and faculty handbooks. It can be the type of furnishings in the student center and the relative age of the available computers. It can be the constant reminder of the institutional logo or published values and principles. Professionalism is learned from all three types of curriculum, perhaps the most from the informal and hidden curriculum.

In Hafferty's (1998) original article, he describes four different domains in which the hidden curriculum exists in medical education: (1) policy development, (2) evaluation, (3) resource allocation, and (4) institutional slang or nomenclature. Each of these is a critical part of allied health education and the necessary alignment of the institution or organization in which it resides. Student success depends on "passing" all three types of curriculum and across all four domains of the hidden curriculum.

In allied health education, policies, procedures, and processes are everywhere, both for the students and for the faculty. They are found in many different places: student-faculty handbooks, school website, human resources, affiliation agreements, and so on.

Evaluations are also everywhere, for the students, the faculty, the program, the administrative team, and the institution. They are both formative and summative. They can be observational or written. As Hafferty (1998) states, they are not simple tools of assessment, but vehicles to convey what is and is not important for the program, school, and organization. They are one component of success or failure. Student evaluations reveal continued growth and development in the profession. For the faculty, evaluations share feedback on their clinical skills and delivery. The program evaluation should provide honest feedback for careful management as needed. Team evaluation should provide a scorecard for effective management. And institutional evaluation is reflected in accreditation and often is linked to federal government reimbursement.

Allied health students tend not to be aware of the complexities of resource allocation in their programs. But they see or feel the need for classroom and facility improvements. Certainly the allied health faculty is aware of resource allocation in their programs as annual budget preparation occurs. The needs for space, equipment, and FTE (full-time equivalents), and the competitive distribution of the institutional resources can influence the thinking of faculty. And this thinking can be passed on to the students. The students can wonder, "What does the leadership of my organization think about my program and its students when we need better classrooms and computers?" Even the location of the classrooms can send a message to learners.

Like Hafler and colleagues (2011), we agree that allied health faculty also are affected by the hidden curriculum, often due to their socialization process as they became faculty members.

3. There are also *differences* in allied health education and the hidden curriculum. The major differences could be categorized into the following:

(a) Wide range of educational training programs (from weeks to years)
(b) Wide range of educational and experiential backgrounds of students and faculty
(c) Expanded exposure to the hierarchy within the healthcare team (other allied health professions and students, medical students, residents, nursing students, all faculty, and attending or supervisory physicians)
(d) More centralized learning environment in laboratory programs
(e) Lower position in hierarchal system
(f) Key role model figure likely allied health faculty or staff

Formal allied health education programs can vary from several weeks (ten weeks for phlebotomy) to multiple years (three years for a clinical doctorate of physical therapy). Students can matriculate to allied health programs as recent high school graduates, or even as postbaccalaureate or graduates. The maturity and experience level of learners can impact how they respond to educational opportunities given their role in a lower hierarchal position relative to the physician group. Patient contact during training can vary widely as well: for example, numerous contacts by the phlebotomy student and no direct contact by the histotechnology student. In each program level, the greatest faculty exposure is often the program director, the clinical coordinator, or the clinical instructor—and these most likely serve as the best role models for these students. Although physicians and medical directors provide leadership to each program through administrative oversight functions, the allied health students and faculty can remain somewhat isolated.

Allied health students and faculty develop their perceptions from the very start of their education, whether in a laboratory setting, a traditional classroom, an x-ray department, or the hospital. They often are met at the front door of the school by their program director, who starts their orientation with the traditional welcome, review of the thick student manual or handbook, brief discussion of the exhaustive list of policies and procedures with emphasis on the don'ts, followed by best wishes and the recommendation to "get to work." The environment of the classroom, the simulation lab, the clinic, and the hospital all tend to be the same on the surface. But both the formal and informal curriculum is delivered in the classroom, via computer, in the simulation center, and then in the clinical practice setting. It is this last location where the exposure to a wide variety of healthcare providers, including the physician staff, is encountered along with *the real patient*. This is the most complex, confusing, and challenging time for the allied health students, with no previous patient exposure or experience, as they are suddenly in this world of healthcare.

The silos in medical, nursing, and allied health education complicate the experience for learners, especially allied health learners. Each discipline prepares its students according to specific paradigms suited for its field, but the students are then placed in an environment with multidisciplinary providers and learners all involved in providing patient care. Learners suddenly have to sort out the relationship among providers at the same time that they are attempting to understand patient care.

Questions arise from the students: Is this real? Is this what I signed up for? How can I fit in with all these professionals? Am I smart enough to do this? In today's team-based care of the patient, we are teaching team-based education. Students are learning that they are valued members of the team, and their goal of quality patient care is the same as the rest of the team.

Clinical experiences and observations are very powerful components of allied health education for the students. This clinical time shapes the professional behavior. It is how students learn to communicate with the pa-

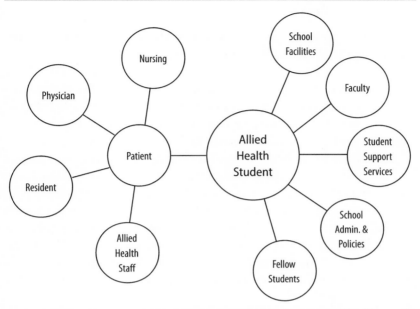

Figure 13.1. The extensive sphere of interactions within education and healthcare delivery systems illustrates the complexity of the hidden curriculum impacting the allied health student.

tient, family, nurse, and doctor. It is how they learn to examine and touch the patient. It is how they respond to the requests of the physician, nurse, colleague, and patient. These experiences shape what the students become. How does a phlebotomy student respond on his first day of clinical rotations when he walks into a patient's hospital room to draw blood, and the patient states that she does not want her blood drawn because she wishes to discontinue treatment? The patient tells the student that she is ready to die. During their first patient contact experiences, students can feel vulnerable and unsure. Textbooks don't typically cover the wide range of situations that students will encounter, and allied health students may not have a preconception of their roles; this is in contrast to medical students, who may better understand the physician's role from past personal experience as a patient and even from popular television shows such as *House* and *Gray's Anatomy*, where the role of the physician, and possibly the nurse, is highlighted, but the responsibilities of the phlebotomist, laboratory technician, and radiography technician are not nearly as visible.

What Are Opportunities for Allied Health Education to Recognize and Teach the Hidden Curriculum?

Teaching and modeling commitment to team-based and patient-centered medicine is both possible and critical to preparing the allied health professionals of tomorrow. There are many ways this can be accomplished. Interprofessional education (IPE) integrated into medical schools and allied health programs with didactic and clinical rotation experiences can address a better understanding and working relationship across professions. Rosalind Franklin University has implemented a comprehensive IPE curriculum across its medical, allied health, and nursing schools, which covers understanding about and with other professions that has the potential to give learners broader and more in-depth exposure across professions, thus building strong team-focused professionals (Aston et al. 2012). Students in their programs begin meeting together and collaborating on projects from the first year of their training.

Before implementing a full IPE program, implementation of a face-to-face professionalism seminar that includes as many professions as possible can contribute to a better understanding of the importance of concepts such as altruism, mutual respect, and honesty. Students from all fields represented in the school, including pharmacy, sonography, nurse anesthesia, and physical therapy, come together for a focused professional program. Short lectures followed by interdisciplinary group discussions facilitated by senior members of the faculty can provide students and faculty with an opportunity to discuss the explicit and observed values in an organization.

This seminar, followed by clinical rotations with faculty-of-student and student-of-faculty evaluations that assess congruities between behavior and stated values, would be beneficial. Faculty preparation of such a course will generate important discussions about the organization's values and help address the impact of the hidden curriculum on the faculty.

Another stand-alone experience that could offer opportunities to close the gap between the explicit and hidden curriculum would be experiences in a simulation center or online simulation experiences that permit students and faculty to be more aware of the hidden curriculum. Working through scenarios that uncover the ways in which the hidden curriculum manifests itself in the classroom and clinical environment could improve the positive impacts of the hidden curriculum, diminish the detrimental impacts, and help address the issue for both faculty and students. Examples might include code response team, seizure response, and cardiovascular surgery. In each of these situations, faculty and students from various disciplines, including medicine, nursing, and allied health, could come together to train. Debriefing by trained facilitators could include explicit discussion of the factors related to the hidden curriculum. Some of these scenarios could also be built as interactive animations online.

Ultimately, imagine preceptors meeting as multidisciplinary teams to plan clinical rotations for all learners together and then engaging with the learners as teams as well as individually. Teams could address sensitive issues such as questioning a doctor's order and working with challenging patients or family members. Could teaching and learning in teams better prepare learners to practice in teams, and could this team approach go a long way in reducing the impact and existence of the hidden curriculum?

Interdisciplinary faculty development opportunities to increase faculty awareness of the hidden curriculum concept and its potential implications would likely be advantageous as well. Workshops could encourage faculty to take an inventory of school, program, and their own individual practices that might be promoting a hidden curriculum. These workshops could become starting points for workshops on course design and evaluation that move toward competency-based and student-centered learning models.

Faculty development opportunities should include non-faculty administrative and support staff members. Open discussions about resource allocation, policies, and pedagogical approaches should occur regularly. Further, administration should review the school and individual programs for potential biases based on lack of diversity of demographics including race, ethnicity, and gender.

In summary, the hidden curriculum does indeed exist in allied health education as well as medical school curriculum, and although there are both similarities and differences, there are opportunities for addressing the issue, most of which would potentially be most powerful if developed and implemented in collaboration.

14: Hidden Amongst Us

The Language of Inter- and Outer-professional Identity and Collaboration

JILL THISTLETHWAITE

Human social contact is fundamentally rule-governed. People seek to act appropriately . . . in terms of the social norms and values of their social groups.
—JOHN C. TURNER (1996, 21), paraphrasing HENRI TAJFEL

In this chapter, I discuss the hidden curriculum and its influence on teamwork and collaborative practice. Interprofessional education (IPE) is promoted as a strategy to help students develop the language and skills of teamwork and collaboration, and to reduce stereotyping and interprofessional conflict through contact and awareness of the impact of professional identity formation. I revisit the work of Allport (1954) and his conceptualization of in-groups and out-groups (terminology frequently employed in describing interprofessional relationships), and consider whether it is still helpful in modern healthcare delivery.

In the twenty-first century, health professionals need to work in teams and looser collaborations to provide optimal care. There are several reasons for this: increasing complexity of long-term and chronic conditions, the aging demographic, super-specialization, and the rise in the number of discrete health professions over the past few decades. As a general practitioner (GP; family physician) of twenty-five years' experience, I have always stressed the importance and necessity of working together with colleagues across professions in both well-defined teams and extended networks. Indeed, in recognition of the imperative for what has variously been called multidisciplinary, multiprofessional, and interprofessional collaborative practice, I am a longtime champion of IPE. To me, it has always made sense that if we are to work together, we must at some point (and indeed at frequent points) in our training learn together to work together.

An extensive literature on IPE and IPCP (interprofessional collaborative practice) informs this chapter (see box 14-1 for definitions), as does my own experience in clinical practice and as an educator. I write from a fairly elevated position in the health professional hierarchy: a hierarchy that has

---

BOX 14-1

Definitions: Interprofessional

Interprofessional education (IPE): Occasions when two or more professions learn with, from, and about each other to improve collaboration and the quality of care (CAIPE 2002)

Interprofessional collaboration: The process of developing and maintaining effective interprofessional working relationships with learners; practitioners; patients, clients, and families; and communities to enable optimal health outcomes (CIHC 2010)

---

many overt and hidden effects on how we work together, how teams form and function, and how our students learn. In my own medical profession, there is a frequent statement reflecting the place of family practice within medicine: I'm *just* a general practitioner. There is both self- and peer deprecation within a single profession (intraprofessional) and between professionals (interprofessional). However, because the word *interprofessional*, without a hyphen, now has mostly positive connotations, I could refer to the darker side between professionals' interactions as *outerprofessional*. This terminology reflects the classic work of Allport (1954/1979), a leading social psychologist of the twentieth century, on prejudice, which introduced us to the concept of the in-group and the out-group. An in-group is "any cluster of people who can use the term 'we' with the same significance" (Allport 1979, 37). We therefore would refer to members of an out-group as "they."

This language is interesting. As a GP, I often refer to some patients as "my" patients. In a GP health center, the doctors may refer to "our" nurses, while other doctors are members of "my" profession. The use of these pronouns seems to reflect a continuity of relationships. For example, medical students attached to a rural community practice for a longitudinal experience (one complete year of a four-year program) often begin to refer to "my patients," while students undertaking more traditional eight-week rotations will refer to "a patient" or "the patients" (Worley et al. 2006). However, this usage may also be seen as paternalistic and possessive. Think how "our nurses" sounds compared to "my nurse." The students' language may simply be reflecting the discourse they hear.

Personally Writing

When I was aged ten, my primary school teacher asked the class what we wanted to be when we "grew up." My mother was a nurse, and I was reading a series of American books about a young nurse progressing through the hospital ranks. I said that I intended to be a nurse. My teacher replied, "I am sure you can do better than that." Subsequently, I became a medical student over thirty years ago, at a time when the medical profession was predominantly masculine and the nursing (and other allied health) profession was mainly feminine. During the first half of my medical degree, the existence of the other health professions largely was ignored in our program. In my clinical years, it seemed that the main interaction between us fledgling professionals was the male medical students' pursuit of female nurses as girlfriends. The health service organization and the university system kept us all formally apart until we were launched on the wards as junior doctors. Senior and experienced nurses had to call us in to write prescriptions, insert intravenous lines, and check on sick patients: all tasks that most would have been perfectly capable of doing themselves with the right education. Some of my peers reacted to this "power" with arrogance and a sense of entitlement; others, like me, were more humble and sought help from these expert colleagues. I thus became used to seeking and giving advice interprofessionally as appropriate. Later, I relished the opportunity to work in a well-functioning primary healthcare team in the north of England. I naively imagined that times were changing—as indeed they were in some places.

Six years ago, now working in Australia, I asked one of "our" more experienced practice nurses for advice. She replied, "You are the doctor, you have to make the decision yourself." The health system and its payment policy in Australia does not allow nurses the autonomy they have in other countries, unless they are practicing in rural and remote areas of the country where there are no medical doctors.

I recently spent time with health professionals in a Southeast Asian country. I was told about a pilot program involving nurses participating in doctors' ward rounds. However, it was proving difficult to expand the initiative because the rounds were held at the busiest times of nurses' shifts. Moreover, many nurses felt unable to communicate within the round because of the hierarchical nature of the clinical workforce and because some doctors did not value the nurses' knowledge of their mutual patients.

Our students and junior health professionals observe such interactions. They hear us talk about teamwork—indeed, they may even learn about teamwork at the university (either uniprofessionally or multiprofessionally) within the formal curriculum. But how often do they observe well-functioning teams in action as part of the informal curriculum? How well do they learn the roles and responsibilities of their colleagues and discuss patient care as collaborating experts in their own field? More commonly, perhaps, they learn in clinical environments predominantly within their professional in-group and attend uniprofessional handovers and ward rounds, influenced by the hidden curriculum of care delivery within their national health service.

Collaboration and Conflict

Our impressions of health professionals affect our attitudes before we start training. We interact with nurses and doctors frequently in childhood, even if we are relatively healthy. We later seek advice about contraception and sexual health. As teenagers, some of us may consult with allied health professionals such as physiotherapists. Our parents may prefer complementary therapists, though if we come from a medical family, this is less likely. Memories of these encounters may influence our career decisions or shape our feelings about who to trust for our future healthcare. In addition, there is no shortage of medical dramas in the media, both real and fictitious. Some of the latter are fairly true to life, but others, needing to heighten narrative tension, are far removed from the mundane day-to-day practice of most health professionals. Nurses and doctors feature predominantly in films and on television; other health professionals rarely get speaking parts.

One dictionary definition of *collaboration* is "working with the enemy." Listening to health professionals talk about their colleagues, one might suppose that there was indeed some enmity among the different professions. Though certain comments may be part of the black humor notoriously employed by the medical profession, or simply playful joking, others are symptomatic of the conflicts occurring in health delivery environments. Allport (1954/1979) famously hypothesized that interactions between members of conflicting groups may reduce prejudice and hostility among them. However, he added that this is possible only if the groups enjoy the same status and there is no power differential operating. Even if, in the clinical environment, nurses and doctors try to act as if no such power imbalance were occurring, in actual practice such imbalances may cause subtle behavior patterns that students assimilate through the hidden curriculum mechanism and perceive as the norm. Although most doctors no longer expect their nursing colleagues to be "handmaidens," and they may *ask* a nurse to do something rather than command, the pattern often is that nurses follow the doctor's request: please give this patient an injection; change this dressing; alter the dosage of the medication, and so on. This becomes an established pattern, so it may then seem odd for a doctor to ask a nurse's advice, as in my personal example.

Exploration of the relationship difficulties between professionals has been undertaken across a number of disciplinary fields, for example, sociology, psychology, and philosophy. This "ology" mix has caused problems of variations in language, epistemology, and theoretical frameworks, similar to those between the professions themselves. Sociologically, the professions jealously guard their knowledge, position, and autonomy. Although medicine is one of the oldest professions, the newer ones, such as nursing and physiotherapy, are now also protective of their space and what makes their in-group different from out-groups. Reeves (2011) has argued from his reading of the sociological literature that the nature of the nurse-doctor relationship is more complicated than it appears at first glance. The subservience that many learners may observe in clinical settings is, in fact, not all it appears. Nurses may seem to be dominated by the powerful physician but, in fact, are guiding the doctors' decisions through covert processes. Moreover, in some settings, senior nurses are making the decisions themselves; but how often do medical students and nursing students who pass fleetingly through the clinical environment recognize this pattern of behavior?

Mind Your Language

Revisiting Allport for this chapter, I was struck by how his examples reflected a time when prejudice was much more overt than it is today, when our laws and societal values in the main deter people from openly expressing racism. However, as we all are aware, such prejudice does still exist, though it is more subtle and subliminal. How applicable are these big themes, such as race and class, to interprofessional relationships? Consider some of Allport's chapter titles: choice of scapegoats; frustration; aggression and hatred; anxiety, sex, guilt; religion and prejudice (Allport 1954/1979). Though there may be some resonance with our daily working life and the experiences of learners, I nonetheless suggest that applying these words to professional relationships generally is not helpful.

Literature focusing on professional interactions often uses language that reflects the potential positivity, but also the risk of collaboration with the "other." IPE and IPCP advocates tend to use positive nouns such as "opportunity(ies)" and "benefit(s)" while describing interprofessional learning opportunities as "value(able)" experiences. We also read: integrated; cohesive; sharing of power, knowledge, skills, responsibilities, and values; shared goals and decision making; reconciliation and negotiation; participative; partnership; flexibility; collegiality; openness; reciprocity; inclusivity (see, for example, D'Amour and Oandasan 2005). In contrast, uniprofessional or multiprofessional learning and working may be described as fragmented, opposing, silos, and hierarchical; or in relation to barriers, stereotypes, and rivalry (see, for example, Hall 2005). Yet there also is a darker lexicon reflecting the dangers inherent in venturing outside our in-groups for intergroup collaboration: side-step(ping), rule-bend(ing), rule-break(ing), role-break(ing), custom-defy(ing), struggle(s), risk(y), danger(ous), threat(ening), vulnerable, tension(s) and difficult(ies), boundary crossing (Brooks and Thistlethwaite 2012). In short, commonly mentioned barriers to IPCP are language itself and professional jargon (Choi and Pak 2007), professional identity (Hall 2005), stereotyping (Choi and Pak 2007), and professional regulation (Lahey and Currie 2005).

Professional Socialization and Identity

I will now consider two of these barriers in more detail: professional identity and its impact on interprofessional contact; and stereotyping.

Our professional language, or jargon, helps us to recognize members of our in-group when we interact with unfamiliar colleagues. Much has been written about students being socialized into their chosen professions and the hidden curriculum impact of role models (positive and negative) on this process. This process happens slowly over time as trainees learn the knowledge, skills, and jargon required to "become" a medical doctor, nurse, physical therapist, and so on. However, there also is an official rite of passage when students graduate and receive not only letters after their name, but a certificate of qualification. When medical students graduate, they also may take a modern version of the Hippocratic oath. This helps set them apart from other professions who do not "profess" in such a way. In the United States, there is also an intermediate ceremony as medical students pass from classroom education to their clinical rotations. The white-coat ceremony, when students put on the white coat or doctors' uniform, has been labeled elitist (see, for example, Veatch 2002), yet it has now been adopted as a feature of other professional courses such as occupational therapy and dentistry.

In the United Kingdom, white coats (traditional medical ones) are no longer allowed in National Health Service (NHS) hospitals due to the risk of spreading infection. As a consequence, many hospital doctors have chosen to wear surgical scrubs or more informal shirts or dresses, because ties and long sleeves are also banned. A UK colleague of mine remarked that this change in dress code appears to have loosened some of the traditional barriers between the professions—it is difficult to distinguish between professions based on dress alone. This may cause some confusion, but it highlights the need for introductions to patients and other staff by name and responsibility.

How we develop professional identities—and our own and others' responses to those identities—is important to consider when working with learners. As we mature in our careers, many of us develop new roles and perhaps changes to our professional identity. Personally, I identify as a medical doctor (family physician), educator, and researcher. How I identify myself to others depends on that other. For credibility in some areas of practice, people need to know I am a medical doctor, whereas in other arenas, I may introduce myself as a health professional educator. Why and how I make these decisions is not always obvious, even to me. I am somehow acknowledging the prejudice (which I may only be imagining) that is attracted to certain roles in certain environments.

Identity and Stereotyping

Social identity theory (SIT), as introduced by Tajfel and Turner (1979), hypothesizes that some of us derive how we define ourselves from our membership in groups. There is pressure "to evaluate one's own group positively through in-group/out-group comparisons" that "lead social groups to attempt to differentiate themselves from each other" (41). Turner (1982) later suggested that we identify with our own social group (the in-group) and may have suspicions and bias against other groups (the out-groups). Stereotyping of out-group members and unfavorable comparisons of their attributes with our in-group helps us establish our sense of self. Turner calls this *intergroup differentiation.*

Allport discusses stereotypes "in our culture" (1979, 189) mainly across racial groupings. His definition is "an exaggerated belief associated with a category. Its function is to justify (rationalize) our conduct in relation to that category" (191)—with "category" for Allport meaning generalization. Even though his era did not contain the information revolution and overload we are experiencing in the twenty-first century, Allport believed that the mass media were responsible for much stereotype formation and maintenance. Formation also is based on early experience, as mentioned earlier, which guides later perceptions (Jost and Hamilton 2005). Hence, we locate the recommendation that students should learn together from early in their professional education and development before stereotyping has a chance to become embedded.

Stereotypes serve as justificatory devices: *ego-justification, group-justification,* and *system-justification* (Jost and Hamilton 2005). Ego-justification manifests as people who feel better about themselves by denigrating others. Group-justification allows members to rationalize discrimination against members of other groups and feel better about their group and the members within it. System-justification provides "legitimacy for institutional forms" of prejudice and discrimination (216). Further, it rationalizes hierarchical structures. Research has shown that low-status groups are stereotyped in more communal, socioemotional terms, while high-status groups (extrapolating here to medicine's place in the health professional hierarchy) are stereotyped in action and achievement-oriented terms: for example, nurses are caring; doctors are diagnosticians.

How we acquire stereotypes is interesting. We obviously develop our attitudes through learning from others: from role models, the hidden curriculum, parents, teachers, peers, the media, and so on. In order to belong to our in-group, to feel wanted and safe, we realize we have to show that we have similar beliefs and values. If we change groups, our beliefs and values may not resonate with our new community. We then have the choice either to change our beliefs and values to fit in; to mimic those of the group while retaining our own, resulting in confusion and dis-ease; or to leave the group.

Most of the time, we probably would not choose to join a group with values that differ markedly from our own, yet sometimes we have little choice (because of migration, marriage, and so on). We may sometimes change groups or, more likely, join an extra group, without realizing the extent of the difference. How often, when changing jobs or joining a new team, do we have a frank discussion about personal and professional values? And if we do, how often do we share such discussions with our students?

SIT has been applied to the interactions that can occur during interprofessional learning: a group of students belonging to one particular health profession (their in-group) compare themselves with one or more groups of other students (the out-groups), undertaking the same activity. Applying SIT, we would expect that to maintain harmonious relationships, the groups must retain a sense of their own distinction. Therefore, some educators argue that IPE activities should take place in the later years of prequalification (prelicensure) programs because, by that time, students already should have a sense of their professional identity and role within healthcare. However, as already noted, other educators believe that interprofessional contact in the earlier years of programs is preferable because it helps later on, and it reduces the impact of the hidden curriculum in clinical placements. This latter belief stems from a different reading of SIT, with the idea that what is necessary for harmonious working is the creation of a common in-group with members from multiple professions—either by bringing these individuals together prior to the formation of any substantive form of in-group identity, or by following the dissolution of preexisting boundaries (see Carpenter and Dickinson 2011 for a review of these arguments).

Professional Contact

Allport's *contact hypothesis* suggests that positive outcomes are possible only if groups are pursuing common goals and the environment is supportive of their working together. However, individual health professionals may set goals with patients that are not agreed on by the rest of the team. Professional priorities may differ, causing confusion for patients and caregivers with the added possibility of one professional saying about another to the patient, "I don't agree we should do that." Such discourse influences any learner who observes such types of interactions. Students soon pick up the language of their tutors—for example, students regularly refer to a patient's lack of compliance. When I have challenged students on their use of this term, it is obvious to me that they have not considered how value laden it is.

The contact hypothesis regularly is referenced as a means of understanding and ensuring that IPE meets its aims of improving relationships and respect between the health professions. However, the original central premise that IPE is the best means of reducing tension and hostility by bringing groups together under appropriate conditions (Brown 1996) sends the message to learners that we should expect hostility within the workplace. A major problem with the contact hypothesis is the issue of generalizability. If a nursing student learns and works with a pharmacy student, and they develop mutual respect, this does not mean that all nursing students at that institution will respect all pharmacy students. It does not even mean that this particular nursing student will feel positive about all pharmacy students or pharmacists in the future. As Brown writes, "Any change in attitudes I experience towards that person cannot be easily extrapolated to other members of his or her group whom I have not yet met" (1996, 182). In particular, it takes time to trust an individual from an out-group who becomes a member of one's healthcare team. However, such trust is less likely to be built if there are subliminal messages that conflict, and hostility is likely.

Allport's ideas are useful to apply to professional contact, if only for discussing similarities and differences in this specialized context. As an example, consider three groups of students from differing professional programs who are brought together for the first time for a learning activity on communication. At the start there is *sheer contact*—physical proximity in the classroom. Unless otherwise engineered, the students sit within their professional groups, sticking with the people they know. The facilitator may mix them up in smaller groups and ask them to get to know each other. But if these students are undertaking a clinical rotation at the same time and in the same working environment, the classroom contact may not progress beyond the superficial unless there is an authentic reason to interact. Some students may enter into *competition*, trying to outdo each other in demonstrating knowledge and skills. There, the skilled facilitator helps bring them to the stage of *accommodation*—becoming at ease with each other while respecting and valuing differences. The fourth stage is *assimilation*. Allport refers to this four-stage passage as a "peaceful progression" (1979, 261) while acknowledging that some groups resist assimilation and hold onto their distinctiveness.

The health professions are groups that tend to be jealous of their professional identities and resist assimilation and acculturation (see Box 14-2) (Wakefield et al. 2006; Baker et al. 2011). Although the concept of *acculturation* is useful when thinking how students may familiarize themselves with the new culture of the clinical environment (hospital wards, operating theaters, and so on), it is not helpful when considering how the professions interact. *Third-culture personality* is a better terminology and aspiration. So the nurse, doctor, and physiotherapist have individual professional identities and cultures (first culture), have contact with other groups (second culture), and learn to work together within this third collaborative culture of healthcare.

Conclusion

The focus on stereotypes and the in-group/out-group discourse is perhaps reinforcing a hidden curricular message that teamwork is a problem because of professional rivalry and other barriers. The premise of IPE and early contact between health professional students is that teamwork processes will be enhanced, and there is emerging evidence that this is the case. Learning outcomes for IPE include communication and the importance of shared language to enhance patient care and safety. Interprofessional educators do recognize, however, that conflict within teams and collaborations are common, and therefore students need to also develop skills in negotiation and conflict resolution.

BOX 14-2

Definitions

Assimilation: The absorption and integration of people, ideas or culture

Acculturation: Assimilation to a different culture, typically the dominant one

Third-culture personality: Retention of basic identity and culture while coming to respect and understand the values of the new group (Benson 2003)

PART V

SPECIAL TOPICS AND APPLICATIONS

This section is intended as a series of case examples on how one can apply the hidden curriculum to a variety of issues related to health professions education. The list of topics covered is not exhaustive, but it is intended to be both broad and eclectic, including how a hidden curriculum perspective shines new light on issues of professionalism (Richard Cruess and Sylvia Cruess, chapter 15); the context of Indigenous health and cross-cultural issues (Shaun Ewen, chapter 16); new models of clinical teaching, such as longitudinal and integrated clerkship training (David Hirsh, chapter 17); social media (Richard Frankel, chapter 18); faculty development (Britta Thompson, Allison Ownby, and Janet Hafler, chapter 19); and how the hidden curriculum operates within a research training environment (Kelly Edwards, chapter 20).

Our intent was to provide examples ranging from topics that have generated a considerable hidden curriculum literature (for example, professionalism), to those where there has been much less exploration using the hidden curriculum as an analytic or interpretive lens. As in other parts of this book, we urge readers not to bracket their thinking (in this instance about applications and examples) to the immediate chapters being showcased. Virtually every chapter in this book contains examples of the hidden curriculum at work. Referring only to the book's opening two chapters, Stern explores medicine's penchant for parable in conveying unseen lessons, along with the impact of physical and organizational structure on the learning environment. Meanwhile, Hundert provides an extensive and highly textured hidden curriculum analysis of the Match.

We conclude this book with a summary chapter by the book editors in which we address two broad goals. First, we review some of the themes introduced in our chapters as well as explore some of the thematic links we found in working with these chapters. Although we did not select either topics or authors for this book with such an intent in mind, one of the great joys in working with this diverse and talented group of contributors is that they have things to say that can (and should) be viewed within the context of things said by other contributors. We hope readers will approach individual chapters with a similar mindset.

Relatedly, we want to alert readers to some of the thematic holes that inevitably emerge in an edited book built around a particular concept. Although we invited authors with certain roles in mind (see comments in part 1 about the Stern and Hundert chapters), we also told authors that they were free to write on whatever interested them about the hidden curriculum. Several of the authors took us up on this invitation, and did so in quite unexpected ways. Finally, our aforementioned word limit made it impossible for authors to exhaustively dissect their topics of choice. As a consequence, we have reserved some space in our concluding chapter to touch on some themes we felt needed additional coverage.

Our second goal, also driven by working with this august body of contributors, was the challenge of where-do-we-go-from-here. Such musings range from how the concept of the hidden curriculum has evolved, and therefore might continue to evolve, to the glaring need for better and more assessment, to how the concept might be applied to other domains of health professions education, as well as how other topic areas might benefit from an infusion of hidden curriculum thinking. Once again, all this is a tall order, and we can do little more than scratch the surface of such issues. However, we hope that readers will come away with new insights into what we believe is a highly effective lens into the cultural undercurrents of what remains a most noble enterprise—the education of future health professionals.

15: Professionalism, Professional Identity, and the Hidden Curriculum

Do As We Say and As We Do

RICHARD L. CRUESS AND SYLVIA R. CRUESS

In a pioneering 1957 study of the sociology of medical education, Robert Merton outlined two separate, but linked, objectives of medicine's educational institutions. He stated that the task of medical education is to "shape the novice into the *effective practitioner* of medicine, to give him the best available knowledge and skills, and to provide him with a *professional identity* so that he comes to think, act, and feel like a physician" (Merton, Reader, and Kendall 1957, 7; emphasis added). Making allowance for the gender imbalance of the day, this quote once more clearly emphasizes the importance of transmitting the culture of medicine with its historical values rooted in morality and service. Merton linked this educational goal to the development of a professional identity, a process that is receiving increasing attention a half century later as the medical profession tries to determine the optimal way of ensuring that medical graduates and trainees become not just skilled physicians, but true professionals (Hafferty 2009; Cooke, Irby, and O'Brien 2010; Monrouxe 2010; Monrouxe, Rees, and Hu 2011; Goldie 2012; Jarvis-Selinger, Pratt, and Regehr 2012).

Many generations of medical graduates have entered practice without formal instruction in professionalism or, indeed, any structured knowledge of what it means to be a professional. Instead, they acquired their values and behavior patterns by modeling their activities on those of individuals respected for both their clinical skills and their professionalism. It has long been recognized that this is an important component of socialization, "the process by which a person learns to function within a particular society or group by internalizing its values and norms" (Oxford English Dictionary 1989). During the years prior to entering practice, students and trainees consciously and unconsciously prepare themselves to fill the social role desired by society—that of the professional. Fundamental to this process are role models who have the capacity to either promote or inhibit the process of professional identity formation (Wright et al. 1998; Côté and Leclère 2000; Cruess, Cruess, and Steinert 2008). Role models function in and help to determine the nature of the learning environment where the transformation from layperson to professional takes place.

The modern "professionalism movement" has arisen because of widespread concerns about the performance of individual physicians and of medicine's professional organizations. There is general agreement that medicine's professionalism is being threatened by a combination of unprofessional conduct by individual physicians, lax regulation by the profession, and healthcare systems that can subvert both professional values and professional behaviors (Cruess and Cruess 1997b; Freidson 2001; Sullivan 2005). The medical profession has responded and, although some have described the response as a defensive attempt to maintain the power relationships inherent in the status quo (Martimianakis, Maniate, and Hodges 2009), there is no question that society, individual physicians, and the profession as a whole will benefit if the behavior of practitioners and their organizations is guided by the values of professionalism (Freidson 2001; Sullivan 2005). An important part of medicine's response to these threats has been to emphasize the teaching and evaluation of professionalism throughout the continuum of medical education.

A frequent question posed to those responsible for teaching professionalism is, "Can professionalism be taught?" The implied assumption is that the characteristics underlying professional behavior should have been developed long before the individual entered medical school (Huddle 2005; Coulehan 2005). Based on our experience, this has not been an easy question to answer. The nature of professionalism, including a working definition, and its history and evolution can be presented to students and trainees, and can be learned. We have termed this the *cognitive base* and suggested that it should represent a key part of any program devoted to the teaching of professionalism (Cruess and Cruess 2009). In Merton's framework, this would fall into the category of transmitting knowledge and skills, a relatively straightforward, uncomplicated task.

Translating this learned knowledge into behavior patterns that will indicate a student is "thinking, acting, and feeling like a physician" is a more difficult and complex undertaking. This task becomes more understandable, and perhaps more manageable, if the question is reframed as, "Can one influence the development of a professional identity?" The answer to this is unquestionably yes. Concentrating on identity allows the focus to shift from "doing" to "being" (Jarvis-Sellinger, Pratt, and Regehr 2012), an approach that has been an objective of medical educators since at least the time of Hippocrates. In addition, there is wide agreement that the influence of the educational program can be either beneficial or detrimental to professional identity formation. It is in this domain that the teaching of professionalism and the hidden curriculum intersect.

Professionalism, Professional Identity, and the Formal, Informal, and Hidden Curricula

When Hafferty (1998) expanded on the concept of what is often loosely termed the hidden curriculum, he identified three categories: the formal, the informal, and the hidden curricula. This classification corresponds to the reality of medical education. It serves to emphasize the importance of these three domains to the learning environment of every teaching establishment. Limiting the analysis to the single term *hidden curriculum* diminishes the usefulness of the exercise, as the three categories provide a structure within which the learning environment can be addressed.

The formal curriculum of each teaching institution is contained in its mission statement and course objectives and outlines. It includes what the faculty believes they are teaching and what they hope will be learned. Professionalism is now part of the formal curriculum in virtually every medical school and training program. Initially, this occurred in response to the perceived threats to medicine's professionalism, but is now an accreditation requirement.

The informal curriculum represents "an unscripted, predominantly ad hoc, and highly interpersonal form of teaching and learning that takes place among and between faculty and students" (Hafferty 1998, 404). It is grounded in a series of interpersonal interactions that occur in multiple sites—corridors and elevators, cafeterias and surgeons' changing rooms, and a multiplicity of personal interactions. It is in these settings that messages are sent that validate the behaviors, values, and beliefs that help individuals to shape their own professional identities.

The hidden curriculum is the result of policy decisions—both those taken and those consciously or unconsciously avoided—that create the organizational structure and culture of the institution. Promotion and remuneration procedures that reward outstanding teachers and role models, or fail to do so, can have a profound impact, as can a culture that does not tolerate poor clinical care or harassment of learners.

In addressing the role of the hidden curriculum in the teaching of professionalism, several things become apparent. First, Hafferty's three categories are at the same time distinct and interconnected. As an example, professionalism for generations was taught almost entirely in the informal curriculum. At that time, it was largely absent from the formal curriculum. In nearly every medical school and teaching program, professionalism now enjoys wide representation in the formal curriculum. Thus, actions taken can move an item from one category to another. Second, in the medical literature, references to the hidden curriculum generally are couched in negative terms, stressing its frequently corrosive nature. Although there are certainly negative elements in the informal and hidden curricula in every educational institution, it must be recognized that virtually every physician entering practice has developed his or her own unique professional identity, and that the impacts of the hidden and informal curricula have often been positive. The informal and hidden curricula have always been present and always will be. The objective is to make certain that their impact is positive. Finally, the influence of the informal curriculum on the process of socialization of medical students, residents, and indeed faculty members, is most significant in the domains of professionalism and professional identity (Hafferty 2009).

How Is Professionalism Learned, and How Is Professional Identity Formed?

Although they are closely linked, there are differences between professionalism and professional identity. Medical professionalism is "a set of values, behaviors and relationships that underpins the trust the public has in doctors" (Royal College of Physicians of London 2005, 14). The emphasis is on the external observations of others, as professionalism is actualized by the demonstration of professional behaviors. This is also true of professional identity, yet there are important internal aspects of the concept of professional identity unique to each individual. Self-perception is equally important—"who I think I am" (Monrouxe 2010, 42).

The explicit teaching of the cognitive base of professionalism is not a mystery. It consists of factual information that optimally should be taught in an integrated fashion throughout the continuum of medical education. Institutionally agreed-upon definitions of *profession* and *professionalism* serve as the basis of both teaching and evaluation, and they include the nature of professionalism, the role that professions play in society, the attributes of the professional, and an outline of the behaviors expected (Cruess and Cruess 2009). The nature of the professional identity of a physician is derived from these definitions. This information should be widely circulated so that a common language is used throughout the learning environment, including the medical school and its affiliated institutions. This material is a part of the formal curriculum, and is both transmitted and evaluated using pedagogic methods favored by the institution.

Acquiring knowledge about the nature of professionalism is an important first step in becoming a professional, but it is insufficient to ensure that learners become professionals. For this to occur, learners must develop "a professional presence that is best grounded in what one is rather than what one does" (Hafferty 2009, 54). Students and residents must participate in the active and passive processes that allow them to personally modify themselves to become doctors. Numerous educational interventions in the formal curriculum are designed to facilitate this process. However, there is a consensus that the transformation of an individual from a member of the lay public to a medical student, to a resident, and then to a true professional involves a host of influences that together socialize each individual student. Many influences that impact the process of socialization are outside the jurisdiction of the faculties of medicine, but students and residents spend a significant part of their lives in learning environments controlled by the profession. Students voluntarily enter this environment because they wish to join the culture of medicine. They move from peripheral to full participation (Lave and Wenger 1991) in a community of practice (Wenger 1998). The formal, informal, and hidden curricula become ever more powerful influences on the evolution of their professional identities. By examining the interrelated activities in the formal, informal, and hidden curricula, it should be possible to have a greater understanding of their positive and negative impact, and through this understanding to make the educational process support the development of a professional identity more effectively.

Figure 15-1 is an attempt to visually represent the complex process through which individuals navigate the various stages of medical education and training. They enter with preexisting identities acquired throughout their lives. These identities include multiple aspects: gender, race, religious and cultural affiliations, sexual orientation, place in the socioeconomic or-

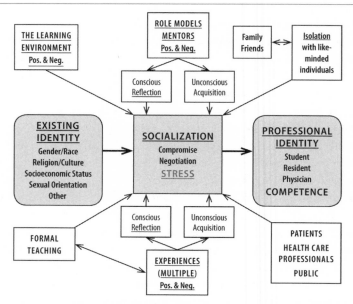

Figure 15.1. A schematic representation of the process of socialization leading to identity formation including the major factors that influence the process.

der, and many other factors unique to each individual. During their educational experience, medical students acquire the identity of medical student (Becker et al. 1961), and during residency this identity is transformed into that of resident. When the individual enters practice, the identity becomes that of medical professional (Helmich et al. 2012). Our understanding of this process has been informed by pioneering early work (Merton, Reader, and Kendall 1957; Becker et al. 1961; Bosk 1979) and refined by recent studies (Hafferty 2009; Monrouxe 2010; Monrouxe, Rees, and Hu 2011; Monrouxe and Rees 2012; Gordon et al. 2012; Veazey, Brooks, and Bosk 2012) including two excellent review articles (Goldie 2012; Jarvis-Salinger, Pratt, and Regehr 2012). The transformation at every stage is not easy. Inevitably, there is conflict between the existing identity and the new one, leading to identity dissonance (Monrouxe 2010). Change requires compromise and negotiation and is accompanied by increased stress levels. Increased competence is a principal objective of medical education and training and, as it develops, it facilitates and supports the confidence that must accompany the emerging identity.

A group of powerful factors help to shape the nature of the identity being formed. They shift among the formal, informal, and hidden curricula depending on institutional policy and circumstance, and many are interrelated. The most powerful factors are role models, experiential learning, and the learning environment. They exert their impact through both conscious and unconscious mechanisms, and are rendered more powerful and effective when they are accompanied by reflection.

Role Models

Role models are "individuals admired for their ways of being and acting as professionals" (Côté and Leclère 2000, 1117) and exert their influence as students engage in "observational learning" (Bandura 1977, 47). The most powerful impact takes place when role models exhibit exemplary behavior and stimulate and facilitate reflection on the behavior (Schon 1987; Epstein 2008; Mann, Gordon, and MacLeod 2009). However, much learning takes place through unconscious patterning of behaviors, both positive and negative, when the reflective process is absent. Unfortunately, instances of unprofessional behavior are common (Wright et al. 1998; Côté and Leclère 2000) and, if tolerated, can fail to "inhibit unprofessional activities in others" (Bandura 1977, 49). Although much of the literature deals with the negative impact of unprofessional or unethical conduct, two things must be noted. First, exemplary behavior is common and, in fact, contributes greatly to the emergence of a proper professional identity. Second, even the most outstanding role models will have instances when their behavior is unprofessional (Cruess, Cruess, and Steinert 2008).

Experiential Learning and Reflection

Professional identity arises from "a long-term combination of experience and reflection on experience" (Hilton and Slotnick 2005, 63). The actual experience of *doing* is an essential component of identity formation, and the provision of opportunities to experience the realities of medical practice becomes fundamental to the curriculum. These must be appropriate to the developmental stage of the learner, and there is a parallel obligation to ensure exposure to all aspects of practice, either in real-life situations or through simulations. Though some of the knowledge acquired through experience remains tacit, "that which one knows but cannot tell," it becomes more powerful and useful if both opportunity and time are provided for reflection on experiences (Schon 1987; Epstein 2008; Mann, Gordon, and MacLeod 2009).

The Learning Environment

Many factors other than role models contribute to the learning environment of educational institutions. If unprofessional behavior in role models, other students or residents, nurses, or support staff is tolerated, learners may consciously or unconsciously determine that this is acceptable, and then incorporate these unprofessional behaviors into their own professional identities (Hafferty and Franks 1994; Gordon et al. 2012). The learning environment is also influenced by those factors that the informal curriculum addresses or fails to recognize. University policies that do not encourage the humane treatment of students and residents, that fail to reward teaching and exemplary clinical care or to discourage harassment or humiliation of learners, and that do not promote respectful interaction between members of the healthcare team will not sustain proper identity formation. If the formal curriculum specifically addresses these issues, it will encourage the development of a professional identity. Unfortunately, learners are frequently exposed to unprofessional conduct, leaving them with the impression that they are supposed to do as their teachers say but not as they do (Brainard and Brislen 2007).

Formal Teaching

Formal teaching can impact professional identity formation by making explicit the objectives of medical education, including the development of a professional identity; by imparting the cognitive base of professionalism; by contributing to the experiences of learners; and by providing structured time for reflection on experience (Cohen 2006; Cruess and Cruess 2009). The inclusion and assessment of material on professionalism and professional identity in the formal curriculum sends a message that it is important (Monrouxe, Rees, and Hu 2011).

Isolation with Like-Minded Individuals

A constant in medical education through the ages has been the use of isolation with fellow students and residents to foster identity formation (Merton, Reader, and Kendall 1957; Becker et al. 1961; Bosk 1979). By living within the culture of medicine with as little distraction as possible, students and residents learn the language of medicine, are exposed to its rituals, come to understand its written and unwritten rules, and are exposed to its hierarchy and their place in it. Working with their peers, they have an opportunity to repeatedly play the role of physician until that role becomes who they are. The process of enculturation that entails absorption of ideals and values, and at least partial assimilation into the ethos of the profession, requires active involvement (Gordon et al. 2012).

Family, friends, home environments, and other outside interests and influences both provide a background to enculturation and impact the process. They can be supportive of the commitment required to become a professional, or they can inhibit the process. These factors in the environment external to the culture of medicine have become extremely important because recent generations of students, residents, and medical practitioners are in the process of readjusting the balance between commitment, personal health, well-being, and lifestyle, in part by redefining altruism (Twenge 2009). This is not a new issue. Merton in 1957 outlined the characteristics of a professional identity. He stated that a professional "should see to it that medical care is available for his patients whenever it is required." He immediately qualified the statement, indicating that "he, too, has a right to a normal life which he shares with his family." (Merton, Reader, and Kendall 1957, 75). The difference, of course, is where to draw the line. A recent issue in medical education and training relates to restrictions on duty hours. Although personal health and welfare is a major issue that must be addressed, the impact on professional identity of what is regarded as a diminished sense of commitment has caused concern (Veazey, Brooks, and Bosk 2012; Ginsberg 2012).

Actions to Take

Given the interrelated nature of the formal, informal, and hidden curricula, it seems logical to address those parts of all three that are amenable to interventions. The following suggestions are aimed at shifting the emphasis from teaching professionalism to facilitating professional identity formation.

1. Make professional identity formation an explicit curricular objective. This involves making all learners aware of the nature of professional identity and how this identity is developed and acquired.
2. Implicit in step 1 is the transfer of a group of activities that heretofore have been in the informal to the formal curriculum. This should make it less likely "that student understandings of professionalism will be negatively influenced by the hidden curriculum" (Monrouxe, Rees, and Hu 2011, 600). Specific issues that should be addressed include ensuring that all aspects of professionalism and professional identity are explicitly addressed in formal teaching, and that real-life or simulated experiences reflecting these aspects are present in the curriculum.
3. Time for reflection on experiences must be built into both the undergraduate and postgraduate curriculum so that learners consciously incorporate the culture of medicine into their ways of doing, being, and feeling. Reflection on even negative aspects of the hidden curriculum can often have a positive impact.
4. Ensure that the influence of role models is largely positive by evaluating their performance regularly using valid tools. Research has shown that it is feasible for students (Todhunter et al. 2011) and residents (Arah et al. 2011) to participate in this process in order to provide evidence-based feedback. Outstanding performance should be rewarded, those requiring help remediated, and those who have shown themselves consistently incapable of modeling good clinical care and a professional identity removed from teaching. Faculty development is a powerful aid in ensuring that faculty members understand professionalism and professional identity (Steinert et al. 2007).
5. Specifically address isolation and stress, important components of the informal curriculum. Some degree of isolation is necessary, and stress is unavoidable as identity dissonance arises from conflicts between the old and the new. All medical schools attempt to provide support for

students and residents. We suggest that this support be framed in the context of identity formation so that everyone understands its nature. Measures based on this understanding should be more effective.

Medicine is a collegial profession, and an important part of professional identity is a sense of belonging. Specific measures, including formal and informal, large and small social events of a welcoming nature, should be held throughout the continuum of medical education. The informal curriculum should contain joyful events.

6. The learning environment should be addressed specifically. Those aspects, almost all of which are within the informal curriculum, that have a negative impact should be addressed. Quaintance, Arnold, and Thompson (2008) have shown that it is feasible to assess the environment, and it has been demonstrated that the environment can be changed (Suchman et al. 2004). The informal curriculum must support the teaching of professionalism and the development of a professional identity.

Conclusion

In an ideal learning environment, the informal and hidden curricula would consistently reinforce a comprehensive formal curriculum that is designed to facilitate the development of the professional identity of physicians. Though this ideal is almost certainly never achieved, it should be the goal to which all medical educators aspire.

16: Indigenous Health and the Hidden Curriculum

A View from the Outside In

SHAUN C. EWEN

This chapter will argue that evidence of unequal treatment (see definition that follows) can be understood and more fundamentally addressed using Foucault's concepts of the *apparatus* and *biopower*. In addition, application of Hafferty's taxonomy of medical curricula foregrounds the medical establishment's focus on the formal curricula to address unequal treatment, thereby exposing the establishment's failure to fundamentally challenge the apparatus of medical schools (in large part, the hidden curriculum) to change or reform. It is the apparatus that controls, enhances, and maintains the exercise of power in medical schools.

This chapter also suggests that historically, medical educators (often also as health professionals) have had significant influence (and self-interest) in perpetuating and sustaining the biopower status quo: that is, the management of the births, deaths, reproduction, and illnesses of a population. This is achieved via the selection and training of future healthcare workers, which, using unequal treatment as evidence, demonstrates how medicine "looks after its own" from a racial and ethnic perspective.

Unequal Treatment and Cultural Competence

Not everyone who seeks healthcare receives the same level of services as others with the same condition or presentation. Indeed, it is now widely accepted that

> Racial and ethnic minorities tend to receive a lower quality of healthcare than non-minorities, even when access-related factors, such as a patients' insurance status and income, are controlled.
>
> The sources of these disparities are complex, are rooted in historical and contemporary inequities, and involve many participants at several

levels, including health systems, their administrative and bureaucratic processes, utilization managers, *healthcare professionals*, and patients. (Smedley, Stith, and Nelson 2002, 1; emphasis added)

Unequal treatment, in the realm of medical education, has been interpreted as a range of cross-cultural and communication issues having their influence within the doctor-patient relationship. Culture, predominantly, has been identified as the culprit: the slippery, difficult-to-name construct that sits at odds with the easily named, defined, scientifically organized and created biomedical world, which, post-Flexner, has been the hallmark of most medical schools, at least in the English-speaking world.

The primary impetus for the cultural competence movement of the last decade has been the demonstration of and publicity surrounding widespread racial and ethnic disparities in healthcare. (Saha, Beach, and Cooper 2008, 1278)

The seemingly unstoppable rise of cultural competence initiatives (and associated accreditation standards [Liaison Committee on Medical Education 2012]) has been hailed as the antidote to such unequal treatment. Cultural competence has "become a byword endowed with almost religious significance, a panacea for the multiple and interwoven problems in health care communication" (Perloff et al. 2006, 835).

Yet, with limited evidence (and perhaps reflecting limited research interest) linking the application of culture within the therapeutic relationship to improved healthcare outcomes for "cultural" groups, the hidden curriculum has become a new target for the old problem. It is this author's experience that the hidden curriculum often is described as at odds with the formal and informal curricula, and, as if grasping at beads of mercury, we wring our hands in despair, claiming that the hidden curriculum now must be to blame for ongoing issues such as unequal treatment and the related underrepresentation of minority groups in medicine.

However, this chapter proposes that recognition of the hidden curriculum, *and acting to reform it*, can change the apparatus (medical school), change the way medical schools create their products (graduates and future health workforce), and ultimately apply Foucault's notion of biopower to address unequal treatment from a whole-of-school approach.

Foucault's Concepts of Apparatus and Biopower

The concepts of apparatus and biopower (at their most general) provide a lens through which to analyze how and why the hidden curriculum may be identified and possibly changed. Foucault (1980) described the apparatus as the "thoroughly heterogeneous ensemble consisting of discourses, institutions, architectural forms, regulatory decisions, laws, administrative measures, scientific statements, philosophical, moral and philanthropic propositions—in short, the said as much as the unsaid" (194).

Foucault's description of the apparatus has strong conceptual parallels with the hidden curriculum and its influence; the unsaid, as much as the said. Foucault described the importance of identifying the relationship between these two elements, because differing relationships between them result in differing discourses and outcomes, along with differing types and impacts of biopower. In relation to biopower and its influence, "The apparatus thus has a dominant strategic function" (1980, 195) and in a medical school context, the hidden curricula of the school *are* the apparatus, producing a particular kind of biopower. The school admits and produces its own subjects (students and, subsequently, doctors) in a process of governance and subjectification. This is not, of itself, a negative thing. Changes to the apparatus will lead to changes in the subjects, and, in this way, health professional factors that may lead to unequal treatment may be more fundamentally addressed than if just the formal curriculum were seen as the sole conduit to change.

In relation to unequal treatment, as mentioned earlier, there has been much focus on the formal curricula (through cultural competence curricula initiatives), with much less focus on the hidden curricula (the apparatus). This leaves the hidden curricula to influence, unabated and unchallenged, and thus the apparatus to continue to influence and produce and reproduce its own subjects, substantially in the mold of those it produced before.

The concept of biopower proposes that medical schools and their graduates are active agents of society and, in their privileged position, they (in part) regulate the births, deaths, and health of the population. However, if we understand biopower as an outcome of the apparatus, it follows that if you change the apparatus, you change the type and influence of the biopower that is produced. Thus, biopower itself is not independent of the apparatus. What biopower affects, and how it is enabled, is a product of the apparatus.

Biopower can be directed to address unequal treatment if the apparatus and related hidden curriculum are attuned to this need.

Health professional factors, which contribute to unequal treatment of patients, do not stem from a lack of expertise in biomedical knowledge. Rather, these factors are related to the personal (mostly unrecognized) biases or prejudices of health professionals. These prejudices stem from the broader societies from which the health professionals are socialized and enculturated, as well as, to a lesser extent, from the socialization that takes place within medical schools themselves. As Perloff describes, "As individualized and emotional as doctor-patient communication can be, it always takes place in a larger society, in which institutional norms, economic realities, and sociopolitical forces impinge powerfully and subtly on physicians and patients" (Perloff et al. 2006, 836).

I argue that we, as medical educators, have focused our remedial efforts on unequal treatment significantly at the level of the formal curriculum, with considerably less focus on the informal or hidden curriculum. This has occurred for at least two reasons. One is a slowly increasing awareness of the role, influence, and existence of the hidden curriculum. The hidden curriculum generally is attributed as being first described by Jackson (1966), then applied in the medical education context by Hafferty and Franks (1994), with an increase in the peer-reviewed medical education and hidden curriculum literature not taking place until the early twenty-first century. A second reason is that the role of medical educators primarily has been constructed around developing and delivering a formal curriculum, not necessarily around reflecting on and changing, if needed, elements of the hidden curriculum, which might be described as institutional. Using Foucault's concepts, the apparatus is largely in place. It chiefly supports the system of relationships that reproduce its own system as it continues to produce a particular form of biopower.

If we change the apparatus, then the new subjects will be in the vision of the new apparatus, not the old, with a concomitant and related form of biopower.

From a critical perspective, the challenge, therefore, is first to identify and describe, and then to challenge and change, if necessary, the hidden curriculum so that the apparatus itself is formally fundamentally addressed and, as a consequence, the type of biopower and its influence is redirected.

Indigenous Health: A Case Study

In many of my discussions with faculty and students in relation to Indigenous health and, by extension, health of underrepresented minority populations, the hidden curriculum most often has been described and understood as a subversive and unchangeable influence on student learning. However, the hidden curriculum is not wrong, not naughty, not lying in wait to undermine our best-laid formal curriculum plan. Just like the formal curriculum, which goes through its quality cyclic reviews and changes, the hidden curriculum should also be subject to review and, if necessary, change. Just because the curriculum is hidden does not mean it is not changeable or addressable. We need to describe it and understand how it is created so we can change it if needed and, perhaps ideally, let it become hidden again so that its influence remains strong. The hidden curriculum thereby becomes the foundation of Foucault's apparatus.

The next section of this chapter describes, from an Indigenous perspective, two elements of the hidden curriculum we can identify and change to fundamentally address the apparatus, so that it seeks to address the health professional factors that relate to unequal treatment.

Student Admissions Policy

Policies that govern student admissions are an integral component of the hidden curriculum. The apparatus, while "consisting of discourses, institutions, architectural forms, regulatory decisions, laws, administrative measures, scientific statements, philosophical, moral and philanthropic propositions" (Foucault 1980, 194) is also, first and foremost, made up of people. One way to modify the apparatus is to change the demographics of people who contribute to the structuring and functioning of the apparatus.

Admission policy needs to be considered on two levels. The first is from a diversity perspective, and with a particular focus on underrepresented minorities. The reasons for this focus generally have been well articulated in the literature but include rights-based arguments, as well as the increased perspectives and experiences that a diverse cohort brings (Cohen et al. 2002; Curtis et al. 2012). Underrepresented minorities and people from underserved communities may also bring a particular commitment and passion to their community and an opportunity to practice parrhesia, or speak freely, to interrupt or influence the apparatus (Ewen 2011).

In Australia, Indigenous Australians constitute 2.5 percent of the overall population, but only 0.2 percent of the health workforce (Australian Institute of Health and Welfare 2011). It was not until 1984 that the first Indigenous medical student graduated in Australia. This can be compared to the United States, Canada, and New Zealand, which had graduated their first Indigenous doctors nearly a century earlier (Anderson 2008). These data may reflect the broader society in which these events occurred, but it is noteworthy that the Indigenous Australian burden of disease is higher than in those settler colonial nations, and life expectancy is significantly lower. Most Australian medical schools now have alternative entry programs to support Indigenous Australian applicants' entry into medical schools. This is an important element of the hidden curriculum, signaling that Indigenous medical students are being encouraged and supported to enter medical school. In 2012, for the first time, Indigenous admissions have now reached population parity, at 2.5 percent (Australian Indigenous Doctors Association 2012). Although Indigenous Australian student recruitment into medical schools has improved, more support and effort is needed to ensure that Indigenous students complete medical school (Garvey et al. 2009; Curtis et al. 2012) so that the graduation rate matches the recruitment rate.

> [I]ndigenous students face significant barriers to participation and success in health education and understanding how to best achieve indigenous health workforce development remains a challenge. (Curtis et al. 2012, 2)

Being only recent participants in the medical education "project," medical schools are not necessarily attuned to or prepared to support the needs of Indigenous students. There also are issues of a delayed pipeline, affecting whether today's Indigenous Australian students are able to be tomorrow's Indigenous faculty, represented at population parity.

In addition to admissions, significantly different student demographics may change or reshape how curricula are developed or delivered, influencing not only student learning but also faculty development through reflection of teaching and learning content, all of which impact the apparatus. For example, in Australia, many curricular representations of Indigenous people constructed them as either the exotic other or the "Indigenous case," and cast them as carrying the burden of disease. Rarely is the Indigenous-related case included simply as part of the *normal* spectrum of diversity in the population. Many Indigenous students I have taught find the burden-of-disease approach reflected in Indigenous cases to be quite stereotypical. It is a worthy question to ask: Would the stereotype (which is reflective of burden of disease) be accepted as the primary Indigenous representation to a cohort of students, all of whom were Indigenous? Would the Southeast Asian case always be linked with tuberculosis if the student cohort were primarily Southeast Asian (Kai et al. 2008)? By taking this well-used approach to developing cases, medical educators are linking a particular ethnic culture with burden of disease. With this linkage also comes the likelihood that students learn to relate stigma and application of a burden-of-disease approach to some cultures. In what is always described as a crowded curriculum, repeating burden-of-disease lecture material as cases in case-based learning examples is not the most effective or creative use of curriculum time. It also reifies the more latent and stereotypical messages of what it means to be an Indigenous person, constructed around disease and deficit rather than wellness and achievement.

The second level to consider regarding student admissions is the skills and knowledge that are required to gain entry into medical programs. Most admissions criteria focus primarily on an applicant's ability to have mastered the foundations of biomedicine: chemistry, physics, and biology. Sociology, the humanities, and related fields rarely are seen as the required foundational knowledge on which students are admitted to the profession. The knowledge and skills that relate to the unequal part of unequal treatment require approaches and understandings from the fields of sociology, philosophy, ethics, humanities, and history, including the history of health and medicine. The very clear hidden curriculum influence on student learning is that these areas of knowledge as viewed by applicants, faculty, admissions committees, and accreditation bodies are not as important or necessary as chemistry, physics, or biology; and this contributes to setting the scene for a continuation of the biomedical hegemony, rampant post-Flexner.

The development over the past decade of an approach to admissions that includes multiple mini interviews (MMIs) for assessing personal qualities of candidates is recognition that the medical profession may demand more than just intellect bent toward biomedicine. MMIs emerged from medical educators' desire to be able to select for personal values and attributes (Eva et al. 2004). However, values on their own—without the conceptual tools for understanding how they developed, and without understanding the social, personal, and cultural processes required to change them—are not that useful in influencing the apparatus in a targeted way. Since the time of Hippocrates, personal and professional values have been a stated part of the vision and commitment for the medical profession. It also may be that by selecting for values, without selecting for knowledge and experience in fields outside of biomedicine, we are in danger of further perpetuating what Esmail (2004) identified in the writing of Vikram Seth when describing issues of institutional racism in the British National Health Service: "If it is only bad people who are prejudiced, that would not have such a strong effect. Most people would not wish to imitate them—and so, such prejudices would not have much effect—except in exceptional times. It is the prejudices of good people that are so dangerous" (1448).

By changing the constituent parts of the medical student body, students and faculty (both demographically and in terms of required basic skills), and beginning with student recruitment, we can see from the examples given here that we may also change the type of biopower that the apparatus produces, such that it becomes aligned with the needs of the communities, which will be increasingly reflected in the student cohort.

Slang

Slang is an important element of the hidden curriculum and is used in ways that often construct learning about "culture" as something different and separate from learning about other elements of the curriculum. "Immersion" is an ideal example of institutional slang. Often, immersion is the name given to a learning experience, frequently off-site, related to learning about the culture or cultures of another population group (Kamaka 2001; Dowell et al. 2001). Using the language of immersion, limited largely to things such as "cultural immersion," obfuscates the reality that most medical training occurs in an immersed clinical setting. Medical educators, using the language of immersion primarily for cultural contexts, construct learning on the wards as being "immersion free," and as such, the professional culture of medicine as fundamentally "normal" (and thus not worthy of critical scrutiny). The corollary of this is that other cultures, other ways of being and doing, are required to be *immersed into,* so as to understand them. The potential unintended consequences of this particular use of slang is that the apparatus, through its interactions, sends messages to students about being "culturally immersed" in an othered experience, ignoring the greater socialization taking place—the immersion into the professional culture of medicine.

When the slang is identified and revealed, it no longer remains hidden, forcing an alternative to be considered. Programs that take students away from the clinical learning environment to another environment, which also is outside of the formal classroom, should be described more accurately within the context of the student learning experience. One approach to learning about Indigenous health and history in Australia is called *On country learning*. It is a phrase used in an Australian context, which refers to the notion of Indigenous sovereignty, of self-determination through "country" and connection to land, and *becomes* the learning environment (rather than describing the learning environment for Indigenous health as "immersion"). Though it is still slang, by more accurately describing the learning approach, I argue that it is good slang, aligning the objectives of the formal curricula with the hidden.

Slang becomes a manifestation of the biopower of the apparatus. The slang is used to reinforce, in this case, the othering of a group. Consider a final example. Since the feminization of medicine, would it be acceptable to describe undertaking the clinical rotation pertinent to women's health as the "women's health immersion," with women being constructed as the exotic other?

Other Cultural Perspectives Related to the Hidden Curriculum

A final and overarching question to consider in this chapter is whether the hidden curriculum is equally hidden to all people. Moreover, are there particular elements of the hidden curriculum that might be more hidden to some than to others? Do some eyes (underrepresented minority) more easily see and experience specific aspects of the hidden curriculum that adversely impact them and their communities?

Given the earlier discussion about the apparatus and its strategic intent to support and protect its own interests, the importance of outsiders should receive significant consideration.

The naive imagination from without deserves a prominent and invited seat at the table. As with all human endeavors, medical education needs the widest possible set of discussants if indeed change is the goal, for self-referentiality, no matter its capacity to fill journal pages and conference lecterns, may very well constitute involution rather than change (Anderson 2011, 34).

If the hidden curriculum is seen and experienced through different lenses by different people, this then becomes another argument for ensuring increased diversity (of student and faculty, ethnicity, gender, sexuality, and age) within the apparatus. Although diversity in gender has been, in the main, addressed in medical student recruitment and admissions in the English-speaking world, diversity in ethnicity and community representation remains a work in progress. Diversity in socioeconomic status also has gained some attention in this context. It remains a truism, however, that to pursue a diversity agenda requires a "mainstream" or a norm from which to measure, or even identify, diversity.

Conclusion

This chapter has focused on two areas of the hidden curriculum that contribute to maintaining the status quo of the apparatus and its relationship to unequal treatment—student admissions policies and slang. These two domains of influence can shape health professional factors that contribute to disparity in health outcomes for patients.

The conceptual tools of the apparatus and biopower challenge us to arrive at certain conclusions related to unequal treatment. I do not know of a single medical school that values oppression, subjugation, or colonization, or has racism as a graduate outcome, or teaches prejudice as a clinical skill. I know of no medical school that wants to graduate clinicians who contribute to ongoing unequal treatment.

Nonetheless, while we say that we value providing the best possible care to all, regardless of diversity, there continues to be strong evidence that suggests our actions as clinicians contribute to unequal treatment, even if unintentionally.

If we are able to uncover elements of the hidden curriculum that are inconsistent with addressing disparities in healthcare, then those elements are no longer hidden. If they are not then addressed, then they lie in the realm of exposed racism and prejudice, both personal and institutional, and should be dealt with as such. Inaction, therefore, no longer can be attributed to the unintentional prejudice of good people. At best, inaction can be attributed to the laziness of the status quo. At worst, it is direct evidence of the very racism and prejudice that those same powers so vehemently disavow.

If we are able to align our hidden curricula with our formal and informal curricula, then the learning experience for students becomes a coherent whole. Given the structure of medical schools and the apprenticeship model of learning, the most difficult sector to control or influence becomes the informal curriculum. However, in a pincer movement, the informal curriculum becomes less able to be an outlier from a congruent formal and hidden curriculum.

Unchanged and unchallenged, the hidden curriculum simply maintains the core of the apparatus, thus condemning medical schools to continue exercising their biopower unchanged and continue contributing to unequal treatment.

Without coherent formal, informal, and hidden curricula, we are in danger of repeating Bloom's observation of a "history of reform without change" (1988, 295), with harmful implications for Indigenous and minority populations.

17: Longitudinal Integrated Clerkships

Embracing the Hidden Curriculum, Stemming Ethical Erosion,
and Transforming Medical Education

DAVID HIRSH

I am reminded of Paul Simon's, "The Sound of Silence" (Simon 1964). In education, the hidden curriculum resides in our words and in our silence. It calls out from our actions and our inaction. The hidden curriculum is mural and intramural. It is, in short, the teachings and the prophecies we learn from our educational context. We have the potential, and I believe the mandate, to shape our educational structures to harness the hidden curriculum to meet our learners' and our society's needs (Frenk et al. 2010). This chapter describes transformative educational models called longitudinal integrated clerkships (LICs), which education designers created intentionally to address the hidden curriculum in medical education. Specifically, LICs may stem the negative hidden curricular effect known as *ethical erosion* (Feudtner, Christakis, and Christakis 1994).

Ethical Erosion

In 1994, when the early work on the hidden curriculum in medical education was emerging, Feudtner and colleagues surveyed students at six Pennsylvania medical schools (Feudtner, Christakis, and Christakis 1994). The authors characterized the negative formative experiences students derived from their participation on house officer–led teams in inpatient venues. These influential forces, the authors concluded, contributed to what they termed students' *ethical erosion*. At the same time, several other works expressed similar concerns (Feudtner and Christakis 1994; Hafferty and Franks 1994; Hafferty 1998; Hundert, Hafferty, and Christakis 1996). In 2001 Coulehan and Williams put a name to these experiences ("vanquishing virtue") as they deftly humanized this discourse of medical education and its impact. They told the story of "Andrea"—the service-minded, mature, thoughtful, and able student who was transformed and, some might argue, quite harmed by her experience in medical school. Such narratives offer one way to understand ethical erosion.

To help seat this chapter's consideration of ethical erosion and its call for educational transformation, I offer a narrative account of the experience of a student called "Daniel." Following the narrative is a review of the domains of ethical erosion reported in the literature that characterize the scope of this phenomenon.

Narrative Characterization of Ethical Erosion

Daniel showed up ready for his clerkship rotation. He had been told he was lucky, and he felt that way. After all, he was well prepared, well studied, loved medical school, and to top it off, he had the famed surgeon assigned as his attending—the surgeon that all his classmates sought out. "They are right—he is amazing," Daniel recounted after his first day in the OR. Sadly, his contact with this potential mentor would be fleeting and rare. Daniel soon learned that his primary work would not be alongside this masterful and engaging attending, but with the residents on that service and the team. "Odd to pay tuition and not have the professor," classmates would say.

After several weeks, the students on the resident team started competing to get their chance to be in the OR—to see "the good cases." Daniel mused, "Why am I saying 'case' all the time?" He sensed that he was getting used to the rhetoric of the resident culture. Beyond the reifying nature of the language, the actions of the team left even stronger feelings.

During rounds one morning, the surgery team's chief resident was called by the emergency department. The chief resident hurriedly told the students, "Apparently there's some huge guy in the ED with a peri-rectal abscess." The day was not especially busy, but the resident noted, "I hate being taken away from work" to see this patient.

Daniel and his fellow student followed the two interns and the chief resident as they jogged off to the ED. The team arrived to find a morbidly obese man lying facedown. Visible from the hallway, the man was alone in the room. The man spoke one word: "Help." The man had a single white sheet over the back of his bare body. Daniel thought to himself that he had not seen a peri-rectal abscess before.

"Student," said the chief resident, addressing Daniel with a blunt gaze, "what do we do for these abscesses?" The resident pulled the sheet back completely as he asked this question, and then duly introduced himself to the patient. Daniel did not know the answer. He also was preoccupied by the man's nakedness. The other student was about to offer a guess when the resident answered for them all, "We lance 'em. Y' know, open 'em. All pus has gotta get out."

The patient—a rural man who had not had regular contact with the healthcare system for years—weighed 386 pounds. The sheet that had covered him, now wet with sweat, had been taken away. The man was unkempt. Straining, and without looking back, the man with his chin on the gurney asked, "What's that mean—'open'?"

"No worry buddy, we'll cure it. We'll let the pus out," was the informed response.

The chief resident pointed to Daniel and the other student. "You hold that cheek and you hold that one," indicating that each medical student should hold one buttock.

Scalpel up, scalpel down. Pop.

A brownish-pink and yellow creamy jet arched out from the abscess . . . onto Daniel's neck, face, and glasses.

The two interns seemed to find this hilarious. They scurried into the hall and bent over laughing—belly laughing—loudly enough to be heard in the patient's room. The chief resident gave one wry (possibly pleased) look at Daniel—wet, stained, and motionless—and smiled. Before bursting into laughter himself, the chief resident quickly walked out to join the interns. The laughter of the three in the hall was audible in the room. "Did you see that student—didn't even move . . ."

"Thanks, doc," the patient said to the two students who remained.

Daniel stood, thinking, "Do I keep holding onto the patient's bottom? Can I let go to wipe my face? Shouldn't we dress the wound?"

This narrative is a true story. The name has been changed, and the events occurred at another institution—not the place where I now work—but the educational concepts the narrative elicits are applicable anywhere. In this chapter exploring ethical erosion and the imperative to transform clinical education structures, the narrative invites several questions: What does Daniel learn? What will he remember? What will the bystanders (the other student and the interns) learn and remember? What power did Daniel have to shape the circumstance before, during, or after the event? What does powerlessness teach, and what does power teach? To what qualitatively different circumstances will these "lessons" be generalized? In what contexts, through what relationships, and by what mechanisms do learners develop an "ethic of care" (Noddings 1984)? And as relates to the professional role, what is the informative power of such experiences compared to coursework, reading, or small-group discussions?

Hidden curricular quanta affect our learners. The literature suggests different ways of measuring ethical erosion. Scholars have used validated tools to shed further light on the forces that play upon every Daniel and every Andrea.

Ethical Erosion and Its Domains

When Hafferty (1998) distinguishes the hidden curriculum from the formal curriculum, he suggests that these forces work at the level of culture. This culture involves the context, what is present and what is missing, and the people who act (or fail to act) in the context. Thus, the hidden curriculum relates to environment as place and environment as a social construct. In this way, the hidden curriculum can be variably influential and can have an impact on learners with positive (affirming or supportive), neutral, or negative (demeaning or undermining) messages. Those effects that negatively impact the professional or human development of the learner constitute ethical erosion.

At the most basic level, the literature on ethical erosion speaks to the students' exposure: students experience, witness, participate in, or simply feel they participated in (or failed to stop) unprofessional or demeaning events during clinical training (Feudtner, Christakis, and Christakis 1994). The structure of the training is implicated (Christakis and Feudtner 1997; Coulehan and Williams 2001). No fewer than three domains characterize ethical erosion stemming from medical training:

1. Students' patient-centeredness: using a validated survey instrument, students show a decline in patient-centered attitudes as a consequence of their medical training especially in the principal clinical year (Haidet et al. 2002).

2. Students' moral development: using a validated survey instrument, students show a diminution of moral development in medical school (Patenaude, Niyonsenga, and Fafard 2003; Bebeau 2002).

3. Students' empathy: using different validated survey instruments, stu-

dents show a decline in empathy during their third-year training (Newton et al. 2008; Hojat et al. 2009).

Even this partial accounting demonstrates the range of validated instruments and studies that characterize ethical erosion (Self and Baldwin 1994; Stern 2006). Fortunately, the structure and venues of clinical education are within our control.

Longitudinal Integrated Clerkships and an Approach to Ethical Erosion

LICs are clinical education structures deployed in the principal clinical year of medical school (typically the third year in four-year schools). In an LIC, learners participate in a single fully integrated clinical experience instead of taking part in the traditional block clerkships (BCs). The international consensus definition states, "An LIC is characterized by being the central element of clinical education whereby medical students: (1) participate in the comprehensive care of patients over time, (2) participate in continuing learning relationships with these patients' clinicians, and (3) meet the majority of the year's core clinical competencies, across multiple disciplines simultaneously through these experiences" (International Consortium on Longitudinal Integrated Clerkships 2007). LICs are well established, are growing rapidly nationally and internationally, and research affirms their educational benefits (Strasser and Hirsh 2011; Hirsh, Gaufberg et al. 2012; Walters et al. 2012; Teherani, Irby, and Loeser 2013).

Notwithstanding its amplitude or valence, the hidden curriculum also can be understood as a force that either is or is not aligned with the formal curriculum. Education planners deliberately designed LICs to realign curricular structure and function in the hope that this would affect the "product" of medical education and at least modulate or ameliorate the effects of the traditional hidden curriculum (Hirsh, Walters et al. 2012). The early LICs needed to address physician workforce (Verby et al. 1991). More recently, educational leaders created LICs to stem ethical erosion (Ogur et al. 2007; Hirsh, Gaufberg et al. 2012; Hirsh, Walters et al. 2012). To transform the structure of clinical training, program developers create LICs to align with the sciences of learning in the domains most likely to foster the outcomes they seek.

Educational Underpinnings

Educational continuity, a concept derived from the learning sciences, was the organizing principle for LICs to stem ethical erosion (Hirsh et al. 2007). This notion of continuity can be divided into three subcontinuities: continuity of the care of the patient, continuity of supervision by experienced and well-chosen faculty, and continuity of the curriculum into a developmentally progressive whole that is more individual-centered (Hirsh et al. 2007). The hope was that through this deeply *relational* construct, students' learning, professional development, and idealism would be fostered. In this context, relational means the explicit creation of curricular structures to support effective and meaningful human connections: student-patient, student-faculty, and student-student work (Charon 2001). Consistent with social learning theory and the principles of workforce learning (Bandura 1977; Lave and Wenger 1991), this model creates meaningful and progressive role development through doing the actual work of physicians in practice and by students' sense of duty and commitment to people (patients, faculty, peers, and self), impelling the learning (Charon 2001). In this way, the meaning derived by the continuity of relationships essentially supports a fourth subcontinuity—the continuity of idealism (the opposite of which is ethical erosion).

Data

LICs have well-documented benefits for students' learning and professional development, and it would seem reasonable to assume the model's alignment with the learning sciences may be part of the reason (Ogur et al. 2007; Ogur and Hirsh 2009; Hirsh, Gaufberg et al. 2012; Walters et al. 2012; Teherani, Irby, and Loeser 2013). It is likely that specifically addressing the gap between the explicit curriculum and the hidden curriculum, and actively working to prevent ethical erosion, may also offer real benefits.

The data that elucidate the impact of LIC design on ethical erosion are inchoate, but they seem to suggest a hopeful effect. In the one-year pilot study of Harvard Medical School's Cambridge Integrated Clerkship and in the three-year follow-up study, the traditional BC students experienced an erosion of their patient-centeredness while the LIC students showed actual improvement, and the difference was statistically significant (Ogur et al. 2007; Hirsh, Gaufberg et al. 2012). The positive effect on patient-centeredness in the LIC group stood in stark contrast to the ethical erosion literature. Naturally, these data beget the question of whether these differences continue in and beyond residency. This issue of the retention of patient-centeredness is currently being studied, and the preliminary results look promising (Gaufberg et al. 2012).

Another validated tool, the C3 instrument, measures students' expressed sense of exposure to the hidden curriculum on three subscales (Haidet, Kelley, and Chou 2005). Hirsh, Gaufberg, and colleagues (2012) demonstrated in their three-year comparison trial that the students in the LIC reported significantly less exposure to the hidden curriculum than did their classmates in the BCs: the subscales "support for students' patient-centered beliefs," "personal experiences consistent with patient-centered actions," and the subscale about the behavior of house staff and attending all suggest that the LIC students' enhanced patient-centeredness may have its origin in the educational environment. It should not be surprising that compared to BC students, LIC students express greater satisfaction in their program and in their learning environment (Hirsh, Gaufberg et al. 2012).

Are there other ways to discern if students' experiences prevent ethical erosion? Perhaps sustaining a sense of advocacy is a measure of resilience against ethical erosion? A qualitative analysis found that in the longitudinal integrated structures of LICs, "[s]tudents reported that their connections with patients over time inspired a sense of idealism and advocacy" (Ogur and Hirsh 2009, 844). Currently, three LIC cohorts and a traditional comparison BC group are being studied four to six years after finishing their programs. Among other differences, the domain of advocacy is noted to be significantly higher among LIC graduates (Gaufberg et al. 2012).

Comparisons of LICs and BCs using validated measures of moral development and empathy have not yet been reported in the literature. Early unpublished data suggests a significant increase in empathy during the LIC, an effect not seen among BC students (Simanton 2012). This remains an area of future research.

Discussion

There appear to be sound arguments to redesign the structure of medical education to stem ethical erosion and better embrace the positive aspects of the hidden curriculum. One approach is to consider the experiences of our learners that we hear, know, and read in the literature (in narrative and survey form). The ethical erosion literature urges transformation from the house officer–led traditional inpatient block rotations. Complementary and overlapping is the literature analyzing the models that have changed clinical education and have benefited students thereby. Although data are nascent, they suggest that LICs are an effective model to address ethical erosion. Some would argue that if LICs merely were equal at fostering learning, but better for embracing the hidden curriculum, this would be enough. Nonetheless, as might be predicted by their aligning the hidden and formal curricula, LICs have shown greater benefits—providing better experiences, advancing learning, improving student satisfaction, and promoting the humanism that students brought to medical school at the outset (Teherani, Irby, and Loeser 2013; Hirsh, Gaufberg et al. 2012; Walters et al. 2012; Hirsh, Walters et al. 2012; Hauer, Hirsh et al. 2012; Hauer, O'Brien et al. 2012; O'Brien et al. 2012; Ogur and Hirsh 2009; Ogur et al. 2007).

Scholars have articulated the value of medical training grounded in educational continuity and relationship-based learning (Holmboe, Ginsburg, and Bernabeo 2011; Bernabeo et al. 2011; Hirsh et al. 2007; Charon 2001; Christakis and Feudtner 1997). But what specific features of LICs lead to these successes? The key is to connect educational redesign to the hidden curriculum—that is, to align structure, context, and desired outcomes.

LICs do not rely on temporary, brief relationships with people, venues, or curricular themes. LICs transform three major structural elements of the educational design, and in doing so, LIC planners are deliberately engaging the potential of the hidden curriculum:

1. LICs enhance the meaningful role of students in the care of patients—patients who see the students as "their personal student," a valued supporter, and important to the care and care team.
2. LICs enhance students' meaningful connection to faculty and other role models (medical and interprofessional) with whom the students care for

patients. Therein the mentoring that proceeds over substantial time is founded on observed practice and a collaborative relationship.

3. LICs foster student-student collaboration rather than competition. Collaboration centralizes the care of patients and learning above other factors such as individual prominence or studying for "the test."

In these ways, the students' needs, the patients' needs, and the system's needs are mutually supported (Hirsh, Walters et al. 2012; Berwick and Finkelstein 2010; Ogur and Hirsh 2009; Worley et al. 2006; Prideaux, Worley, and Bligh 2007). Put another way, when LICs align the hidden curriculum with the formal curriculum to advance learning and stem ethical erosion, they may be succeeding because with the LIC structure, each student's "soul meets role" (Palmer 2004).

To be sure, the exact mechanisms that account for LICs' successes are still to be determined. Going forward, as researchers use validated tools to analyze resilience, well-being, depression, burnout, relational attachment, or humanism, we may uncover other LIC strengths. Nonetheless, future work should attend as well to the critical questions of why and how LICs deliver their formative benefits.

Conclusion

In this chapter, the negative potential of the hidden curriculum is captured under the rubric of ethical erosion. Narrative and literature-based reviews bring the risk to light. Although LICs offer one remedy, we are pressed to explore even more deeply what aspects of LICs are the forces at work. Scholars suspect the answer lies in creating meaningful learning relationships and meaningful roles for students—to ensure learning is situated in dynamic discourse and role development that affirms the students' ideals at the same time students come to requisite skill training. It would not be enough to posit that LICs are just the current best model, because continual improvement of medical education and system improvement should be the goal (Berwick and Finkelstein 2010). On the other hand, to adhere to traditional models of medical education that have either failed to address ethical erosion or that may, in fact, be the source of ethical erosion, is to betray the spirit, intent, and mandate for medical education.

We educators should no longer whisper or tolerate sounds of silence. Medical education leaders must give voice to the value of and values that arise from LICs and other educational models structured to attend to the hidden curriculum.

18: Tweets, Texts, and Facebook Requests

Social Media and the Hidden Curriculum in Medical Education

RICHARD M. FRANKEL

In 1988 my colleague Catherine Pettinari, a linguist, published a book (her PhD thesis) on the relationship between the operating room discourse she recorded in a series of cholecystectomies and residents' written documentation of those surgeries in their chart notes (Pettinari 1988). Among other things, Pettinari noticed that the notes of new trainees almost always appeared in the form of a narrative, whereas the notes of more advanced trainees were reduced to lists or descriptions. Pettinari was struck by the absence of narrative in the more "advanced" residents' notes and the attenuation of communicative richness that resulted. Although the label "hidden curriculum in medical education" had yet to be coined, what Pettinari witnessed was without question part of the implicit socialization process of graduate medical education in surgery that reduced the narrative thread of medical practice to its stripped-down functional equivalent. Her research also is an instructive example for thinking about how social media is shaping the ways in which information is encoded and managed in medical education today.

Now, twenty-five years after Pettinari's study, a broader cultural transformation is affecting entire generations of users as they compress their lived experience into SMSs (Small Message Service), 140-character tweets or text messages, or social media sites such as Facebook. To be sure, narrative still is alive and well in medical education and still is a major vehicle for teaching interviewing skills and clinical care processes in the classroom and at the bedside (Fortin et al. 2012). At the same time, social media's growing influence in transmitting meaning and values in medical education is barely understood and appreciated by faculty, most of whom use it completely differently from those they are training.

My goal in this chapter is threefold. First, I present background information on the increasing use of social media by all segments of society, but especially Millennials, those aged eighteen to thirty-two, which includes most medical students, residents, and fellows. Second, I explore generational differences in social media usage as analogous to relationships between "immigrant" and "native" groups. Finally, I describe a case in which a medical student's inappropriate use of social media led to a cross-generational effort to communicate with his classmates about the risks and challenges of using social media in professional training.

Background

Within minutes, and long before it appeared on network television, millions of people around the world knew that Representative Gabrielle Giffords had been shot and severely wounded on January 8, 2011. The incident went viral on the Internet and social networking sites, and details about the shooting and the psychiatric history of the young male assistant emerged rapidly. In another incident, a student at Rutgers University committed suicide after compromising photos of him were posted to a social networking site. Again, the story went viral and became an international topic of conversation. Finally, a Canadian teenager named Justin Bieber, hungry to break into the music business, posted some of his songs on YouTube and, in the course of eighteen months, went from being unknown to having millions of dedicated (mostly adolescent female) fans, eventually selling out a concert in Madison Square Garden in twenty-two minutes!

What these examples have in common is the increasing use and importance of electronic social media to instantly receive and send information with the click of a button. In essence, the use of social media represents a new type of learning and language exchange based on the instant availability of small amounts of information. Little currently is known about how medical students use social media during their education and what effects, if any, this is having on what and how they learn.

What Is Known about Students' Use of Social Media

It is widely known that Millennials, a group that includes medical students, residents, fellows, and some junior faculty, use social media almost continuously. Recent estimates put the number of users of Facebook at over 1 billion, with approximately 166 million in the United States alone (www. insidefacebook.com). One observer of this generation wrote, "Millennials cast a big, wide-open net across their lives pinging and poking friends on social networking sites, instant messaging and e-mailing, blogging and posting, uploading and downloading—all instantly and incessantly" (Fine 2010, 21). This method of communication has supplanted other forms of interaction, including the telephone and even email, which are more commonly used by older faculty.

Posts by Millennials on Facebook range from factual to intimate. Medical students and residents often favor texting rather than paging to communicate during clinical rotations (Contemporary Pediatrics Staff 2012). These "digital natives" are developing styles and modes of communication that are often quite foreign to their faculty (Prensky 2001a). Much like the "generation gap" and "failures to communicate" that characterized student unrest in the 1960s, many medical school and residency faculty report that students' use of social media is worrisome, and raise professionalism and patient care issues (Chretien et al. 2009). At the same time, but perhaps less in the limelight, medical trainees regularly use social media to gather, share, and act on information more quickly and efficiently than at any other time in history, and this factor has major implications for the hidden curriculum of medical education.

Social Media and the Cultural Divide between Students and Faculty

The author of an article titled "Digital Immigrants, Digital Natives" argues that there is a "digital divide" that separates Millennials from Generation Xers or Baby Boomers (Prensky 2001a, 2001b). On one side are digital natives, Millennials born after 1980 who are surrounded by digital media to such an extent that it may have altered their brain structures so they differ from those of previous generations (Erickson et al. 2010). Digital natives thrive on receiving and processing information from multiple sources simultaneously. They are able to analyze situations and data by multitasking and parallel processing of information. They also prefer looking at graphics before reading a text rather the reverse, which is characteristic of Baby Boomers and Gen Xers. Digital natives also prefer random access (such as hypertext) to linear search strategies. They function best when networked with others, and thrive on instant gratification and frequent rewards. And they prefer games to "serious" work (Prensky 2001a): a recent *New York Times* article pointed out that there are 40 million active users and 75 million paid and ad-supported downloads of the game *Angry Birds*, the majority being Millennials and digital natives. It is estimated that 200 million minutes a day are spent worldwide by users inside the game (Anderson 2012)!

On the other side of the digital divide are digital immigrants, those born before the advent of the digital age. They reveal their non-native status through a "Digital Immigrant Accent" (Prensky 2001a, 2) that manifests it-self in several ways. For example, digital immigrants would rather print out a digital document to edit rather than editing it online. The telephone is their preferred mode of communication rather than texting, tweeting, or in-stant messaging (IM). Digital immigrants approach using hardware or soft-ware by reading and following step-by-step written instructions, and often wind up frustrated when the instructions don't produce the desired result. "Digital Immigrants don't believe their students can learn successfully while watching TV or listening to music, because they (the Immigrants) can't" (Prensky 2001b, 1). Digital natives rarely read and follow written instruc-tions, and instead use trial-and-error and intuitive methods to find their way through a program or game.

Exploring the Digital Divide

In a pair of recent meetings sponsored in 2011 by the American Academy on Communication in Healthcare (AACH) and the American Association of Medical Colleges (AAMC), my colleagues and I presented a workshop titled "A Click Is All It Takes," in which we explored the reality of the dig-ital divide between Millennials, Gen Xers, and Baby Boomers. One of the exercises we used was based on a revision of a generational quiz posted by blogger Penelope Trunk:

Generational Quiz

1. Do you have your own web page? (1 point)
2. Have you made a web page for someone else? (2 points)
3. Do you IM your friends? (1 point)
4. Do you text your friends? (2 points)
5. Do you watch videos on YouTube? (1 point)
6. Do you remix video files from the Internet? (2 points)
7. Have you paid for and downloaded music from the Internet? (1 point)
8. Do you know where to download free (illegal) music from the Internet? (2 points)
9. Do you blog for professional reasons? (1 point)

10. Do you blog as a way to keep an online diary? (2 points)
11. Have you visited Facebook in the last week? (1 point)
12. Do you communicate on Twitter? (2 points)
13. Do you use email to communicate with your parents? (1 point)
14. Did you text to communicate with your parents? (2 points)
15. Do you take photos with your phone? (1 point)
16. Do you share your photos from your phone with your friends? (2 points)

Finding your group:

0–8 points = Digital Immigrant
8–15 points = Straddling Both Worlds
16 or more = Digital Native

Revised from http://blog.penelopetrunk.com/2007/06/25/what-generation-are-you-part-of-really-take-this-test/

At the beginning of the workshop, the participants, who were diverse in terms of age, position, and social media use, were asked to fill out the quiz and sort themselves into three groups according to their point totals. Predictably, there was a strong correlation between academic rank (a proxy for age) and group identification. Most, but not all, professors and senior administrators (Baby Boomers) fell into the digital immigrant category. Some middle-level faculty and administrators straddled both worlds (Gen Xers). Almost all the students, residents, fellows, and instructors (Millennials) identified themselves as digital natives.

The second part of the workshop was a series of dialogues among the groups designed to explore values and attitudes about social media in medical education. The digital immigrant group felt strongly that social media was a hindrance and not worth it for them to invest in. One participant said, "I'm digitally challenged. If I have a question about how to use social media or anything else having to do with technology, I ask my teenager who can figure it out in a tenth of the time it would take me." Digital natives felt that social media was an integral part of their lives and how they learned best. This group was grateful for rapid access to information and the ability to communicate instantly with colleagues and friends. They also felt that social media was a huge benefit to their education, especially in terms of time efficiency and access to online resources. One participant reflected, "By listening to a lecture on streaming video, I can save time driving to campus, parking, and driving home. I can also speed up or slow down the pace of the lecture to suit my learning needs, and I can pause or rewind if I don't understand something." Straddlers felt that there were some benefits but also some real challenges to using social media. One straddler commented, "I think social media is great, but I'm already overwhelmed with a thousand other things vying for my attention, and I'm not sure this one is worth the time and effort it would take to become proficient." Clearly, whether you see social media as a facilitator of or barrier to learning, in reduced or expanded form, depends at least in part on whether you are a digital native or a digital immigrant.

The final portion of the workshop was devoted to a large group dialogue about "crossing the digital divide in medical education." Millennials were quite active and made lots of suggestions for increasing the uses of social media in their education. For example, they suggested that many technical skills could be taught virtually, and that smart mobile devices and portable EMRs could be used to monitor patients' medications and progress. This group also suggested that tweeting was a much more efficient way of communicating important information than more intensive information-transfer strategies such as email, text, or telephone.

Response to the Millennials' suggestions was mixed. Some straddlers and digital immigrants thought that the suggested innovations might not work very well because of logistical and security concerns. Others felt that the Millennials' use of tweets and texts was disrespectful and shallow. The tone of these conversations felt very much like an argument between a group of young entrepreneurs (Millennials), wanting to try out new ideas, and senior management (Gen Xers and Baby Boomers) countering with all the reasons they wouldn't work! In any event, the conversation seemed to instantiate an aphorism attributed to Anaïs Nin, "We don't see things as they are, we see them as *we* are."

An unusual feature of the generational divide in social media use is that the digital natives (students), for the most part, are in a younger, less powerful generation than the immigrants (faculty). As was pointed out in both workshops, it is the digital immigrants who control how medicine is taught and the digital natives who must follow the rules set down by those with less expertise and different norms, values, and expectations than they. Not surprisingly, non-experts making the rules for experts is sometimes a cause of tension and misunderstanding. At the same time, it can also be an opportunity for growth and community learning.

Social Media in Medical Education: Notes of a Digital Immigrant

I am a professor of medicine and geriatrics at Indiana University School of Medicine (IUSM) and also the statewide competency director for the school's professionalism competency. I am a Baby Boomer, having been born in the 1940s, and I am definitely a digital immigrant. I never learned to play video games, bought my first smartphone a couple of years ago, and have never used Twitter. I consider the computer an essential tool of my professional life, but I use it for little other than work. I have never taken an online course or prepared an online lecture. If I have a problem with my smartphone or my computer, I seek help from my adolescent children. When it comes to social media in medical education, I have very little relevant experience and suspect this is also true of many of my colleagues. What I do have experience with is the process of physician formation and the elements of behavior that traditionally define medical professionalism, some of which are relevant to social media use (HIPAA violations, plagiarism, cutting and pasting of medical records, and so on), and some of which have yet to catch up with this rapidly expanding medium.

As ill prepared as I may be, I and others who are responsible for teaching and maintaining professionalism are increasingly being called upon to deal with questionable uses of social media by medical students. IUSM has had a competency curriculum since 1999, and in 2011 published guidelines for social media use (Indiana University School of Medicine 2011). Cases of unprofessional behavior are brought before the student promotions committee (SPC), which decides whether students will be allowed to remain in school, put on probation, or dismissed. As a condition for remaining in school, students who are flagged for unprofessional behavior must remediate their deficiencies to the satisfaction of the competency director and the SPC. In an average year, approximately two dozen professionalism cases come before SPC, the majority of which involve behavioral issues such as acting out, personal or professional boundary violations, and cheating or plagiarism. Over the past five years, two to three SPC cases per year have involved inappropriate use of social media.

A Click Is All It Takes . . .

Matthew Strausburg (name used with permission) is currently a fourth-year student at IUSM. In October of 2011, one of his classmates came to the school administration with a concern about having read a highly offensive "doctor joke" posted on Mr. Strausburg's public Facebook page that included the tagline "IUSM Medical School Class of 2013." The student was concerned that the school's reputation might be put in jeopardy if members of the public happened to access this page. Although technically outside of the school's formal jurisdiction, members of the administration felt this behavior was serious and unprofessional enough to warrant an Isolated Deficiency (ID) in professionalism, which automatically triggered an SPC "progress hearing."

At the hearing, Mr. Strausburg was deeply embarrassed and remorseful about what had happened. After extensive discussion, the committee voted to allow Mr. Strausburg to remain in school after remediating the deficiency. The remediation plan called for several actions: reviewing the literature on social media use by medical students, crafting letters of apology to those affected by his actions, and writing a reflective essay on what he had learned from his experience. In his essay, Mr. Strausburg shared that he was unaware of the risk he had taken when he uploaded the joke to his Facebook page, which he thought was unrelated to his status as a medical student. This was a lesson he now wanted to communicate to others who might have similar beliefs. Recognizing that as president of his class, he could influence others, he offered to use his experience and office as a service to the community to raise awareness about the risks of using social media. Mr. Strausburg's offer turned out to be a perfect opportunity for everyone in the community—students, faculty, and administration—to learn.

SCOPE is IUSM's weekly community-wide online newsletter. In addition to newsworthy items, it also publishes a column titled Mindfulness and Medicine (M&M), which features short vignettes that bring attention to issues of professional values and behavior. Many of the columns also contain a commentary by a student or faculty member. Given his interest in educating others, I asked Mr. Strausburg to consider writing an M&M column about the risks of social media. Following are that column and a portion of the commentary written by Gabriel Bosslet, MD, an IUSM pulmonary/critical care physician and social media researcher.

A Student Reports

I recently posted an offensive and tasteless "doctor joke" for my friends to see on Facebook. Another medical student who viewed it thought the posting was highly unprofessional and put the school in a potentially negative light so brought it to the attention of school administrators. As a result of my actions I was required to make an appearance before the student promotions committee and face the possibility of dismissal for behavior unbecoming a medical student.

As a result of this experience I have become acutely aware of the attractions and dangers of social networking and its potential to do harm. Since a case in which a student at Rutgers committed suicide after compromising information about him was circulated on social networking sites I have come to realize that I have a responsibility to recognize that one click of the mouse is all it took to jeopardize my entire future as a physician.

—MATTHEW STRAUSBURG, MS II

Commentary

This story is one that is becoming more and more common given the explosive popularity of online social networks. A whole body of literature is developing around the effects that online social networks have on physicians, professionalism, and the patient-doctor relationship. We are only beginning to grasp the potential impact of social networks in medicine. It is clear, however, that some of the challenges for professionalism, ethics and medical education have already become apparent.

Did you know?

- A 2009 study of deans found that 60 percent reported incidents where students had posted unprofessional content online. Some of these postings included patient information, inappropriate language, depictions of intoxication and sexually suggestive material.
- Another recent study found that most medical students' Facebook accounts listed personally identifiable information, and only one-third had their security settings as private.

- More than 50 percent of employers currently search Facebook and other social media sites prior to hiring applicants. This includes physicians.

One could argue that Facebook profiles are private spaces and that what one does in one's "off-duty" time is one's own personal business. Consider, however, the "Kevin Bacon effect." For a person with only 50 Facebook friends, assuming that each also had 50 friends, 2,500 "second-degree" friends would potentially have access to his or her profile. Physicians are held to higher standards of moral and ethical behavior than most other professions and this applies to online behavior as well as that of non-virtual realms.

The negative consequences of online professionalism lapses can be severe and are treated just like other professionalism transgressions by IUSM administration, as the student report above illustrates. The IUSM Professionalism Team has put together *"Guidelines for use of online social networking for medical students and physicians-in-training"* to help students and residents avoid the above situation. These best-practices guidelines are a tangible list of do's and don'ts for those who routinely use online social networks. Check them out, as a click is all it takes!

SCOPE 15 (5), Indiana University School of Medicine, Feb. 4, 2011

Following the student report's publication, email traffic to the *SCOPE* website increased, and there were many positive comments complimenting Mr. Strausburg on his willingness to sign his name to the column. More important, what began as a potentially adversarial remediation process wound up as the team effort of a Baby Boomer, a Gen Xer, and a Millennial. In addition to the column in *SCOPE*, the Professionalism Team hit on the idea of using orientation week as a target of opportunity for affecting the informal curriculum teaching about social media. In August 2011, and again in August 2012, Mr. Strausburg voluntarily addressed the incoming class, describing what he had done, the impact it had on him, and the lessons he learned from the experience. His presentation carried tremendous weight with the incoming classes so that as of this writing, there has not been a single incident of inappropriate use of social media in the class of 2015 or 2016!

A Concluding Thought

It is undoubtedly true that social media is a reduced form of communication. To some (digital immigrants), this represents an impoverishment of being and doing; one that robs the initiator and the reader of the richness of everyday life and conversation. To others (digital natives), the ease and efficiency of reducing communication to its essentials represents a kind of freedom from ritual and routine that is time saving and direct.

In this chapter I have tried to make the case that there are two general worldviews about social media use held by trainees and faculty. Each has implications for understanding the hidden curriculum of medical education. On the one hand, social media may limit the content of information drastically, as compared with other forms of communication. On the other hand, it may connect individuals and groups much more efficiently and provide greater flexibility in responding to requests or the need for action. Michael Polanyi, in his work on personal knowledge, points out that context is a critical component of making meaning and achieving understanding (Polanyi 1974). One important question, as yet unaddressed in studying the effect of social media on the hidden curriculum of medical education, is the implicit contextual knowledge that medical students and trainees bring to its use. When they clash, the gulf between these two worldviews can be enormous and may cause significant distress, depending on whether you are a student or seasoned medical educator.

Many questions remain to be answered about the role of social media in the informal curriculum of medical education. In the end, there is much to be said for creating a rich dialogue *across* generations using questions about social media as the focus. Stories, knowledge, values, and attitudes embedded in tweets, texts, or Facebook requests may be difficult for digital immigrants to embrace because we have not grown up or lived in the digital world. Similarly, long phone conversations and emails are a waste of time for digital natives because they have always been part of that world. Our task as medical educators is to understand both the content and the *context* of how our trainees are using social media in their education, not to judge them out of hand because they don't do things the way we do or were taught.

In the end, our ability to transcend the digital divide may be the only way to ensure that our trainees, and generations to come, will be able to practice effectively and humanely. The greatest lesson that has come from research on the hidden curriculum is the importance of observing what and how medical trainees learn in and out of the classroom. Social media will continue to exert a profound effect on both the formal and informal education of physicians, and we would do well to watch and learn the most effective ways to use it in educating tomorrow's physicians and helping them use it to good effect.

19: The Hidden Curriculum for Faculty

Betwixt and Between

Britta M. Thompson, Allison R. Ownby,
and Janet P. Hafler

Medical school faculty have complex roles (Harden and Crosby 2000) as both purveyors and receivers of the hidden curriculum. To date, the medical literature on the hidden curriculum in medical education has focused almost exclusively on medical students rather than on faculty (Hafferty and Franks 1994; Haidet and Stein 2006). Recently, the role of faculty development to help faculty decode the hidden curriculum has been discussed (Hafler et al. 2011). In this chapter, we will explore both the formal and the hidden curriculum for faculty, and propose how a comprehensive faculty development program might begin to help faculty understand how they are purveyors and receivers of the hidden curriculum.

What Is the Formal Curriculum for Faculty?

When they enter academic medicine, most faculty are formally provided with information about what it means to be a successful faculty member. This formal curriculum includes information provided by the institution through its mission, vision, and value statements; offer letters; a faculty handbook; promotion and tenure documents; and written expectations of the faculty member's percent effort for teaching, research, and clinical responsibilities. These formally stated expectations of what it means to be a faculty member also include requirements such as annual institutional review board (IRB) as well as Health Insurance Portability and Accountability Act (HIPAA) trainings.

Some schools schedule faculty development activities, such as a new faculty orientation where faculty members may hear about expectations for promotion within the institution, or workshops to enhance a faculty member's teaching skills. Even though a formal curriculum for faculty often is part of an institution's faculty development program, faculty also hear stories from colleagues about what really counts toward success. In addition, faculty observe their environment, for example, who is promoted or what types of meetings are scheduled at what times. These informal conversations and experiences provide insight into how the formal curriculum is enacted, and the broader institutional cortex in which that curriculum functions.

What Is the Hidden Curriculum for Faculty?

The formal curriculum provides the institutionally sanctioned rules and procedures for faculty, but the hidden curriculum includes the actual practices under which these sanctioned rules and procedures are operationalized. The hidden curriculum for faculty is multifaceted and is associated with socialization processes; with the varied contexts that intersect faculty life (learners, the institution, and the environment); and with the multiple roles of faculty (teacher, researcher, clinician, and administrator). Preferably, faculty come to realize the complexity of the hidden curriculum one layer at a time; once one layer is decoded, another layer may emerge for its own decoding. Once faculty identify examples of how they are subjected to the hidden curriculum, such as weekend meetings that affect work-life balance or the influence of pharmaceutical marketing practices, other examples emerge.

For this chapter, we will focus on illustrations of the hidden curriculum as it affects faculty: faculty awards, service expectations, promotion and tenure practices, as well as faculty as purveyors of the hidden curriculum. Although the formal curriculum may state that teaching, research, and patient care are all equally important for the promotion and tenure process, faculty quickly learn what their school truly values. Take, for example, two MD faculty being considered for promotion (see case example) and how the hidden curriculum may function within this domain of faculty life.

Case Example

Two female assistant professors in the Department of Internal Medicine are preparing their promotion packets. Both are clinicians (MD) with similar patient care responsibilities and are eight years post-fellowship.

- Dr. Research is a clinical investigator who occasionally lectures to medical students in the preclinical curriculum. She teaches medical students, residents, and fellows while attending. Most of the evaluations of her teaching have been average; however, a few have been quite poor. In addition to her teaching, she has received an R01 for her clinical research. She also has seven publications that include one review article and six peer-reviewed research papers in scientific journals.

• Dr. Educator is a clinician educator who has had a large teaching load as a small-group facilitator and as a large-group facilitator-lecturer to medical students in the preclinical curriculum. She teaches medical students, residents, and fellows while attending. She has been the clerkship director for the Department of Internal Medicine for the past three years, and has received outstanding evaluations from all the learners that she instructs and directs. In addition to teaching and clinical service, she has six publications that include two review papers, one case study, one book chapter, and two peer-reviewed curriculum models published in *MedEdPortal*.

As is his custom, the chair meets with both faculty for a pre-review to ensure the readiness of each. To Dr. Research, the chair indicates that he is pleased with her progress and is happy to put her up for promotion. He tells her not to worry about her poor evaluations, stating, "It is not important, since you have an R01 and published peer-reviewed papers in scientific journals." He goes on to say, "The promotion and tenure committee won't really care about the quality of your teaching. The R01 and peer-reviewed articles carry the most weight in their decisions."

When the chair meets with Dr. Educator, he thanks her for her large teaching load and comments that he is pleased with the quality of her teaching. He notes that although she has a large teaching load, she does not have any grants. He goes on to say that the she does not have any publications, and that "the only publications that really count to the promotion and tenure committee are peer-reviewed journal articles in scientific journals." He adds, "Although I am really pleased with your progress, I'm concerned that if I put you up for promotion, it will be denied. Let's wait another year. In that time, I want to see at least one peer-reviewed paper, and I also want you to try for a K01 or some type of NIH grant. Let's hope that by this time next year, you will have achieved the things that really matter for your promotion."

Additional areas in which the formal and hidden curriculum may provide differing messages to faculty are awards and service activities. The formal curriculum may indicate equal commitment to the tripartite mission of the institution (teaching, research, and patient care), yet the number, types, dollar value, and fanfare linked with various faculty awards associated with each mission often may suggest that one area is valued above another. For example, teaching excellence awards may be fewer in number, have limited or no monetary reward, and have little fanfare associated with the dissemination of the award when compared to faculty awards in research or patient care (Wright et al. 2012). Service expectations also are rife within the hidden curriculum. At some institutions, faculty who generate substantial research or patient-care dollars may be able to "opt out" or "buy out" of service on time-intensive committees such as medical school admissions. At another institution, the administration may publicly endorse global health initiatives, but may require faculty to take vacation time to participate in these initiatives.

Faculty are the purveyors of the hidden curriculum to the learners they teach while simultaneously being subject to, and a part of, the hidden curriculum at their institution (department, school, affiliated hospitals, health sciences center) and the larger environment (national organizations, accrediting bodies, licensure committees, healthcare system) (Hafler et al. 2011). Figure 19-1 represents the complexity of the hidden curriculum for faculty as hidden curriculum transmitters and receivers within the institution and the larger environment in which they work. Although the numerous examples of the hidden curriculum content that faculty purvey to learners are outside the scope of this chapter, these examples are detailed in other chapters of this book.

Interestingly, the influence of learners on the hidden curriculum has remained largely unexplored. For example, students can become an important vehicle of the hidden curriculum, dissuading faculty from implementing or sustaining nontraditional methods of teaching through their lack of buy-in or support and their insistence that faculty continue more traditional teaching methods (DaRosa et al. 2011). Such inattention or related lack of enthusiasm sends a powerful hidden curriculum message to faculty that satisfaction and buy-in from students are more important than potential learning outcomes associated with an educational innovation or the latitude to try new teaching methods.

As figure 19-1 indicates, faculty are transmitters and receivers of the hidden curriculum to and from the larger environment, which includes, but is not limited to, national organizations such as specialty organizations or

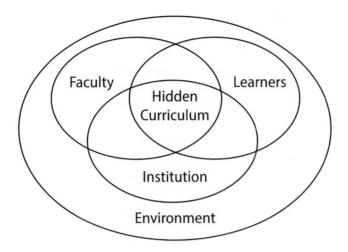

Figure 19.1 Representation of the complexity of the hidden curriculum for faculty with the intersection of learners (medical students, residents, fellows), the institution (department, school, affiliated hospitals, health science center), and the environment (national organization, accrediting bodies, licensure committees, healthcare system).

medical education organizations, accrediting bodies, licensure organizations, and the larger healthcare system. It is important to recognize that the larger environment provides an additional context in which faculty can transmit and receive the hidden curriculum. However, a discussion of the complexity and the number of components associated with the hidden curriculum in the larger environment is beyond the scope of this chapter.

Faculty purvey the hidden curriculum to other faculty and to the institution through participation on faculty committees and their daily interactions with faculty colleagues as well as others in the institution. For example, faculty who teach in the clinical setting may discredit or diminish what students have learned during an introduction to clinical skills course, such as relationship-centered care, by saying things such as "That's what you may have learned, but that's not how things really work in the real clinical world," or by telling students that they "will not ever really need to use the basic sciences that they learned in the 'real world.'" Likewise, when physicians belittle one specialty in front of students, faculty, or others, this teaches a hidden curriculum of specialty stratification (Thompson et al. 2010).

At first glance, these examples appear to focus solely on students, but they also send powerful messages to the faculty who teach these courses

(Ownby et al. 2011). Faculty also influence the hidden curriculum for other faculty through their service or leadership on various institutional committees. As discussed previously, faculty who serve on promotion and tenure committees within departments or at the college or institutional level can perpetuate the devaluation of teaching contributions and scholarship by denying promotion to faculty on clinical educator tracks even though they have met all the written expectations for promotion. Research regarding the influence of faculty on the hidden curriculum for other faculty and the institution is an important area for further exploration.

Faculty Development to Address the Hidden Curriculum

The goal of faculty development is to empower faculty members to excel in their roles, enhance skills, and improve the vitality of faculty (Steinert et al. 2006; Wilkerson and Irby 1998). Faculty development programs provide faculty with a sense of belonging, engagement, and relatedness (Steinert et al. 2009). Traditionally, faculty development has been delivered through workshops, short courses, seminar series, and longitudinal programs (Steinert et al. 2006). Virtually all of these activities address the formal curriculum of the institution, such as its mission, values, and formal procedures. These activities also have been driven by the need to socialize new faculty to the institution and its culture, help faculty develop discrete teaching skills, professionalize teaching within academic medicine, develop educational scholarship, sustain academic vitality, and prepare faculty for the promotion and tenure process (McLean, Cilliers, and Van Wyk 2008). Other important topics include developing career and personal goals, preparing for negotiations (for resources and support), enhancing networking opportunities through positive role models, mentoring and coaching, formative evaluation of progress toward promotion and tenure, and networking opportunities (Pololi et al. 2002; Kuhn, Abbuhl, and Clem 2008; Levine et al. 2011).

Nonetheless, and within this range of foci, very few publications in the area of faculty development address the hidden curriculum for faculty, with one notable exception (Hafler et al. 2011). Although the words *the hidden curriculum* were not used, Wilkerson and Irby (1998) proposed a framework for comprehensive faculty development including professional development, instructional development, and leadership development, as well as organizational development. The following paragraphs provide examples of how faculty development programs might address the hidden curriculum within each of these four frameworks.

Wilkerson and Irby (1998) discuss that faculty development should help faculty effectively identify their role within the institution and socialize them to the profession of academic medicine. Although faculty usually are made aware of what being a successful faculty member means as part of the formal curriculum, we propose that faculty should be supported with a faculty development program that can address the hidden curriculum. This could include an established network of experienced, knowledgeable, and nurturing faculty who will help faculty members understand the realities of how the mission, values, formal expectations, and procedures of the institution are practiced on a daily basis (Pololi et al. 2012; Pololi, Cooper, and Carr 2010; Trowler and Knight 1999).

Instructional development for faculty traditionally has focused on helping faculty master teaching skills such as instructional design, assessment, and feedback. Focusing on assessing and rewarding or remediating faculty as role models of professionalism can provide an opportunity to help faculty consider the hidden curriculum that they are teaching (Todhunter et al. 2011). We suggest that faculty developers might provide opportunities for faculty to identify their role as transmitters of the hidden curriculum for learners and reflect on the unintended messages they are conveying about the profession of medicine.

Leadership development for faculty traditionally has been limited, but the role that faculty leaders play in the hidden curriculum can be significant. Leadership includes formal positions such as dean, chair, division chief, and residency program director, as well as less formal positions such as curriculum committee member. Faculty development can help faculty leaders become aware of their pivotal role in the hidden curriculum and develop ways to effectively acknowledge and address the hidden curriculum for faculty, learners, the institution, and even the environment (Souba et al. 2011).

Finally, faculty development must include organizational development. Existing faculty development literature suggests addressing the hidden curriculum at the organizational level through methods such as encouraging collaboration and collegiality among faculty, emphasizing the relational aspects of the culture of academic medicine, providing opportunities for faculty to reflect on the meaningfulness of their work, building confidence and hope among faculty, and recognizing and disseminating successes of faculty (Levine et al. 2011; Pololi et al. 2009; Pololi et al. 2012; Wilkerson and Irby

1998). Institutions can begin to address the hidden curriculum for faculty by implementing a clinician educator track, "counting" educational scholarship as equal to basic science research, implementing an educator portfolio system, and ensuring alignment of department values and mission with that of the institution.

In this chapter, we have defined the formal and hidden curriculum for faculty and explored the complex role that faculty play as both purveyors and receivers of the hidden curriculum for learners, other faculty, the institution, and the environment—the betwixt and between for faculty. We have also suggested how a comprehensive faculty development program can help address the hidden curriculum for faculty in four areas: professional development, instructional development, leadership development, and organizational development. A dearth of research exists regarding the influence of the hidden curriculum on faculty; much more needs to be studied in this area. As one author suggested more than two decades ago, "[O]ur inquiries ought to probe beneath the veneer of supposedly self-evident and self-justifying assumptions and practices and enable us to expose the contradictions and possibilities inherent" (Cornbleth 1990, 55).

20: What Does the Culture of Research Teach Next-Generation Scientists?

KELLY EDWARDS

A recent incident on campus brought to mind the hidden curriculum in research. It was, on the surface at least, a minor incident, hardly notable except with regard to how incidents like this are signals to us on faculty and in leadership positions that our daily practices may not seem to align with spoken rules and standards. The incident was this: a student in an advanced-level science course gave a presentation about a research issue and used several slides found on the course website produced by the professor. The slides were borrowed and used without attribution, simply incorporated into the student's talk and overview of the research issue. The professor was dumbfounded, witnessing what she took to be bald plagiarism. When confronted, the student could not see that he had done anything wrong. His response? "I see you faculty borrowing slides from each other all the time."

What happened here? We have rules about plagiarism in the student handbook (buried amid 200 pages of other detail). Each summer, we also have required classes on the responsible conduct of research. These courses often are taught, and not so incidentally given our focus on the hidden curriculum, in large lecture halls with examples that may or may not resonate with the research trainees, eager to get back to the lab—the "real work" of research. Overall, what is happening is the implicit education that occurs when our students, ever diligent observers of their role models on how to succeed in the world of academic medicine, see behavior that we do not take time to explain or discuss. Faculty do indeed borrow slides from each other, ideally with permission, and, where appropriate, with attribution. However, understanding the difference made by permission and acknowledgment in the process of using other people's work is an essential part of the practice.

In this chapter, I examine a few such disconnects between our formal research ethics curriculum and our hidden curriculum in research practice, as reflected in our actions and choices. The formal curriculum in research ethics, in general, is limited to two requirements. First, students—actually anyone—conducting research with human subjects must complete human subjects training. Many researchers accomplish this requirement through the highly regarded CITI online program (Collaborative Institutional Training Initiative). The second opportunity kicks in for trainees on federally funded research grants, through NIH (National Institutes of Health) or NSF (National Science Foundation). These individuals are required to complete a course in responsible conduct of research each year of their funding. Now, I am an ethics professor who also is a federally funded researcher, and I am 100 percent behind making ethics and integrity an essential part of research training and practice. That said, I often think that the fastest way to kill an ethics topic is to make it mandatory. Because students and other researchers have to go get the certificate showing they have completed the training so they can be eligible to receive the grant funding, trainees often see these mandatory courses and classes as *the thing* that stands between them and their funding or research work.

Given the time, stress, and pressure, trainees and researchers bang through the online course as fast as possible (to CITI's credit, the site warns you if it detects you are moving through the material too quickly) to get through to the reward—a certificate of completion that they can present to our principal investigator (PI) and the funding agency. Did trainees absorb anything? Did they understand how the general topics and issues relate to their individual specialty or project? Did they have a dialogue with their research group about how they will handle issues when they arise? All too often, the answer is no. Trainees "just get through" the required training and move on to the "real work," the research itself. These shortcomings have been noted, and NSF has shifted to requiring that a portion of the training be done in person rather than online. Regardless of method, the gap remains between explicit messaging (there are rules to be agreed to) and implicit messaging (there are everyday judgment calls in the daily work of research that the rules do not address directly).

Research misconduct is defined as a lapse in scientific and ethical standards (National Institutes of Health n.d.). The challenge the hidden curriculum creates is what happens when scientific standards themselves, as enacted within our institutions, create a culture that we would not aspire to, professionally or personally (Goering et al. 2008). One of the most recent and pressing examples is the federal regulation that de-identified specimens or data sets that are not considered human subjects and therefore do not require further consent or recontact for research (Office of Human Subjects Research Protections n.d.). However, and given this exemption, we now risk significant disconnects between what the original research participants might think is happening with their data or specimens and what actually ends up happening. In some instances, lawsuits have been initiated and settlements negotiated, despite the fact that no laws were broken (Harmon 2010).

For the most part, researchers are neither misguided nor bad people. The official criteria for research misconduct constitutes an admonition that is difficult to argue with: "Do not lie, cheat, or steal." Most, if not all, researchers would certainly agree with these rules. That said, the actual work of research involves a remarkable number of everyday judgment calls that require a much more nuanced rule book. When does cleaning up an image for publication become fabrication? Does leaving one set of results off the paper because they pull the analysis in the "wrong direction" constitute falsification? What happens when a key insight comes from reviewing a prepublication version of a manuscript from a competitor lab? In 2002 Martinson and de Vries distributed an anonymous survey to over 3,000 scientists to assess the prevalence of various misbehaviors. The results showed that although serious misconduct in the form of falsification, fabrication, or plagiarism does occur, it is more common to find everyday issues, such as failing to present data that contradicts one's own previous research; changing the study design, methodology, or results in response to pressure from a funding agency; or dropping observations or data from a study based on a gut feeling that they were inaccurate (Martinson, Anderson, and de Vries 2005).

At research institutions, we live in a world where real pressures and competing values create tensions in our work. How one negotiates those tensions is a testament to what kind of culture develops at that organization or in that research group. Is it a publish-or-perish culture—or perhaps, publish first before the other lab does? In a federal funding environment where the payline (for example, percent of grants awarded) hovers around 7 percent, competition to be not just good, but the best, is fierce. This competitive environment shapes our culture, our judgments, and our practices, and the trainees we work with are soaking it up.

Those of us working within this research climate find ourselves in such a predicament. The pressures of research—to compete for increasingly smaller pots of money, to distinguish yourself or your group among a crowd of stars, to get the paper out before the other group does—can work against some of our best behavior. In this chapter, I call attention to some highlights from our culture of research practice and point to ways students and trainees can

---

BOX 20-1

A Sampling of Hidden Curriculum Issues in Research Culture

- The IRB is a necessary evil or hurdle to get through.
- If we qualify for waiver of consent or exempt status, we are home free.
- Publish or perish—the only outcome that matters is impact-level peer-reviewed publications.
- Science is objective.
- Ethics is "soft" and subjective.
- Credit and recognition are more important than outcomes and real-world impact.
- Facts speak for themselves. "Findings emerge."
- Don't admit failure. Don't show your vulnerabilities.
- Suffering is the way to truth.
- Industry-sponsored research is not to be trusted.
- Put the PI or lab director on every paper.
- There is not enough time to stop and explain. Better to ask forgiveness than permission.
- Students will figure it out. And if they do not, they will not succeed in science.

---

resist (and still keep your position!). Though there are numerous cultural practices within the research realm having to do with authorship practices, data management, conflicts of interest, and so forth, I chose four that I have seen influence trainees as they strive to find a path forward within academic research.

Research Culture Message One: If the IRB has signed off, all issues of research ethics have been addressed, and we are home free.

For many researchers, following the rules and policies of the institutional review board (IRB) is essential. IRBs were mandated by federal regulations regarding the protection of human subjects in research in 1974. IRBs are there to make sure that participants are sufficiently informed about what will happen in the research, that the risks they are being asked to assume are not out of proportion with the potential for benefit, and that individuals or populations are not taken advantage of inequitably in research (that is, that one group benefits at another group's expense). Federally funded projects require IRB review and approval before funding is released. Because of this, IRB applications are submitted at the outset of a project, and all relevant protocols are mapped out in detail for the review committee. Reviews can take anywhere from a month to a year, depending on the complexity of the project, with investigators often developing a love-hate relationship with the IRB during the review process.

On the one hand, the requirement of approval creates a bureaucratic hurdle between researchers and their research and can be incredibly time-consuming. Often, there are frustrations in that the IRB may not actually understand what the science requires, or perhaps does not understand the special needs of a given population (Ranjbar 2012). Some have noted an "IRB paradox" where the process of going through the IRB can encourage deceit among investigators just eager to get approval, and may justify small deceptions based on the belief that the IRB does not understand what is really in this population's best interest (Keith-Spiegel and Koocher 2005). On the other hand, once IRB approval is in hand, this is a magic green-light moment for the research to begin. Nonetheless, and back to our earlier point about the hidden curriculum, all too often, this green light signals an end to any further ethical considerations.

The challenge of leaving all the moral determination to an external body is that this takes the judgment out of the research context and thus leaves the researchers unaware of other ethical dimensions of their work. At its worst, and given the amount of legal jargon that is required to include in a consent form, it can feel like the IRB is protecting institutional interests rather than those of the human participants. Requests (or demands) for revisions and clarifications are emailed, corrections are made, and rarely is there dialogue or understanding about the underlying values or implications. As discussed earlier, many judgment calls arise in the course of conducting research that require more ethical deliberation. Even though secondary analysis of de-identified data does not require IRB review (because it is not considered human subjects research), do we not have some kind of obligation to communicate with past participants and let them know about additional studies that are heading in a very different direction from the original study?

Further, the IRB process requires a complex eighteen-page consent form. How can I be sure participants understand what the study will entail, given this blizzard of detail? Moreover, how much of that form involves the participants, and how much is for institutional protection? Should I ask permission of the family before I publish their genetic sequence? For these real-time judgments, we encourage lab meetings or the use of growing research ethics consult services to promote dialogue about what the considerations are for the decisions (McCormick et al. 2013). The bottom line is this: IRB review and the regulations regarding research with human subjects provide the floor of behavior, but it is up to the culture of science, along with the more localized cultures of individual research labs, to strive for excellence within our practices (Fullerton et al. 2010). Further, for a culture of science to develop in a more morally robust way, it takes open dialogue and exchange between research team members and leaders (Sharp 2002).

Research Culture Message Two: Science is objective.

Medical students learn this perspective from their basic science coursework buttressed by multiple-choice exams and the necessity of passing the Board exams. The resulting worldview that embraces data-as-truth has implications not only for patient care, but for the work of research as well.

One such implication of scientific objectivity is the perception that scientists cannot be advocates. This cultural message has created much confusion among trainees. Graduate students and postdocs motivated toward socially responsible work, and by a desire to have their work count, have done some remarkable things partnering with nonprofits and community-based organizations. That said, going to present at the port authority about the environmental health impact of the shipping industry can feel quite risky to those of us within the academy because of a perception that we are advocating for a position in a political setting. Will our research be forever called into question because we have been seen consorting with those outside the academy? Are we introducing bias and subjectivity into our research?

In a world where objectivity reigns, those are some of the most dreaded claims you can have held against you. The basic message, which can be both explicit and implicit, is that it is best to choose a traditional research track, publish in peer-reviewed journals, get a good job, continue to secure funding, then get promoted, *and then, and only then*, should you consider stepping out and doing more unconventional things. Publish in a community newsletter? Speak at a town hall? These can be considered volunteer or service time, but they are not considered integral to our traditional notions of research (Nicholson and Ioannidis 2012). What if students are considering research careers outside of academic research? This can feel like a failure. Nonetheless, as more and more of our trainees are going into diverse careers outside of the traditional research academy (Fiske 2013), we will need to expand deeply held notions of what it means to be a scientist or researcher.

A troubling implication of these cultural messages is that we are cultivating habits and practices, ways of doing science, that actively discourage or discredit the types of communication that need to be taking place if we are to rein in these traditional sources of noise and cross-messages. Wonderful models and exceptions to the dominant practices do exist. The recent head of the National Oceanic and Atmosphere Administration and an internationally respected leader in research, Jane Lubchenco, regularly speaks on the need for scientists to engage more actively with the social issues of our time. She, along with the American Association for the Advancement of Science, provides workshops and guidance for researchers on how to use their expertise, their credibility, and their understanding of the evidence to inform public policy deliberations. Rather than remove our expertise from these domains, it is important to know how to use expertise appropriately so the real advocates can do their work. Other important innovations include student-run organizations such as Forum on Science, Ethics, and Policy (Knight 2004) where the students take the lead on keeping socially engaged research front and center.

Research Culture Message Three: Guard your intellectual property.

As mentioned earlier, competition is fierce within the sciences. This often translates to holding your cards close to your chest, along with your data, your results, your failures, and your research strategies. Trainees are asked to uphold confidentiality and not discuss experiments or developments with anyone, even other students in their cohort. These admonitions run counter to NIH goals for data sharing and collaboration. Even though the stated goal of federally funded research is to lead to advances in human health, this kind of isolation and competitive behavior can be counterproductive in challenging ways. Failed experiments are repeated over and over around the world because we are not communicating about them despite there being three journals of negative findings (all of which, not so incidentally, remain minor in terms of their impact scores). Nonetheless, and given the incentive structure that remains firmly in place (rewards for lead author publications in prestigious journals and more funded grants), there are few tangible rewards, and perceived risks and losses, for more collaboration and open sharing. In these ways, researchers are astute readers of their environment and are being highly responsive to the existing structure. If we want to shift practices to align with the stated goals of publicly funded research, we will need to shift reward structures as well.

There are alternatives emerging. The open science movement (Open Science Federation) is experimenting with open lab notebooks online in an effort to accelerate discovery and creativity (Bradley and Neylon 2008). The Human Genome Project, notably, was completed ahead of schedule because of a mandated data-sharing approach from all labs participating in the sequencing (National Human Genome Research Institute 2003). The NIH currently requires that all sequences from genome-wide association studies be posted in dbGaP (National Institutes of Health 2008). This collection of de-identified data sets has been accessed multiple times and is slowly making an impact on research, particularly in the tool and methods development realm (Walker et al. 2011). However, much of the buzz on the street is that these data sets are exceedingly difficult to use for meaningful human studies, given the diversity of annotation used and variations in data quality. Disincentives discussed earlier remain strongly in place, and it is still best to negotiate with the investigator directly for collaborative sharing options rather than access through this public source. Mandates to share, like our mandates to train in ethics, are not always as effective as changing the culture.

Research Culture Message Four: The heavy hitters are untouchable.

If you bring enough grant dollars into an institution, your behavior is inscrutable. Trainees can get caught in this system, and cynicism about integrity can develop if it seems that power-through-dollars trumps the integrity or virtues of a mentor running a research group. We have seen senior researchers publish articles written by industry interests as honorary or ghost authors (Wislar et al. 2011). With indirect rates upwards of 56 percent (81 percent at the high end), the cost to an institution is significant if it loses a well-funded researcher. Pressure to get studies through IRB review or to figure out ways to do controversial work are high when it means keeping the lights on at the institution.

It is clear from studies on the impact of responsible conduct of research education that role models are the single most powerful influence on behavior and attitudes of trainees (Fisher et al. 2009). With that in mind, research organizations would do well to showcase role models who are modeling behavior the organization, profession, and community would value. Developing a regular news column and finding ways to visibly and meaningfully recognize and amplify research leaders and groups that are performing best practices for team development and research integrity can be an important counter to the other messages transmitted and received throughout the system (Yarborough and Hunter 2013).

Changing the Culture for Research Ethics and Integrity

As the four cultural phenomena just described suggest, researchers clearly are responding to the rules, regulations, and reward structures within the federal and local organizational systems (Martinson et al. 2010). And yet, these very structures are creating tensions within research practices and perhaps leading our young trainees down a limited or crooked path. Mandating ethics training when there is a lapse is less effective (or not at all effective) than developing a culture of integrity throughout (Tavare and Godlee 2012; Yarborough et al. 2009). On the one hand, I do understand the predicament of funders and institutional leaders: if we do not require ethics training, then we risk appearing not to have standards (at best) or that the field comes to lack moral grounding altogether. On the other hand, there is something about requiring ethics and integrity training—something mandated for all trainees on NIH and NSF grants, and any researcher conducting human subjects research—that makes this mandatory training seem onerous or like a hoop to jump through on your way to the real work of research.

Of course, rather than stand-alone, tick-the-box kinds of programming, the most effective research integrity programs are integrated into the labs or departments where the trainees are doing their work (Council on Graduate Schools 2009). This integration both assures tailored content and involves senior leadership and practicing researchers in the discussions of integrity. This, obviously, is only as helpful as the messaging that is shared by said senior leadership. When the response to peer-review practices is that "it is just a flawed system," this does not give trainees a moral barometer by which to test their own future decisions.

Alternatively, when training sessions are able to draw on the implicit moral structure of scientific responsibility and reasoning, trainees can learn a coherent approach to difficult situations in their own research careers (Deming et al. 2007; Fryer-Edwards 2002). Further, lab directors and senior personnel should make visible the rationale behind their decisions (Sharp 2002). What was negotiated with the company before the PI agreed to take on the industry-sponsored trial? What is the justification for including the recruiting physician as an author on the paper? If faculty and leaders can turn everyday judgments into opportunities for transparency and discussion, we may actually come to see those judgments in a different light. In this way, working with trainees can help research investigators think past the response of "we have always done it this way" to reconsidering certain practices if, in fact, they do not have a justifiable public explanation that fits. If a certain faculty member is unable to see another way forward, having faculty peer-peer conversations to share alternative approaches and ways to think about an issue can be highly effective toward evolution and change (more effective than the ethics professor telling them so). In this way, we can take advantage of the shifting cultures and practices, and leverage some of our research champions who do see things differently. Required courses often focus on "awareness of issues" or rules, but we need to start teaching *all* dimensions of ethical practice—including how to think through difficult decisions, how to weigh competing claims, and how to take action that often requires moral courage. These principles can enhance our culture of research:

- Integrating ways of knowing (disciplines or stakeholder perspectives) will get us closer to the "truth."
- Engaging stakeholders will help us get to real-world impact.
- Accountability to publicly funded research initiatives means we should align incentives and rewards to real-world impact.
- Sharing is a faster way forward.
- Failure is part of the process.
- Transparency leads to more credibility, not less.

The Next Generation of Work on the Hidden Curriculum

Concluding Thoughts

FREDERIC W. HAFFERTY AND JOSEPH F. O'DONNELL

The nineteen chapters that form the heart of this book provide us with a rather extraordinary and literally groundbreaking look into the hidden curriculum (HC) of health professions education. Although there is an emerging literature on the HC and health professions education, particularly in medicine, this is the first time that HC materials covering theory, methods, and application have been brought together in one volume. As noted in the introduction, and in addition to this concluding section, this book unfolds across five thematic areas: (1) Working within the Framework: Some Personal and System-Level Journeys into the Field; (2) Theoretical Considerations; (3) Methodological and Assessment Approaches; (4) The Hidden Curriculum and Health Professions Education; and (5) Special Topics and Applications.

Although the editors came to this project with certain preconceived notions about contributors and the topics they might cover, contributors were told that they were free to explore the HC in whatever directions they saw fit—and they did so with great élan. The contributors also worked within a rather restrictive word limit, something we imposed to provide readers with the largest possible number of HC voices and perspectives. As such, whatever shortcomings exist in this book, either in the topics selected or their coverage, are the fault of the editors.

These qualifications are important as readers look either backward or forward through this book. Not all topics relevant to the HC and health professions education appear in our table of contents. As we worked on this book, we quickly realized that we easily could have compiled a sister volume covering additional themes and materials that surfaced during our editing work. Such is life. Readers also should not take the part headings of this book too literally. Although we do have formal sections on HC theory (how to think about it), HC methods and measurement (how to measure and track it), and HC applications (how to apply it across a variety of domains), readers should not be lulled into thinking, for example, that chapters in the methods section are void of theory or that chapters covering applications have nothing to say about methods. Insights into theory, methods, and application appear across all chapters making up this book. The product is a nonlinear compilation through the HC, and we hope that readers will treat it as such.

In addition, we strongly encourage readers to explore the dense network of interrelated themes and issues that weave their way through this book—many of them unanticipated by the editors. Using the book's first six chapters (parts 1 and 2) as examples, we believe it is telling that all of them deal (in different ways) with issues of identity formation and professionalism—themes that also receive considerable coverage through this book, but particularly in chapters by Rabow (chapter 11); Thistlethwaite (chapter 14); Cruess and Cruess (chapter 15); Hirsh (chapter 17); Thompson, Ownby, and Hafler (chapter 19); and Edwards (chapter 20). These six chapters also deal, in different ways, with issues of role models and modeling, along with concerns about the rise of the corrosive presence of student abuse and mistreatment, the rise of student cynicism, and the loss of student idealism and empathy—themes that appear throughout this book (see, for example, Rutberg and Gaufberg [chapter 9] and Rabow [chapter 11]). Interesting to us was the fact that four of the opening chapters also address the null curriculum, and thus showcase early how this underappreciated and relatively unexplored aspect of the HC fits into the overall framework of HC analysis. Another example of an overarching concept—interprofessional education and the HC—can be found in material ranging from Stern (chapter 1) through Hughes and Kuper (chapter 3), Wright-Peterson and Bender (chapter 13), and Thistlethwaite (chapter 14).

Moving to a few more chapter-specific examples, Stern's (chapter 1) material on parables and the HC nicely dovetails with Hundert's observations on student narratives, which link us, in turn, to additional material by Rutberg and Gaufberg (chapter 9) and by Balmer and Richards (chapter 10) on student narratives; Martimianakis and McNaughton's work (chapter 8) on discourse analysis as a methodological tool; and Frankel's (chapter 18) examination of social media and the HC. Meanwhile, Wear and colleagues (chapter 5) and Lempp and Cribb (chapter 6) tackle issues of power, hierarchy, and occupational stratification—themes that can be found across a variety of other chapters in this book, such as Hodges and Kuper (chapter 3), Taylor and Wendland (chapter 4), Rabow (chapter 11), Thistlethwaite (chapter 14), and Edwards (chapter 20); as well as Martimianakis and Mc-Naughton (chapter 8) and Ewen (chapter 16), which both use the Foucauldian concept of biopower.

Meanwhile, Taylor and Wendland (chapter 4) has thematic links to Lempp and Cribb's (chapter 6) framing of the potential tensions that can exist between the "breadth" of the HC (variations across curricula) versus its "depth" (the foundational logic of what makes medical knowledge "special"); Martimianakis and McNaughton's (chapter 8) discussion of the unintended consequences of conducting an HC inquiry; and Rabow's (chapter 11) insistence that curricular discordance is a central element of professional formation and growth, and thus disjunctures in the learning environment should not always be a target for eradication (which is not the same thing as saying that the HC may sometimes function as a positive force). In short, we strongly encourage readers to be proactive in constructing their own thematic map linking the various concepts and issues raised by the chapter authors.

In spite of all this connectedness, there are issues and themes of critical importance to any grounded understanding of the HC and health professions education that remain underexplored in this book. One example will have to suffice. In chapter 16, Ewen explores issues related to Indigenous populations and the HC. Underrepresented minorities, particularly matriculates who come from marginal social, ethnic, or cultural backgrounds, often find themselves to be the ultimate outsiders in their school-based social networks. In terms of both access and opportunities, they often lack the cultural and insider know-how that would allow them access to insider ways of navigating their educational environments. Barriers can be formidable and unrelenting as medical educators conveniently believe that all trainees receive the same educational experience simply because all matriculates must take the same classes or have met some homogenizing admissions threshold.

Nothing, of course, could be further from the truth. Everyone does not "get" the same medical school experience, the (formally claimed) "undifferentiated" nature of undergraduate medical education notwithstanding. Nor will all students encounter, or be forced to navigate, the same HC. As noted by Haidet and Teal (chapter 7), there are multiple hidden curricula circulating throughout a given educational environment—not one. What Haidet and Teal do not say, but Ewen does, is that what remains hidden both for minority applicants and matriculates is more pervasive, and less systematically accessible, than what is hidden for the privileged, with healthcare, particularly medicine, remaining a highly stratified seat of entrenched privilege. Here, too, we should note that Ewan's work on the HC and Indigenous populations provides additional insights into related phenomenon such as structural and institutionalized racism (Steinecke and Terrell 2010).

Finally, and as readers already may have noticed, we are using a slightly different HC nomenclature in this chapter. Authors in this book were given free reign to use whatever terminology they wished, but we believe readers will find it helpful, at least within this concluding chapter, to differentiate between two broad HC categories. The first is the hidden curriculum as a *particular type of curricular influence*—along with what it is and how it differs from other types of curricula. The second is the HC as a *broad categorical label*—as when somebody refers to "the hidden curriculum of medical education." In this latter framing, writers usually assert that there is a domain of learning and influence that exists outside (or alongside) the formal curriculum. Using such a broad and sweeping brush can be quite helpful at times. However, the editors of this book also do not find this kind of either/or thinking to be particularly useful when analyzing the *various types of social action* that may underpin some particular aspect of health professions education. In this instance, we are talking about *certain types* of curricular influences versus *other types* of influences, and thus greater specificity is needed. Therefore, and in this chapter only, we will use the acronym HC when talking about the big picture, and thus the other-than-formal curriculum as a general category of influences such as referring to a distinctive approach (an HC approach) to thinking about issues of health professions education. Conversely, we will use the full term *hidden curriculum* when we are making a specific point about a particular type of influence.

The remainder of this chapter is divided into three sections. The first (Issues Raised) covers some of the HC issues that surfaced for the editors as they worked with the various chapters that comprise this book. The second (New Directions) focuses more specifically on new possibilities in HC theory—again raised by working with the contributing authors. The third (Closing Thoughts) tackles two issues near and dear to the editors' hearts. The first of these explores how to identify and work with what we consider to be a *hidden* HC literature, and the second focuses on a need to build a critical mass, particularly among faculty, to support using the HC as a tool for building reform with (as opposed to without) change.

Issues Raised

Numerous issues have been raised about the HC of health professions education across the preceding chapters, and although the editors claim no authoritative voice in their decision to focus on certain topics rather than others, we do want to devote a modicum of reflective space in this closing chapter to a small number of issues that caught our HC attention while working on this book. Nonetheless, we also realize that our choice of topics and issues may not be what readers need or want to hear as a *first word* on the HC. For this reason, we hope that readers will begin this book with the introduction and thus with its broadly framed look at HC history and issues before diving into individual chapters. Ultimately, we hope this book, taken as a whole, will fuel some disruptive changes in your own work and that, if inclined, you will share your insights, observations, questions, and (yes) criticism with the editors. We would very much like to hear from you.

Issue One: Lexicon

Over the years, a variety of scholars have sought to capture both the formal and the other-than-formal aspects of educational life. In doing so, they have deployed an extraordinary array of concepts to fit their needs. For example, the formal curriculum has been described as the *manifest curriculum*, the *intended curriculum*, the *stated curriculum*, and the *curriculum on paper*—with this being only a partial list. For all practical purposes, and regardless of the actual term used, these essentially are functional equivalents and thus can be treated as synonyms.

An even longer list of concepts has been created to capture the other-than-formal aspects of educational life. Examples include the *curriculum in action*, the *covert curriculum*, the *creditless curriculum*, the *experienced curriculum*, the *hidden curriculum*, the *informal curriculum*, the *latent curriculum*, the *learned curriculum*, the *null curriculum*, and the *tested curriculum*. Again, the list is partial. In this case, however, the terms are not equivalents. There are, for example, important differences between the null curriculum (that which is conveyed when things are *not* said or done) versus the *taught curriculum*, which might be used (depending on the author) to target the difference between what a given faculty member actually does teach versus what that faculty member said she or he was going to teach.

Although the authors in this volume were told to use whatever terms or framings they felt would best convey the points they wished to make, we would be less than forthcoming if we did not mention our own preference for certain key distinctions. As noted in the introduction, we ground our own approach to HC analysis within the tripartite distinction of the formal, the informal, and the hidden curricula—along with the very consequential (in terms of social action) differences that are contained within these three domains of learning. A key issue here is what is meant by the term *hidden*. If readers were to journey to some of the original HC writings from the 1960s and 1970s, they would encounter a somewhat radical and relatively Marxist-flavored literature on educational life—along with some very detailed reasons that authors chose to use the descriptor "hidden." During this period of early work, scholars tried to capture a set of influences that fell outside the awareness of the social actors in question. Thus, when investigators pointed to how underlying messages were built into the structure or daily practices of grade school education, and how these messages functioned to "teach" obedience and conformity, or how schools functioned to replicate the class structure of society or interests of the power elite, their use of the term *hidden* was both descriptively and analytically accurate. Schools did function in such a way, and teachers, administrators, parents, and children often had little (or no) idea about the latent messages that had been woven into the structure, process, and overall content of the formal educational enterprise.

For these (and related) reasons, it is both awkward and analytically sloppy to speak about a curriculum that is hidden and yet also manifestly obvious to all involved. In a similar fashion, just because people share a common, yet informal, understanding of "how things work around here," this does not make these understandings part of the formal (and thus the intended and stated) curriculum. So what do we call a social dynamic that is neither hidden nor formal? Our answer is that we need an intermediary concept where social actors act on the basis of shared understandings of how things are supposed to be, yet not have those understandings be considered part of the formal order of things—something like the *informal curriculum*.

In the introduction, we mentioned one example drawn from everyday life—namely, the social processes by which virtually all automobile drivers come to learn that there is a very real and functional difference between the official, posted highway speed limit and the "actual speed limit." If we take the official, posted speed limit as our formal curriculum, it would be analytically distorting to frame the real, enforced speed limit as belonging to some hidden set of messages that drivers somehow or mysteriously discover. Similarly, we can point to a rather large popular literature on the "unwritten rules" of a variety of domains of social life, including sports from baseball to golf (see, for example, Bernstein et al. 2008), the music business (Daley 1997), PhD research (Petrie and Rugg 2011), and even social relationships (Grandin and Barron 2005). In all instances, the literature describes how participants in these different social arenas come to learn what *really* is expected of them versus what *formally* is stated in some rulebook "governing" that activity.

Is *informal* the best concept to use in all of these intermediary instances? Absolutely not. However, and as just noted, it does not serve any analytic purpose to take knowledge, skills, or values that are shared by all and label them "hidden" just because, technically speaking, they are not formal.

One example of an informal curriculum at work in the world of health-care is *workarounds* (Halbesleben et al. 2008). Further, and to underscore this point, we will assume, without additional foregrounding, that most readers will know *exactly* what this term means. The fact that many work-places are awash with shared understandings about how work is *optimally* or *most expeditiously* accomplished—as opposed to the more formal and centralized rules governing how that work is *supposed* to get done—is part of the reality of everyday work. Workarounds are not formal, but neither are they hidden. And calling workarounds part of the hidden curriculum, when we can be analytically precise, is being descriptively shoddy.

A second point about HC terminology that appears throughout this book, but has its most detailed rendering in chapter 7 by Haidet and Teal, involves the frequency with which we refer to hidden (or informal, null, tacit, and so on) curricula as if we were talking about a singular and homogeneous set of influences—when this is not really the case. The variety of learning environments that make up health professions education are awash with a chaotic jumble of hidden, tacit, informal, and null messages. Untangling these messages is a major challenge for both students and faculty in understanding the scope and power of professional formation. Singularities may work as category labels, but when it comes to capturing the granularities of what is going on in nursing, or physical therapy, or dental education, referring to *the* hidden curriculum or *the* anything usually is not helpful.

In this regard, we wish to reiterate that although we are not particularly dogmatic about what terms people use to capture the other-than-formal dimensions of social life, we are catholic just so long as the term(s) used are not misleading or do not otherwise distort what is going on. Similarly, we are not dogmatic about singulars versus plurals, just so long as observers realize that the learning environments found across and within health professions education are awash with a variety of informal, hidden, and null messages and thus also are awash with elements of disarray and disagreement. Organizations rarely speak in one voice, and even formal pronouncements may harbor nuanced or crossed messages—and this before we even get to the differences between what organizations say and what they actually do. All this clutter and chaos is just one of the reasons that discordance and gaps are the rule rather than the exception in organizational life.

Messiness is the norm.

Alignment is more rhetoric than reality.

Finally, we want to briefly touch on *hidden agendas* as a methodological issue, a topic also mentioned in this book's introduction. Social life is awash with individuals and organizations whose words or actions are intended to deceive. A variant would be a statement of goals or aspirations, but where there is no real intention of delivering on these "promises." Organizational mission statements, for example, often have been criticized as being more like propaganda than like authentic marching plans.

Although duplicity and deception may be omnipresent, hidden agendas are not the same thing as hidden curricula. Moreover, this type of social action essentially falls outside the boundaries of HC analysis—at least at first blush. This is not to say that administrators never lie to faculty, or that faculty never intentionally deceive students, or that students never "game" their superordinates. However, when we are conducting an HC analysis, the primary issue at hand is the congruence or discordance among the variety of curricula (formal, informal, hidden, null, and so on) that exist within a given educational environment. Interjecting deception into the picture, however important this may be to understanding the full range of factors influencing a given dependent variable, moves us into a different analytic arena than that occupied by HC analysis. Although hidden agendas may operate as one source of discordance, perhaps better framed as a "false concordance," we consider issues of duplicity to stand more in the analytic wings than at center stage when traversing the curricular landscape.

Issue Two: Methods

We genuinely are excited by the diversity of methodological approaches for biopsying the HC contained in this book. They range from the detailed quantitative approach outlined by Haidet and Teal (chapter 7) to the more qualitative approaches of discourse covered by Martimianakis and Mc-Naughton (chapter 8) and the narrative analysis of Rutberg and Gaufberg (chapter 9), to the more survey-oriented approach outlined by Balmer and Richards (chapter 10). Given the paucity of methodological approaches within the HC literature as a whole, we consider the decision to include a dedicated methods section, and to showcase different methodological techniques for dissecting the HC, to be one of the most important features of this book.

This assessment array notwithstanding, the editors do want to add a few more surface details about how one might go about analyzing and understanding both the formal and the other-than-formal dimensions of educational life. We begin with the postulate that whatever our intended focus or preferred interpretive framework (hidden, informal, and so on), it is highly likely that we will uncover an array of formal and other-than-formal curricula as we move into data collecting. Moreover, it is also likely that we will find these curricula playing off one another in complex and synergistic ways. Given this amount of diversity and degree of interdependency, we believe that it is methodologically sound, as well as conceptually advisable, to *first* anchor one's investigation within the formal curriculum. As readers will see as they move through the examples provided in this book, most other-than-formal curricula detailed in these pages operate in consort with, and in response to, the formal curriculum. As such, readers may find it helpful to imagine the various types of other-than-formal curricula that operate within educational milieus as a type of *shadow curriculum*. As a general rule, therefore, we believe it is extremely difficult to make sense of what is going on within these other-than-formal dimensions of educational life without having first dissected the formal curriculum as a baseline or point of reference.

This call to begin one's analysis with a thorough understanding of the formal curriculum has a pragmatic side as well. For example, many health professions schools claim that they provide their trainees with an integrated curriculum. A few even assert that their curriculum is "fully integrated" (perhaps implying that other schools have achieved only "partial integration"— whatever oxymoronic image that is supposed to conjure up). Nonetheless, few schools have taken the time and effort to identify in detail (which, for us, means not only the pieces, but all of their interconnections) the full range of influences that drive teaching *and* learning in the arena of health professions education. Curricula mapping is one possible tool in achieving a true systems-level view of education, but once again, the devil is in the details (Harden 2001; Cameron et al. 2012). Constructing a detailed accounting of what one does, along with how the pieces fit together (or not), is a difficult undertaking. Moreover, and as we detail in our introduction, significant curricular events can be left off maps—with some of these now "non-events" rendered invisible by the very success with which they have become incorporated into the curriculum.

Nonetheless, mapping is an important tool, not just to set the baseline from which to view the other-than-formal pieces of the pedagogical puzzle, but as a way to directly explore the possible interconnections and the disjunctures between the curriculum faculty believe they deliver and the curriculum students believe they are receiving. For example, Plaza and colleagues (2007) asked both faculty and PharmD students to generate graphical curriculum maps and to rank the relative importance of each domain in their maps in order to explore the "intended/delivered" versus the "experienced" curriculum. In this study, the investigators found appreciable concordance between the intended/delivered and the experienced curriculum—something they would not have found had they not looked at both sides of the curriculum picture. This article also serves as a wonderful example, given our previous discussion about terminology, about how one set of terms (for example, intended/delivered versus experienced) can work just as well as others (for example, formal versus hidden) in exploring a given issue.

The final reason for beginning one's examination with the formal before moving to the other-than-formal aspects of educational life relates to a technical and often underappreciated point in writings on the HC. Strictly speaking, references to the HC as a positive or negative influence do so *in terms of* the formal curriculum. Thus, a school may claim (formal curriculum) that it is in the business of creating "physician leaders." Having identified this focus, we then might want to examine the full range of formal educational activities taking place within a given educational setting—including what faculty are taught via faculty development programs—to see how this intended focus ("leadership") is supported or undercut within the overall educational milieu. We *then* would move to examine how other (hidden, informal, null, and so on) types of influences might either support or undercut this stated focus on leadership. There is, however, nothing within the HC framework mandating that a focus on leadership, or any other issue for that matter, is or *should be* considered a positive aspiration. Perhaps a school's stated goal is to produce "pharmacy despots" or "clinical gods"?

However distasteful such an end point might sound, adopting an HC perspective means exploring how things taking place within the rest of the educational milieu might function to support or undercut that goal. For all practical purposes, the stated goal, from an HC perspective, is value neutral. It is neither good nor bad, positive nor negative. In this sense, the "value" or impact of the other-than-formal dimensions of educational life come into play only when we examine whether that goal is being supported or undercut by these other dimensions of the learning environment. In short, the HC is a positive influence when it supports the formal curriculum, even if one feels that the goals of the formal or intended curriculum are distasteful or otherwise questionable.

None of the preceding discussion, however, should be taken to mean that one *must* begin all inquiries with the formal curriculum. After all, one may stumble upon some other-than-formal aspect of organizational life and have this serve as an investigatory launch point. Nonetheless, and however one might choose to explore the tacit dimensions of learning, never to examine what the organization says is happening would be a major analytical mistake.

An example of how one might begin one's probe at the level of the *formal* curriculum is found in a recent *Academic Medicine* study reporting that relatively few US medical schools formally embed issues of race, ethnicity, underrepresented minorities, health disparities, the "health of the public," or similar themes in their mission statements (Grbic et al. 2013). If we are interested in exploring this apparent void using an HC perspective, we would move beyond mission statements to explore the variety of additional ways in which underrepresented minorities, and so on, might appear in formal organizational statements of "what we do" and "what is." Once this is completed, and having done so exhaustively, we next would turn to an equally detailed look at the other-than-formal aspects of a given school's learning environment that may contribute to this void. Perhaps we find that mission statements are the exception rather than the rule, and that US medical schools are peppered with formal statements and structures supporting the place and presence of underrepresented minorities in their schools. Alternatively, we may not only find an absence of such formal materials, but also learn from students that they see all kinds of tacit messages in their learning environments that imply that underrepresented minority patients are less valued than majority patients or scripted to receive certain types of treatment interventions rather than others. Whatever the outcome, we never will see the big picture unless we are willing to troll deeply within *both* the formal and the other-than-formal dimensions of educational life as we seek answers to the complexities of these social environments.

Finally, readers should not interpret the wealth of methodological details and insights contained in the aforementioned chapters as an edict that research into the other-than-formal aspects of educational life *must* be exemplars of exactitude. One of our favorite studies on the HC of undergraduate medical education was conducted by Naheed Dosani, a (then) McMaster University undergraduate medical student (Dosani 2010). Dosani's approach, although simple in its directness, was a highly effective probe into the less obvious aspects of medical school life. In preparation for a presentation on the HC, Dosani went to the Internet and asked his peers across Canada to answer the following question: "What things have you learned in medical school that you weren't supposed to?" He then compiled his peers' responses into a David Letterman–style Top Ten List, much to both the pleasure and the consternation of his audience. Although Dosani's question certainly is not the only portal into the HC, it was revealing and thought-provoking. In summary, even though methodological sophistication has its upsides, there is no sin in being unassumingly direct.

Issue Three: The HC as a Positive (and Negative) Force

Across this book, contributors have devoted a healthy degree of attention to the fact (and it is a fact) that the hidden curriculum can function as a positive as well as a negative force. Indeed, most organizations hope (and expect) that there will be an appreciable alignment between their stated mission and goals and their actions.

Such expectations notwithstanding, there are a few qualifications that need explication. The first is the likelihood or possibility of alignment. Organizations are complex creatures. Among their many functions, organizations send out a constant stream of messages, and do so to an equally diverse set of audiences—both external and internal. Some of these messages are intended. Others are not. Some are formally delivered. Others come via more indirect or tacit routes. Some are recognized (by the organization), while others fly beneath the organizational radar—until, *perhaps*, they bounce back as others demand to know exactly what the organization had in mind when it said or did not say, acted or did not act, in this way or that. The sheer volume of these messages, coupled with the fact that what is said can be quite different from what is heard or learned, underscores the relative difficulty of achieving alignment.

A simple exercise may illustrate this point. Take your index fingers, hold them in front of your face, and then bring the tips together. Although the act itself may be reasonably straightforward, there is only one way—or plane—that permits these two objects to be in alignment and therefore connected. Alternatively, there are a vast number of planes that contribute to misalignment.

A second and also previously mentioned point is that whatever its valence, the HC is deemed positive or negative in terms of the formal curriculum. If the HC supports the formal curriculum, then it functions in a positive manner. If it does not, then it operates in a more countervailing manner.

There is, however, a more fundamental and underappreciated issue within the HC literature having to do with the HC being seen as a positive or negative force. By its very nature, the HC has the potential to stand in opposition to the sanctioned and authoritative voice that operates within a given domain of social life—which in our case is the life-space of health professions education. Within this context, the formal curriculum is the stated, intended, and most significantly, the *authoritative* voice of the organization or group in question. Although the HC need not always be negative, and thus something to be overcome or countered, it has the potential, by definition, to be an *alternative* or even *antithetical* framing to that being offered up by the powers that be. This antagonistic potential is part of what makes the HC irreverent, insidious, threatening, and often dismissed as fictional and irrelevant by those powers. Quite literally, the HC is a curriculum that is *not-in-their-voice*.

The fact that the HC can literally stand in opposition to the official version of things has great import for those who want to do work in or on the HC, whether that be through writing papers, conducting studies, or giving presentations on health professions education. Although what you say may resonate as spot-on for some, it may literally offend others, particularly those in positions of power, and thus those who create the mission statements, course curricula, competencies, and so on. The notion that there may be *other* ways of looking at things—and that these *other* ways may be more foundational to what *their* trainees learn about what it means to be a nurse, physical therapist, dentist, or phlebotomist—is not a value-neutral message. In many cases, HC work can biopsy things that *will be* embarrassing. In turn, the investigator, writer, or speaker *will* be viewed as impertinent—at best, for those who create the formal curriculum *will* feel attacked, misunderstood, or slighted.

Readers are welcome to (re)visit our all-too-real case example in the introduction, where one of us sought to interject an HC perspective into a group that had been charged with reforming the curriculum at a particular medical school. The surface response (as detailed in our introduction) was to "be quiet." What was not said in the introduction, but probably was contemplated by at least some of the faculty in that curriculum reform group, was that the nudge in question was not a "team player," or perhaps was even a "troublemaker." Be forewarned.

New Directions and Challenges

As we look forward in time, there are multiple examples in this book of how we might take the HC in new directions and into new arenas of investigation. For example, the chapter by Hodges and Kuper on the reform of Canadian medical education is a study(ies)-in-waiting on several levels. If "addressing the HC" has become one of Canada's ten reform initiatives, how will this policy directive be implemented (if at all) both in terms of reform design (what is to be done) and reform implementation (what do these design initiatives actually look like as they unfold on the educational shop floor)? At minimum, we need to ask how one might visualize, at a national level, what it means to "address the HC." Even more important is how we might view such an initiative across Canada's seventeen medical schools or even within the nine provinces in which these schools are located. If nothing else, the opportunity to conduct a comparative analysis of the HC across these various social and political constituencies would be a substantive methodological undertaking. Similarly, Day and Benner's (chapter 12) insights into nursing's struggle to recalibrate its theory-over-practice instructional paradigm and the identification of nursing's signature pedagogy (situated coaching) beg for investigations into how this shift is occurring. After all, focusing on differentiating between pronouncements versus implementation and experience is key to approaching issues form an HC perspective.

Numerous other chapters and examples in this book suggest future initiatives and research possibilities for the HC. Moving no further into this book than its first two parts (Working within the Framework; Theoretical Considerations), Stern's (chapter 1) focus on parables as a window into the HC; Hundert's (chapter 2) extended case study of the Match; Taylor and Wendland's (chapter 4) focus on how we create our own invisibilities; Wear, Zarconi, and Garden's (chapter 5) focus on assessment practices; and Lempp and Cribb's (chapter 6) emphasis on the structuring effects of the HC with respect to power, authority, status, prestige, and occupational stratification all point to important change and research issues. Whatever the particular topic, issue, or foci, the ultimate goal is to better understand how learning environments are both structured and experienced, and to move beyond what the school or faculty say they deliver into the realm of context and culture. Ultimately, we seek to better understand the dynamics and complexity that envelop the social and structural relations that make up the educational milieu.

The remainder of this chapter is divided into three sections. First, and in addition to the previous examples, we will highlight three additional examples of how we might employ the HC as an analytic tool. Second, we will share some thoughts on how readers might identify and work with a substantial, yet unrecognized piece of the HC landscape—namely, work that draws upon HC principles yet does not employ an HC lexicon. Finally, and in an afterword, we want to return to a vignette detailed in the introduction on being a solitary HC voice in a group charged with "curriculum reform." Here, we will add some closing thoughts on the need to move from an N of 1 to a critical mass of HC advocates in the service of orchestrating reform with change.

Our first example, or challenge, is a recent AAMC report identifying a range of new competencies for undergraduate medical education (Englander et al. 2013). Graduate medical education has had its list of six core competencies for nearly fifteen years, but this is the first time that undergraduate medical education has *substantively* moved into the competency arena. How might an HC lens help with both framing and implementing these competencies? We will offer a few thoughts.

Our second example is a rapidly unfolding arena of health professions education—interprofessional education (IPE). Here, we build on one of our own chapters, by Jill Thistlethwaite (chapter 14), and challenge educators to think more broadly not only about the variety of messages that students can encounter as they move through their IPE experiences, but also about the variety of laws and organizational policies that govern who gets to do what within different healthcare settings. We have been talking about IPE for decades, yet studies continue to document deep-seated cultural divides not only between healthcare occupations, but also within many of these same occupational groups (Resnick 2013). In the 1990s, we learned that simply adding more ethics courses did not necessarily make medical students more ethical (Hafferty and Franks 1994). We suspect that adequately addressing contemporary issues of teamwork and interprofessional training will not be accomplished solely by adding more IPE courses to the pedagogical fire. Issues of context, along with occupational and workplace culture, will have to be addressed as well.

Our third example has us visit the arena of medical ethics and ethics education and, therefore, brings us back full circle to a topic area first explored in 1994 by Hafferty and Franks—this time with some new thoughts in mind.

Our fourth set of new directions and challenges focuses on issues of professionalism and professional formation. Currently, these two topics form the bulk of the HC literature, at least within medicine, and both topics appear prominently throughout this book. Because of this attention, we wanted to include some closing thoughts about using the HC as a lever for change around these issues.

In our last New Directions example, we turn to the aforementioned *hidden* HC literature to challenge readers to be more inclusive in their thinking by exploring how they might identify articles or books that adopt an HC perspective, even if the authors do not formally label their work as belonging to this genre of analysis.

Finally, in an afterword, we explore the dangers of being a solo HC voice in a wilderness of "curriculum reform."

New Directions A: Competencies and Undergraduate Medical Education

In 2013 the AAMC identified a set of fifty-eight competency standards that extend across eight (the original ACGME six plus two) domains of medical training (Englander et al. 2013). The AAMC sees these domains and their respective competencies as applicable to "any health care profession" and as something that can "provide a single, relevant infrastructure for curricular resources" (Englander et al. 2013, 1088). These are the original ACGME competencies:

(1) *patient care* ("provide patient-centered care that is compassionate, appropriate, and effective for the treatment of health problems and the promotion of health");

(2) *knowledge for practice* ("demonstrate knowledge of established and evolving biomedical, clinical, epidemiological, and social-behavioral sciences, as well as the application of this knowledge to patient care");

(3) *practice-based learning and improvement* ("demonstrate the ability to investigate and evaluate one's care of patients, to appraise and assimilate specific evidence, and to continuously improve patient care based on constant self-evaluation and life-long learning");

(4) *interpersonal and communication skills* ("demonstrate interpersonal and communication skills that result in the effective exchange of information and collaboration with patients, their families, and health professionals");

(5) *professionalism* ("demonstrate a commitment to carrying out professional responsibilities and an adherence to ethical principles"); and

(6) *systems-based practice* ("demonstrate an awareness of and responsiveness to the larger context and system of healthcare, as well as the ability to call effectively on other resources in the system to provide optimal health care"). (Englander et al. 2013, 1091–92)

To this core, the AAMC has added two competencies (Englander et al. 2013, 1092):

(7) *interprofessional collaboration* ("demonstrate the ability to engage in an interprofessional team in a manner that optimizes safe, effective patient-and-population-centered care"); and

(8) *personal and professional development* ("demonstrate the qualities required to sustain lifelong personal and professional growth").

To date, the domain receiving the most HC attention in the medical education literature has been professionalism. Although most of this literature focuses on the role of the HC either in promoting or retarding things like professional formation and student-based professionalism (rather than on professionalism as a competency per se), this literature remains the single best example of how we might think about an intersection between the HC and other competency domains. There is, however, a story worth recounting here, even in its truncated version, given the fact that it illustrates how competencies as formal curricula can intersect with the HC and do so in unanticipated ways.

Beginning in the 1990s, medical educators began to roll out a variety of strategies to promote professionalism—all with the best of intentions (Hafferty and Levinson 2008). These included new definitions and assessment tools, as well as new professionalism codes, charters, competencies, and curriculum. The HC rub was that these formally embedded initiatives created a certain amount of confusion, along with a certain degree of anger and cynicism, among trainees (Brainard and Brislen 2007; Finn et al. 2010). It was easier, it turned out, to create definitions, assessment tools, codes, charters, competencies, and related formal course material than it was to change the structure and culture of clinical practice. As a consequence, students found themselves subject to an array of countervailing messages as they moved between the classroom and the clinics. Moreover, students felt unreasonably singled out when they discovered that although they were the objects of professionalism assessment initiatives—faculty were not. In short, students felt lectured at, unduly targeted, singled out, unreasonably scrutinized, and subject to a variety of double standards. As a result, students began to push back against the "p-word." In one instance, students effectively lobbied to have the term banned from that school's educational lexicon (Goldstein et al. 2006).

This ongoing interplay of the HC and professionalism provides us with a pedagogical morality tale in which clinical practices that largely had gone unchallenged or uncriticized for decades, and thus appeared "normal" and essentially taken for granted by both practitioners and trainees, were challenged by the advent of these now formal professionalism curricula. Practices long viewed as "quite reasonable" or "entirely appropriate" no longer appeared so admirable or worthy of positive-role-model status. In turn, students felt caught in the crosshairs of these older, culturally sanctioned practices and these newer standards. We believe that similar conundrums may await the introduction of other competencies. Before we turn to an example, we need to reemphasize that none of this tension is unequivocally "bad"—at least from a sociological perspective. Yes, it is messy, and yes, this messiness may generate considerable rumblings or even cynicism within student and faculty ranks, at least in the short term. However, the long-range consequences of this messiness may be quite positive. In order to move forward, we *must* be willing to place our educational practices and learning environments under a critical lens, and the HC offers us one such tool to this end.

So, how might we think about competency domains such as interprofessional collaboration and personal and professional development (because these are the two newest domains) from an HC perspective? If we take the actual four competencies (7.1–7.4) for interprofessional collaboration and the eight (8.1–8.8) for personal and professional development as our formal curriculum (because these are the stated and intended standards), what might we find if we were to go out today and explore the hallways, exam rooms, and surgical suites of a given medical, nursing, or pharmacy program, for example, to see what the behaviors related to these two competencies might look like as they actually are practiced within the context of medical work, nursing work, and so on? Because we will be dealing with the topic of IPE in what follows, let us take (randomly) one of the eight personal and professional development competencies (in this case, 8.3: "manage conflict between personal and professional responsibilities") for a brief run-through.

Based on our previously outlined steps for launching an HC inquiry, we would begin by examining the formal curriculum and do so at two levels. First, we would look at what the AAMC has to say, about personal and professional development in general, and also about the specifics of the competency in question (8.3). Next, we would move to the organizational level to see what the medical or nursing school says it is doing to help trainees manage conflict between personal and professional responsibilities. As an additional step, we would examine how this formal curriculum dovetails with other formal statements (policies, programs, practices, and literal curricula) about personal and professional development. Do they all say the same thing? Do they all deliver the same message? All this information would fall into our formal curriculum box.

Next, we move from *saying* to *doing*, and thus how the AAMC and individual training programs operationalize personal and professional development—along with what is seen as arenas of (1) personal responsibility, (2) professional responsibility, (3) conflict between them, and (4) the appropriate management of any such conflicts (as the four domains of 8.3). Here, we begin to enter the realm of the informal curriculum. Different schools, after all, may see matters of personal and professional responsibilities, along with their conflict and resolution, in differing ways. We may even find, like our speed-limit example, that informal or tacit "rules" about these matters actually hold more sway more than the formally stated rules. Finally, although the formal standards will continue to exist, and although someone can always drag them out and say, "Here is what the AAMC says about personal and professional development," there still is the matter of how schools choose to interpret those standards *and* what the AAMC (and particularly the LCME) accepts as evidence of meeting those standards. After all, what schools offer as "proof" that they are meeting standards, and what the LCME accepts as evidence of meeting those standards, may not actually dovetail with the "letter of the law."

The level of informal group practices take us further onto the shop floor of medical education practice, and thus into the realm of how educators actually teach to this standard, and, in turn, what learners come to think constitutes adherence to these standards. What *is* going to happen for students when they are told that they are expected to (1) identify personal and professional responsibilities, (2) recognize when there is conflict between these two realms, and then (3) manage that conflict? Further, what are they being told (via the formal curriculum) about what constitutes—and does not constitute—"conflict"? What are they being told about what falls within the category of "personal" versus "professional"? Will schools tell students directly and intentionally, or will there be some other-than-formal vehicles used to transmit the school's normative culture? Moreover, what will students see being role modeled by faculty, and what will students interpret as successful conflict management, given what they learn to see (via professional formation) as a conflict versus the absence of conflict? And to add yet another layer to this picture, what are schools telling faculty with respect to any of this? Will schools initiate faculty development programs around this competency? If so, how will the "letter of the competency" be rolled out in this setting?

Finally (although there certainly are other issues), how does the school identify its responsibilities with respect to this competency? Will schools see themselves as having a responsibility to "minimize conflicts" within learning environments? If so, what steps will they take to do so? Conversely, will they see themselves as responsible solely for teaching students to acquire skills to "manage the conflicts" already present? Or, perhaps, will schools see their responsibilities as limited to admissions and to identifying applicants who have an exceedingly high "conflict management potential"? The permutations are endless, and no doubt we will see a variety of organizational responses to this new standard. Variability aside, our HC point is that whatever the organizational response, that response (or responses) will send a set of messages to faculty and students about what it means to "manage conflict between personal and professional responsibilities," and that these messages will exist and function *outside* of the formal standards themselves (for example, the formal curriculum). Finally, the same general range of issues and questions exist for any of the other domains and their related competencies identified by Englander and colleagues (2013). There are numerous possibilities for research on the HC and a competency approach to health professions training.

New Directions B: Interprofessional Education

Because the array of things that we might say about the HC of IPE is lengthy, we will be relatively circumspect in our comments. First, whatever the complexities of educational life and identity formation within one's given occupational home, these forces become even more complex and nuanced once we begin to talk about multiple occupational groups and their intersections. Nonetheless, and with these all-too-real complexities notwithstanding, an HC perspective should be tremendously helpful in understanding the continuing evolution and impact of formal IPE training and how these efforts intersect with the already established in-house educational activities (formal, informal, hidden, and null) taking place within those individual health occupations. Moreover, an HC perspective should be of additional help in understanding how the complexities of work settings, awash as they are with interoccupational dynamics, function as a source of additional informal and hidden learning as trainees are placed within the "real world" of clinical care.

One HC issue that comes to the fore when thinking about IPE is how one healthcare group comes to learn about its other healthcare brethren. Once again, we argue that one should never stop (at least from an HC perspective) with how a particular health occupation formally is cast and characterized—be that (1) by its "home" occupational group, (2) by the other occupational groups in question, or (3) by whatever formal interprofessional training context might be relevant to our inquiry. Revisiting the methodological roadmap we outlined in our earlier competency example, we initially need to determine first the formal content across these three domains and then the degree of congruence (or lack thereof) among them. Perhaps all three are in alignment? More likely, this is not the case. Instead, we may find that although the formal curriculum of a given occupational group says a great deal about itself, it says very little about the other health occupations involved in the interprofessional segment of the curriculum.

Even more likely, we may discover that the only manifest content about the skills and occupational identity of the other IPE partner groups comes within the context of whatever formal IPE is being offered. What trainees are left with, then, is an overall set of messages through which students hear a little bit of "good stuff" within their formal IPE training about what these partners can bring to the table in terms of things like patient safety or quality of healthcare, yet virtually nothing (in a formal sense) about these same groups within their own occupation-specific training. Overall, the meta-message students (and faculty, for that matter) receive is that all this learning-about-the-other must not be so important if the IPE part of their training is the only place where they hear anything about "the other." Stated in HC language, what we may discover is a null curriculum operating at full steam.

Moving on with our HC approach to IPE training, because it is highly unlikely that we would find the formal curriculum infused with disparaging content about other health occupations, it is critically important from an HC perspective to augment our journey into the formal curriculum of IPE with a detailed look at how occupational identity (one's own and others') is conveyed within the informal and the hidden curricula. Most likely, trainees will encounter a variety of messages about the value (or lack thereof) of other types of healthcare workers within the more informal or tacit domains of their learning environments. In some instances, they will see exemplars of teamwork and occupational cooperation within some clinical settings. In other instances, exactly the opposite will be the case. The formal curriculum of IPE notwithstanding, we believe trainees continue to learn a great deal more about the value of interprofessionalism and teamwork within the informal and hidden curriculum than they do within formal IPE training. There is literature on the HC and IPE (Whitehead 2007; Weaver et al. 2011; Reeves 2013), but it is small, and there are considerable opportunities for new work.

New Directions C: Ethics

Although ethics training is not highly profiled in this book, the fact remains that the first widely cited article on the hidden curriculum and medical education used ethics and ethics teaching as its analytical fulcrum (Hafferty and Franks 1994). Although there have been many subsequent articles on ethics and the HC, a number of ethics and HC issues are left to be explored. With this caveat in mind, we offer readers one example of how to go about identifying an HC issue within this domain, and we do so using an instance where the HC is *not* part of the analytic framework. As such, we are offering readers an example of a *hidden* HC article, and thus an article where the concept does not appear in the body of the article (a topic we will cover in more detail in the closing section of this chapter).

To this end, we will use a recently published commentary by Mueller and Hook (2013), "Technological and Treatment Imperatives, Life-Sustaining Technologies, and Associated Ethical and Social Challenges." The commentary covers four articles in the July 2013 issue of *Mayo Clinic Proceedings* and argues that physicians often feel under a technological or a treatment imperative when providing medical care to patients. In other words, if a treatment option is available, physicians often feel duty-bound to employ that option. Similarly, if there is a technological resource, something that one might use for diagnostic or treatment purposes, many physicians feel compelled to employ that technology. Discussions about technological imperatives have appeared both in medicine (Burger-Lux and Heaney 1986; Koenig 1988; Rothman 1997) and in sociology (Sewell and Phillips 2010).

Although the Mueller and Hook commentary and related articles discuss a range of ethical issues concerning various patient care situations, and although the commentary specifically does raise the issue of treatment and technological imperatives, what remains unexplored in these articles is any sense of how and why physicians might come to feel so compelled, or more specifically, whether trainees are either formally taught or informally learn some version of "If you have a hammer, all options are nails." Perhaps trainees receive formal instruction on their "duty to do something"? Similarly, perhaps they are explicitly taught, "When in doubt, treat" or "Employ the most advanced technological resource available"? Though possible, we doubt this is the case. Likewise, we also believe it is rather unlikely for us to find language similar to these directives in formal documents such as course descriptions or competency standards. Rather, we suspect that trainees pick up such imperative-lessons during the course of their training in a tacit or subliminal manner as they pay attention to and internalize what is happening around them, including what they see other role models doing or not doing.

The issue before us is not to solve the question of treatment and technological imperative concerns, but rather to point out that when we see (or read about) such normative patterns of behavior, ways of knowing, or particular value orientations, we need to ask, "How is it that healthcare providers act this way—or that?" Similarly, we can ask, "How is it that providers come to learn or internalize these behaviors, knowledge, and values?"

In asking such questions, we begin to move more into an HC framework. If we find out that such lessons are conveyed via the formal curriculum, then we have one answer. It may not be the only answer, but it is an answer. If such lessons are not formally conveyed, then we need to look elsewhere. This takes us into the realm of the other-than-formal curriculum, one aspect of which may be tacit or otherwise hidden. Bottom-line message: just because an article never mentions the hidden curriculum, this does not mean the concept or lens is irrelevant to what is going on.

New Directions D: On Being an HC Stranger in a Strange (allegedly non-HC) Land

In the introduction to this book, one of the editors (Joe) recounts a tale of HC woe—and personal rejection. Joe had been placed on a faculty committee charged with guiding "curricular overhaul" at his medical school (also see Balmer and Richards, chapter 10, for additional insights into how an HC lens can open up different ways of framing and understanding curriculum reform). In spite of his repeated suggestions to colleagues about how the committee might reframe issues from an HC perspective, other committee members remained decidedly unreceptive to his entreaties. Instead, their overhaul crosshairs were resolutely focused not on the school's overall learning environment, but on the more restrictive landscape of its formal curriculum. Joe functioned as a solitary HC soporific, an N of 1, and ultimately a less-than-critical mass.

Joe's story, although unique in its particulars, resonated with his coeditor (Fred). Although Fred never had the chutzpah, or integrity, to directly lobby his colleagues to recalibrate their mental models of medical education, he too had experienced faculty life as an HC stranger in a strange land—and a land where, according to the messages conveyed by faculty actions, there was no HC. Although Fred had written an early paper on the HC and medical education with his then dean (Hafferty and Franks 1994), his faculty-peers expressed little interest in considering such a framework when it came to redesigning the learning environment at his school. He too found himself functioning as an N of 1, a less-than-critical mass.

Although one of the editors (Joe) is inherently more optimistic than the other (Fred), we both genuinely believe that an HC framework offers faculty and students a viable tool for reforming the learning environments that make up health professions education—and does so in a manner that promotes reform with change. We also believe that at least four factors need to be operating in some conjoint fashion to reach a viable HC activation point. In describing these elements, we also wish to acknowledge the work of Tom Inui, Rich Frankel, Deb Litzelman, Tony Suchman, Penny Williamson, and others at Indiana University, where the principals used the tools of appreciative inquiry and hidden-informal curriculum lens to engineer a cultural shift in the learning environment of their medical school (Suchman et al. 2004; Cottingham et al. 2008). They tackled the problem first.

Our first element is leadership. No leader—no reform with change. More specifically, the leader must be both HC-savvy (must understand the underlying logic and methodology of HC inquiry) and HC-committed (must be—and must be seen—as an "HC true believer"). Indiana had such a leader. However, even though an HC-savvy and dedicated leader is necessary, it is not sufficient. At least three other elements also must be in play.

The second element is a critical mass of similarly sophisticated and true HC believers. Moreover, it helps if some members of this cabal hold positions of formal authority (dean of admissions, dean of student affairs, dean of education, and so on). Indiana had such a team, both in the formation of a critical mass and as holders of key authority positions. However, as leadership positions changed, and as the original members circulated out of key positions, the direction and momentum of change began to shift as well. Tending to the hidden dimensions of organizational life is an ongoing proposition.

Third, and much as we hate to say it, there needs to be a visible commitment of resources, particularly financial resources, associated with any HC reform initiative. In medical education, and we suspect health education in general, the coin of the realm is $$$. Funding, whether it is funded research or funded programs, means status and power in the health professions.

Funding also means the ability to acquire other symbols of power and influence, such as space. However, funding cannot come from just any source. HC initiatives cannot be fueled by the reallocation of internal resources and thus viewed by community members as a source of impoverishment for somebody's pet (and loved) programs. Indiana had considerable external funding to launch its reform initiatives. Indiana had an initial and appreciable source of external funding. The degree to which this initial funding was replaced or augmented by other funding sources (including internal) is not known to the editors.

The final element is stories—stories about the school, but stories that must be told from within an HC framework. These stories can be positive or appreciative inquiry stories; stories about countervailing messages received by faculty and students; or even stories of essentially nondescript, mundane, or more equivocal events that are taking place within the community. Medical schools, like all organizations and communities, are awash with accounts and stories about what it means to be an insider or member, how one satisfactorily makes the transition from outsider to insider status, and how the community responds to disruptions of its taken-for-granted understanding of things. In short, all groups have an oral culture. In some instances, stories circulate among the group as a whole. In other instances, certain stories will circulate more restrictively among members of particular subgroups within the community.

Our point here is that although these stories are essential to the functional integrity and well-being of any social group, they often are viewed by community members as "simply stories" and thus stories without any deeper purpose or meaning. As such, stories told about what happens to people—particularly unwitting outsiders—who violate "local norms" may be viewed as having little meaning other than to pass along some surface account of humor or woe—as opposed to an organizational or community morality tale conveying important messages about what happens to those who violate community values and norms. In the context of the present discussion, what has to happen is that some of these stories need to be relabeled and recognized as HC stories and thus stories that convey important messages about the community and how it *really* operates; and if some of these subterrestrial meanings are rather antithetical to formally stated community values and objectives, then these conflicts need to be recognized as well.

An example might be helpful. One of us recently received a group-faculty email from the dean of education at a medical school, in which the dean described a situation he felt needed to change. The basic situation was that students were hearing one set of facts from one faculty member and a second, and contrary, set of facts from another—all in the same course. Knowledge and understanding aside (Which "fact" was right?), the manifest problem for students came at exam time when students became confused about how they should answer a given exam question on the topic or "fact" in question. The long-standing response from the school to students on this issue (and it was a long-standing problem) was for students to answer the question depending on which faculty member had written the question. If faculty member A had written the question, then the right answer was X. If faculty member B had written the question, the correct answer was Y.

However grateful students might be for having a definitive answer to their rock-and-hard-place dilemma, the school did lose an important opportunity for broader structural changes, had the situation been approached as a *possible* HC problem. First, the problem was one of long standing and did exist in more than one course. Similar situations had been around for over two decades. Second, what were students learning as a result of these practices? We can imagine at least two sets of possible lessons: those at the course level, and those at the level of how administration chose to respond to long-standing student concerns.

At the course level, and because many of these conflicts occurred between basic science (PhD) and clinician (MD) faculty (with each telling students that the other did not know what he or she was talking about), students were learning (at minimum) that the science and practice of medicine can be at considerable loggerheads—regardless of what the medical school had to say about the close and interdependent nature of science and medicine. Parenthetically, although the countervailing message of discord may have ultimately been an important lesson for students to learn, it was not a part of their formal curriculum. Further, students were learning that their school community was not all that community-like, that faculty did not necessarily coordinate what they were teaching, and that school pronouncements about colleagueship and mutual respect were little more than rhetoric posing as professionalism.

At the level of the school (and thus at the level of the administrative response to the situation), students learned that faculty could do or say almost anything without recourse, and that student concerns or complaints carried little weight. Finally, and even more fundamental, students learned that the "truth," or the "correct answer" to the exam question (Was it what faculty A said? Or faculty B? Some mixture of the two?) was not an important issue, at least for the school. Instead, what students learned was that the best way to resolve such a conflict or disagreement was to dance around the conflict, not to confront those directly involved (faculty), and that exam questions will hardly ever be changed except (perhaps) for the *most* egregious of circumstances (and that this situation was not one of them).

By not framing this situation as an HC problem, faculty lost the opportunity to explore at least two major issues: (1) what students were learning from this set of practices, and (2) once identified, whether *other* aspects of the learning environment also were contributing to this set of tacit or indirect messages. Perhaps, for the sake of this discussion, there *were* several additional educational practices where students came to learn the same set of messages outlined earlier. As such, addressing one vehicle, such as the problem or transgression just outlined, though still important, may not solve the overall problem because the other "reinforcing" practices now will continue to be unidentified and therefore unremediated. Moreover, students and faculty will now "see" that when a given problem is identified, and when it is addressed, the approach to take (in a normative sense) is piecemeal, thus sending out yet another set of messages about how the school actually (as opposed to rhetorically) views the structure of its educational enterprise. From an HC perspective, answers rarely come from focusing on the stimulus or event that percolates to the surface. They almost always lie within a network or system of precipitants.

Afterword: On Encountering a Hidden, Hidden Curriculum Article

As readers exit this book, we hope you will maintain the broadest possible take on the HC as a conceptual lens and analytic tool. When we opened this chapter, we referred to the HC as a heuristic device for obtaining a reasonably quick, valid, and most important, a contrarian look into the social and organizational fabrics that make up health professions education. In an earlier section of this chapter, we also noted that education scholars have used a broad array of terms to capture the formal and other-than-formal aspects of educational life. Some are synonyms. Others are not. We hope you will use whatever nomenclature best serves your purposes.

As we take our leave, we do so with one additional caveat or warning. Although there is a growing literature on the HC and health professions education, there are other literatures that draw on an HC framework, or that tackle HC issues, yet never employ an HC interpretive framework or lexicon. This is not a shortcoming of these publications. One does not have to talk the HC talk to walk the HC walk. Nonetheless, a consequence of this lacuna is that when one does a keyword search using HC terms, none of these works will be identified as an "HC publication." In short, and in addition to all of the other HC issues covered in this book, what we are talking about here is a rather large *hidden* HC literature.

In addition to individual articles (examples follow), there are whole literatures that might be considered, to one degree or another, as "HC friendly" or "HC inclined." For example, there are literally thousands of articles that reveal a mind-numbing degree of variability in healthcare practices, be that by setting, by provider type, by patient demographics, and so on. These data often can be chilling, particularly from a patient-safety or quality-of-care perspective. So where does the HC intersect with this body of work? Short answer: Everywhere. Medical, nursing, PT, and pharmacy students *all* learn their craft within this cacophony of practices, and thus tacitly encounter a broad variety of messages about what it means to be a good practitioner and to carry out good-quality healthcare.

In the end, and often with great cynicism, trainees see it all—undertreatment, overtreatment, cost-prohibitive treatments, experimental treatments, iatrogenic-producing treatments, provider-centric (as opposed to patient-centered) treatments, and so on—and they often do so while hearing those practices characterized (explicitly or implicitly) by someone (often someone in authority) as "good-quality healthcare." In turn, those engaged in carrying out such work practices often are held up to trainees (again, either explicitly or implicitly) as "good role models." Given the important function of apprenticeship training in healthcare, we need to be much more vigilant about how articles on different aspects of healthcare delivery *also* convey important things to us about the HC of medical and health professions education.

Broad categories aside, there are many specific instances of hidden HC articles. One example is "Professionalism in Medicine: Results of a National Survey of Physicians" (Campbell et al. 2007). This article is a national study of physicians in six specialties that sought to "ascertain the extent to which practicing physicians agree with and act consistently with norms of professionalism" (795). The investigators found that although physicians were likely to affirm a variety of professionalism principles, their self-reported behavioral adherence to those norms or principles was an altogether different matter. Once again, we ask what messages trainees might receive about the meaning of professionalism or what it means to be a professional from role models who believe one thing and yet act in a different manner? At root, the Campbell article is very much an HC study, yet the term *hidden curriculum* and other associated terms do not appear in this article. Nor are study findings discussed in terms of their impact as education issues.

Another example directly involves an educational setting. In this study, Klatt and Klatt (2011) asked "How Much Is Too Much Reading for Medical Students? Assigned Reading and Reading Rates at One Medical School." The authors found that faculty were assigning students a staggering amount of reading, ranging from twenty-eight to forty-one hours per week (with hours being determined by the amount of material divided by an externally validated reading rate). From an HC perspective, we might ask, "How did students make sense of this practice? Were faculty being mean? Were they just oblivious? Did one faculty have any idea what other faculty were assigning?" More to our HC point, "What message(s) did students glean from having to operate under such a reading deluge?" The list of possible answers, particularly to this last question, requires that we question students directly. Whatever we might learn about the more tacit or even hidden messages buried within such a practice, one thing we do know is that concepts such as hidden, informal, and null curricula were *not* part of this article. As such, and like the Campbell study, you will not find this article by doing an HC keyword search. Nonetheless, it very much is in the HC genre.

Hidden HC works are not limited to healthcare. A quick visit to Amazon.com will uncover literally hundreds of books that promise to provide readers with some backstage, inside, secret, or hidden insights into one issue or another, with results limited only by one's keyword imagination. There are a multitude of *insider's guides* for getting into schools like Harvard or landing a job at a Big-4 accounting firm. There are books about the *unwritten rules* of sports, social relationships, and organizational life. There are books about the *invisible* aspects of the universe, mathematics, the US Constitution, and intuition. Then there are books that tell you *what they don't teach you* at X, Y, or Z school. Popular magazines also are rife with articles on such topics, including a recent publication in *Forbes* on "nine dangerous things you were taught in school" (Hagy 2012) ranging from (1) "the people in charge have all the answers," (4) "what the books say is always true," (7) "standardized tests measure your value," to (9) "the purpose of your education is your future career." This last publication is written within a classic

HC framework regarding primary school education, yet the term *hidden curriculum* never appears in the article.

Finally, and returning to healthcare, readers may encounter (probably by accident) books that do formally employ the HC as an interpretive tool, but without the term appearing in the title or book description. This is the case for Prentice's *Bodies in Formation: An Ethnography of Anatomy and Surgery Education* (2012) even though she formally devotes an entire chapter to HC issues. Then there are books with an almost perfect HC title (for example, Kansagra's 2011 *Everything I Learned in Medical School Besides All the Book Stuff*), but where the term never appears. Neither of the books just mentioned will be identified on Amazon.com using "hidden curriculum" in a keyword search.

If there is a moral to this afterword, it is to be HC-savvy. Some publications will tell you, in no uncertain terms, that they are about the HC. Others will only hint at the possibility, perhaps via an otherwise-worded title or by virtue of one's study design (like the Campbell article). Then there are publications about health professions education that, at a first or even second glance, have nothing to do with the HC, and yet something is there, scratching at the surface, sending out its silent message.

Perhaps Sherlock Holmes said it best in the 1892 short story "Silver Blaze" (Doyle). Holmes and Watson were investigating the disappearance of a famous racehorse named Silver Blaze when Holmes happened to notice the behavior of the watchdog on the night in question.

[Gregory, Scotland Yard detective:] "Is there any other point to which you would wish to draw my attention?"
[Holmes:] "To the curious incident of the dog in the night-time."
[Gregory:] "The dog did nothing in the night-time."
[Holmes:] "That was the curious incident."

Contributors

Dorene Balmer, PhD, RD, is associate director of the Center for Research, Innovation and Scholarship in Medical Education at Texas Children's Hospital and associate professor in the Department of Pediatrics, Section of Academic General Pediatrics, at Baylor College of Medicine. Dr. Balmer started her professional career as a nutritionist at the Children's Hospital of Philadelphia. Fascinated by the "clinical classroom" in which she worked, she pursued a doctoral degree at Temple University, a postdoctoral research fellowship at the University of Pennsylvania, and an education generalist position at Columbia University's Center for Education Research and Evaluation. In her current position, Dr. Balmer supports and collaborates with pediatric faculty, residents, fellows, and other stakeholders engaged in education research and other forms scholarship. She is the 2009 recipient of the Pediatric Academic Society's Helfer Award, which recognizes creative, scholarly work in pediatric education. Dr. Balmer regularly shares her passion for qualitative inquiry in medical education through professional presentations, publications, and national organizations.

Claire E. Bender, MD, MPH, is a consultant and professor in the Department of Radiology as well as dean of the Mayo School of Health Sciences. She received her undergraduate degree at Nebraska Wesleyan, her medical degree at the University of Nebraska College of Medicine, and completed residencies in internal medicine and radiology at Mayo Clinic, Rochester, Minnesota. She received her master's degree in public health from the University of Minnesota. Dr. Bender is chair of the Mayo Clinic Rochester Education Committee, Allied Health Professional Academic and Promotions Committee. She has chaired the Career and Leadership Development Committee, Diversity Committee, Personnel Committee, and been a member of numerous Mayo Clinic and Department of Radiology committees. Dr. Bender also participates in several medical organizations outside of Mayo Clinic and serves on the editorial boards for *American Journal of Roentgenology* and *Radiology*, and she reviews articles for several other journals. Dr. Bender also developed the Radiography Program at the Mayo School of Health Sciences, and has served on the boards of the Joint Review Committee on Education in Radiologic Technology and the American Registry of Radiologic Technologists.

Patricia Benner, RN, PhD, is the Distinguished Visiting Professor at Seattle University College of Nursing. She led the Carnegie Foundation for the Advancement of Teaching National Nursing Education study titled "Educating Nurses: A Call for Radical Transformation." She is author of *From Novice to Expert: Excellence and Power in Nursing Practice* and *Clinical Wisdom and Interventions in Acute and Critical Care* with Pat Hooper Kyriakidis and Daphne Stannard. She hosts a faculty development website, EducatingNurses.com.

Alan Cribb, PhD, is an applied philosopher based in the Centre for Public Policy Research, King's College London. His major methodological interest is in the development of an interdisciplinary applied philosophy and, in particular, in building links between perspectives in applied philosophy and empirically grounded analyses of policy and practice. He has pursued this interest in relation to a number of substantive themes, including public health and professional ethics as well as work on medicines and prescribing. In recent years, his personal scholarship and collaborations have focused on (a) the changing nature of healthcare and education relationships; (b) science studies and the sociology and ethics of translational research; and (c) aims and methods in applied and interdisciplinary ethics. Previous research includes theoretical work on philosophy of social science and empirical research on the experience and management of chronic illness, particularly cancer.

Richard L. Cruess, MD, is professor of orthopedic surgery and a member of the Centre for Medical Education at McGill University. He graduated with a bachelor of arts from Princeton in 1951 and received his MD from Columbia University in 1955. An orthopedic surgeon, he served as chair of orthopedics (1976–81), directing a basic science laboratory and publishing extensively in the field. He was dean of the faculty of medicine at McGill University from 1981 to 1995. He was president of the Canadian Orthopedic Association (1977–78), the American Orthopedic Research Society (1975–1976), and the Association of Canadian Medical Colleges (1992–94). He is an Officer of the Order of Canada and of *L'Ordre National du Québec*. Since 1995, with his wife Dr. Sylvia Cruess, he has taught and carried out independent research on professionalism in medicine. They have published widely on the subject and been invited speakers at universities, hospitals, and professional organizations throughout the world. In 2010 McGill University established the Richard and Sylvia Cruess Chair in Medical Education.

Sylvia R. Cruess, MD, is an endocrinologist, professor of medicine, and member of the Centre for Medical Education at McGill University. She previously served as director of the Metabolic Day Centre (1968–78) and as medical director of the Royal Victoria Hospital (1978–95) in Montreal. She was a member of the Deschamps Commission on Conduct of Research on Humans in Establishments. She graduated from Vassar College with a bachelor of arts in 1951 and received her MD from Columbia University in 1955. Since 1995, with her husband Dr. Richard Cruess, she has taught and carried out research on professionalism in medicine. They have published extensively on the subject and been invited speakers at universities, hospitals, and professional organizations throughout the world. She is an Officer of the Order of Canada, and in 2011 McGill University established the Richard and Sylvia Cruess Chair in Medical Education.

Lisa Day, PhD, RN, CNE, is assistant professor at Duke University School of Nursing. Dr. Day was a consultant on the first phase of the Robert Wood Johnson Foundation–funded project, Quality and Safety Education in Nursing (QSEN), and is coauthor, with Patricia Benner, Molly Sutphen, and Vickie Leonard, of the landmark publication *Educating Nurses: A Call for Radical Transformation.* She provides faculty development workshops for schools of nursing worldwide.

Kelly Edwards, PhD, is associate professor in the Department of Bioethics and Humanities and core faculty for the Institute for Public Health Genetics at the University of Washington School of Medicine. She is also an acting associate dean in the University of Washington Graduate School. She received an MA in medical ethics and a PhD in philosophy of education from the University of Washington–Seattle. Her work incorporates communication and public engagement as an ethical obligation for clinicians and scientists. She is director of the Ethics and Outreach Core for the NIEHS-funded Center for Ecogenetics and Environmental Health, co-director of the Regulatory Support and Bioethics Core for the Institute for Translational Health Sciences (CTSA), and lead investigator with the NHGRI-funded Center for Genomics and Healthcare Equality.

Shaun C. Ewen, PhD, is an Australian Aboriginal academic at the University of Melbourne. He is professor and director of the Melbourne Poche Centre for Indigenous Health. He has an undergraduate degree in applied science (physiotherapy), a master's degree in international studies, and a doctoral degree in medical education. In his decade of clinical experience, he worked across Australia, Africa, and Europe, in contexts including remote, rural, and urban clinics. His master's research focused on the South

African Truth and Reconciliation Commission, and he undertook a year as a visiting researcher at the University of the Witwatersrand, Johannesburg. His doctoral research focused on perceptions and practices of cultural competence at the University of Otago, Christchurch, School of Medicine. He is the inaugural associate dean (Indigenous Development) in the Faculty of Medicine, Dentistry and Health Sciences, The University of Melbourne, a senior position created to ensure the faculty embeds Indigenous values and perspectives across its core work. He has research interests and expertise in Indigenous health, cultural competence, and values in medical education.

Richard M. Frankel, PhD, is professor of medicine and statewide director for professionalism competency at Indiana University School of Medicine. He is director of the Mary Margaret Walther Center for Research and Education in Palliative Care and associate director of the Indianapolis VA Center of Excellence in Implementing Evidence-Based Practice. He is a qualitative health services researcher whose interests include face-to-face communication and its effects on quality, safety and outcomes of care; and more recently, using approaches from the positive social sciences to change the culture of academic health sciences centers. He has been a medical educator for the past thirty years and was the co-program director of the internal medicine residency program at Highland Hospital–University of Rochester. He also served as vice president for research at the Fetzer Institute, a mind, body, and spirit foundation in Kalamazoo, Michigan.

Rebecca Garden, PhD, is associate professor of bioethics and humanities at Upstate Medical University in Syracuse, New York. She received her doctorate from Columbia University's Department of English. Committed to cross-disciplinary conversations, she has published in journals ranging from *New Literary History* to the *Journal for General Internal Medicine* and *Disability Studies Quarterly* to the *Journal of Clinical Ethics*; and she teaches the health humanities, disability studies, and bioethics to nursing and medical students, residents, and hospital social workers, as well as arts and sciences undergraduates. She is executive director of the Consortium for Culture and Medicine, an interinstitutional and interdisciplinary research and education collaborative.

Elizabeth H. Gaufberg, MD, MPH, is a double-boarded internist-psychiatrist and associate professor of medicine and psychiatry at Harvard Medical School (HMS). Dr. Gaufberg's work spans the undergraduate, graduate, and continuing education stages of physician professional formation. She is director of the Cambridge Health Alliance (CHA) Center for Professional

Development, director of the psychosocial curriculum for the CHA Internal Medicine Residency Program, and Patient-Doctor III Site Director for the HMS Cambridge Integrated Clerkship. Dr. Gaufberg cofounded the CHA Medical Humanities Initiative and is a founding editor of *Ausculta-tions*, the award-winning CHA employee literary arts journal. Dr. Gaufberg holds several national leadership roles in medical education including the Jean and Harvey Picker Director of the Arnold P. Gold Foundation Research Institute for Humanism in Healthcare. A Gold Foundation Professorship has allowed her to pursue a longitudinal research study on graduates of the HMS Cambridge Integrated Clerkship. Her innovative curricula on professional boundaries, the stigma of addictions, and the hidden curriculum are in use in hundreds of medical training institutions worldwide. In her personal life, Elizabeth Gaufberg is married to Slava Gaufberg, a CHA emergency physician and residency program director. Together they are raising four teenaged daughters.

Frederic W. Hafferty, PhD, is professor of medical education; associate dean for professionalism, College of Medicine; and associate director of the Program for Professionalism and Ethics at the Mayo Clinic. He received his undergraduate degree in social relations from Harvard in 1969 and his PhD in medical sociology from Yale in 1976. He is the author of *Into the Valley: Death and the Socialization of Medical Students* (Yale University Press); *The Changing Medical Profession: An International Perspective* (Oxford University Press) with John McKinlay; and *Sociology and Complexity Science: A New Field of Inquiry* (Springer) with Brian Castellani. Forthcoming books include an edited volume, *The Hidden Curriculum in Health Professions Education* with Joseph O'Donnell (Dartmouth College Press), and *Understanding Professionalism* with Wendy Levinson, Katherine Lucy, and Shiphra Ginsburg (Lange). He is past chair of the Medical Sociology Section of the American Sociological Association and associate editor of the *Journal of Health and Social Behavior*. He currently sits on the Association of American Medical College's Council of Academic Societies and the American Board of Medical Specialties standing committee on Ethics and Professionalism. His research focuses on the evolution of medicine's professionalism movement, mapping social networks within medical education, the application of complexity theory to medical training, issues of medical socialization, and disability studies.

Janet P. Hafler, EdD, is professor of pediatrics and assistant dean for educational scholarship at Yale University School of Medicine. As the leader for educator development in the Teaching and Learning Center, her responsibilities include the creation and implementation of medical education programs for teaching faculty, students, and residents. Throughout her career, she has nurtured a climate where faculty, students, and residents are exposed to cutting-edge literature, and has focused on assisting them to explore innovative ways to effectively promote learning in both the classroom and clinical settings. Dr. Hafler runs an active research program applying qualitative research methods in medical education. She collaborates with and mentors faculty on the elements of qualitative research in the field of medical education and medical care. She has published more than 100 book chapters, curriculum materials, and original articles in medical education and clinical journals. She serves as visiting professor internationally and is invited to present regularly at professional meetings.

Paul Haidet, MD, MPH, is professor of medicine, humanities, and public health sciences at Pennsylvania State University. Dr. Haidet received his bachelor of science in 1987 and his MD degree in 1991 from Penn State. He completed a residency in internal medicine at Penn State Milton S. Hershey Medical Center in 1994, and completed the Harvard Faculty Development Fellowship in General Internal Medicine at Beth Israel Medical Center in Boston, Massachusetts, in 1998. He received his MPH degree from Harvard School of Public Health in 1997. Dr. Haidet served as a general internist at the Michael E. DeBakey Veterans Affairs Medical Center and as a researcher at the Houston Health Services Research and Development Center of Excellence and at Baylor College of Medicine from 1998 until 2009. In 2009 he moved back to Penn State in the role of director of medical education research. Dr. Haidet's career has focused on relationships in healthcare, including patient-physician, student-teacher, practitioner-practitioner, and individual-organization. He served as president of the American Academy on Communication in Healthcare (www.aachonline.org) in 2011. His current work focuses on the role of improvisation in medical communication and the importance of this concept for building productive relationships.

David A. Hirsh, MD, is associate professor in medicine at Harvard Medical School and Director and cofounder of the Harvard Medical School Cambridge Integrated Clerkship. Dr. Hirsch graduated summa cum laude with a BA in history from Dartmouth College in 1988 and received his MD from the University of Virginia in 1992. His scholarship and academic contributions span multiple areas including "educational continuity," medical education transformation, longitudinal integrated clerkships, OSCEs, professionalism, and humanism in medicine. He has received numerous local, national, and international honors and awards for his teaching, academic work, clinical practice, and public service. He has cofounded a thriving community health center in metropolitan Boston, and he served from 1995 to 2009 as medical director of the City of Cambridge Healthcare for the Homeless Program. With colleagues, he cofounded the international Consortium of Longitudinal Integrated Clerkships. He serves as a visiting professor of education and educational consultant across North America and on a global scale. He continues to practice primary care women's health in Cambridge, to mentor student and faculty research, and to teach courses in all four years of the Harvard Medical School curriculum.

Brian David Hodges, MD, PhD, is professor in the Faculty of Medicine and Faculty of Education (OISE/UT) at the University of Toronto, the Richard and Elizabeth Currie Chair in Health Professions Education Research at the Wilson Centre for Research in Education, and vice president of education at the University Health Network (Toronto General, Toronto Western Princess Margaret, and Toronto Rehab Hospitals). He leads the AMS Phoenix Project: A Call to Caring, a five-year initiative to rebalance the technical and compassionate dimensions of healthcare. Dr. Hodges's research focuses on using Foucauldian-inspired discourse analysis to study the nature and construction of various aspects of health professional education and practice: competence, assessment, professionalism, and globalization. He is currently undertaking a three-year SSHRC-funded project together with colleagues at McGill University to study the discourses of excellence, diversity, and equity in Canadian medical school admissions processes. He is an active teacher and speaker, both in Toronto and internationally, on qualitative methods, discourse analysis, and various dimensions of competence, assessment, and globalization.

Edward M. Hundert, MD, Dean for Medical Education, is director of the Center for Teaching and Learning, and senior lecturer in medical ethics at Harvard Medical School. Over the past thirty years, he has held professorial appointments in psychiatry, medical ethics, cognitive science, and medical humanities, and served as president of Case Western Reserve University, dean of the University of Rochester School of Medicine and Dentistry, and associate dean for student affairs at Harvard Medical School. Dr. Hundert co-chaired the Institute of Medicine's National Summit on Health Professions Education and has written dozens of articles and chapters on topics in psychiatry, philosophy, medical ethics, and medical education as well as two books. Dr. Hundert is a psychiatrist and has degrees in mathematics and the history of science and medicine from Yale; in philosophy, politics, and economics from Oxford; and in medicine from Harvard Medical School. He has served on the boards of the Association of American Universities, the Association of American Medical Colleges, the Liaison Committee on Medical Education, and the Rock and Roll Hall of Fame. He currently serves on the board of TIAA-CREF. He has received numerous teaching, mentoring, and diversity awards, and for six consecutive years was voted "faculty member who did the most for the class" by Harvard Medical School graduates.

Ayelet Kuper, MD, PhD, is assistant professor and clinician-scientist in the Department of Medicine at the University of Toronto, a scientist at the Wilson Centre (University Health Network/University of Toronto), and an internist based at Sunnybrook Health Sciences Centre, where she attends on the general medicine inpatient wards. She received a bachelor of arts in 1994 from Harvard, a master's degree in 1995, and a doctorate in medieval and modern languages in 1997 from Oxford as a Rhodes Scholar. In addition, she received her MD in 2001 and an MEd in 2007 from the University of Toronto. Her research program considers the relationship between currently accepted knowledge production modalities in medicine and medical education, the legitimacy and/or limitations of particular subject areas within mainstream health professions education research, and the implications of those limitations on the practice of medical education. She is currently supported in conducting her research as an AMS Phoenix Fellow and as a Canadian Institutes of Health Research (CIHR) New Investigator.

Heidi Lempp, PhD, is senior lecturer in medical sociology at King's College London School of Medicine, Department of Academic Rheumatology, and is a visiting research fellow at King's College London Institute of Psychiatry, Department of Health Service and Population Research. She completed her PhD (sociology) in 2004 in undergraduate medical education, University of London. Her current research interests focus on the interface of physical and mental health in inflammatory rheumatological autoimmune diseases, patient and carer involvement in research, the psychosocial impact when living with long-term conditions, and health service research. She continues to supervise and teach (1) undergraduate medical students, for example, novel special study modules in art and medicine, and patient involvement in research; and (2) postgraduate students in qualitative or mixed-method studies and their research projects. Her special interests in patient and career involvement in research have provided opportunities to contribute to research for the improvement of services for patients, their families, and healthcare staff in the delivery of mental and physical healthcare in a range of low- and middle-income countries.

Maria Athina (Tina) Martimianakis, PhD, is assistant professor in the Department of Paediatrics and a Cross Appointed Scientist at the Wilson Centre for Research in Education, University of Toronto. She directs the Office of Medical Education Scholarship in the Department of Paediatrics, which oversees faculty and resident development in scholarly educational practice. She holds a master's in political science from Wilfred Laurier University; and a master's of education with a focus on health professional education and a doctorate in higher education, both from the Ontario Institute for Studies in Education–UT. Her research explores the intersection of governance and faculty experiences and draws from a combination of critical sociopolitical traditions. Theoretically, she studies the material effects of discourse, particularly the ways in which professional identity is constructed through discursive relationships. Tina's current research projects include the exploration of how discourses of collaboration manifest in interprofessional dynamics; how discourses of integration are used to rationalize different and competing educational activity; and the effects of globalization on the field of medical education. Her previous research focused on the ways in which contemporary collaborative knowledge-making rationales contribute to the regulation and formation of subjects in interdisciplinary positions in medicine and engineering.

Nancy McNaughton, PhD, is associate director and director of research with the Standardized Patient Program in the faculty of medicine at the University of Toronto. She holds a master's of education and a PhD in higher education from the Ontario Institute for Studies in Education. She is a critical qualitative researcher and health professional educator who is trained in the sociology of education. She consults, collaborates on research, and is invited to present work internationally. She also designs and delivers curriculum, evaluation programs, research projects, and remediation activities for a wide variety of health professional trainees and practicing professionals. For the past five years, Dr. McNaughton has been faculty for the courses on qualitative research theory and methods as well as simulation research with the Wilson Centre for Research in Education. She holds appointments as an education research scientist with the Centre for Ambulatory Care Education, at Women's College Hospital, affiliated scholar with the Wilson

Centre for Research in Education, and academic educator with the Centre for Faculty Development in the Faculty of Medicine at the University of Toronto. Her current research program focuses on affect, emotion, and acting at the intersection of human simulation and health professional education.

Joseph F. O'Donnell, MD, is senior advising dean and director of community programs, professor of medicine and of psychiatry, and senior scholar of the C. Everett Koop Institute at the Geisel School of Medicine at Dartmouth. He received his AB from Harvard College in 1969 and his MD from Harvard Medical School in 1973. He did his internal medicine training at Dartmouth (1973–76) and trained in medical oncology at the National Cancer Institute in Bethesda, Maryland (1976–78). He began serving as chief of oncology at the Dartmouth-affiliated VA Medical Center in White River Junction, Vermont, in 1978 and joined the dean's office at Dartmouth Medical School in 1985. Active in the teaching of medical students and residents, Dr. O'Donnell was selected as one of the initial cadre of master educators at Geisel, and was the first recipient of the Holly Sateia Award for his enthusiastic and effective leadership in advancing diversity and community at Dartmouth College. His particular interests are in education for prevention, end-of-life care, moral growth in medical students, professionalism and humanism, the use of the humanities and arts in medical education, the doctor-patient relationship, and professional formation. He has edited *Oncology for the House Officer*; *A Life in Medicine: A Literary Anthology* with Randy Testa; *Finding Hope and Compassion: Inspiration for Doctors, Nurses, and Other Caregivers Coping with Illness, Disability, or Suffering* with Bill Beetham and coauthors; and *The Hidden Curriculum in Health Professions Education* with Fred Hafferty (Dartmouth College Press). He is past president of the Association of American Medical College's Northeast Group on Educational Affairs. He was an associate editor for *Academic Medicine* (1997–98). He served as associate editor of the *Journal of Cancer Education* (2003–6) and also as editor-in-chief (2006–13). He has chaired the Governor's Advisory Panel in Cancer and Chronic Disease in New Hampshire and consults and presents nationally and internationally. He has been called the "heart and soul" of the Geisel School of Medicine at Dartmouth.

Allison R. Ownby, PhD, is assistant dean for faculty and educational development at the University of Texas Medical School at Houston (UTHealth Medical School at Houston) and is associate professor in the Department of Pediatrics. She graduated with a bachelor of arts from the University of Iowa in 1993, a master of arts in political science from Rice

University in 1999, a PhD in political science from Rice University in 2001, and a master's of education in curriculum and instruction with an emphasis in health science education from the University of Houston in 2004. Dr. Ownby provides educational expertise in curriculum design and development, learner assessment, and program evaluation for the undergraduate and graduate medical education programs at UTHealth Medical School at Houston. Additionally, she is involved with faculty development in the areas of educational theory and practice, including curriculum design, program and learner assessment, the use of standardized patients in residency training, and team-based learning as an instructional method. Her research interests include exploring the hidden curriculum for faculty and how faculty development initiatives may assist faculty in negotiating the hidden curriculum as well as the role of social capital in pursuit of education within health science education institutions.

Michael W. Rabow, MD, is professor of clinical medicine in the Division of General Internal Medicine at the University of California–San Francisco (UCSF). He completed fellowships at UCSF in general medicine and in medical education research and is board certified in internal medicine and palliative care. He directs a leading outpatient palliative care comanagement program, the Symptom Management Service, at the UCSF Helen Diller Family Comprehensive Cancer Center. His research covers topics in palliative care, family caregiving, end-of-life care education, professional development, and the hidden curriculum. He has written and taught widely about family caregiving and communication with patients and families around serious news and existential issues at the end of life. Dr. Rabow is a member of the UCSF Academy of Medical Educators and serves as the director of the Center for the Study of the Healer's Art at the Institute for the Study of Health and Illness at Commonweal. He is assistant editor of the best-selling general medicine textbook *Current Medical Diagnosis and Treatment.*

Boyd F. Richards, MD, is assistant vice president for education research and evaluation and professor of medical education (in pediatrics) at the Columbia University College of Physicians and Surgeons. Formerly, he was director of the Office of Curriculum and professor in pediatrics at Baylor College of Medicine. Since earning a PhD from Indiana University in instructional systems technology in 1984, Dr. Richards has focused his administrative, service, and research activities on many different aspects of medical education. These activities include educational scholarship in academic promotions, teaching academies, clinical performance examinations, problem-based learning curricula, team-based learning interventions, program evaluation, performance assessment, and programs for improving faculty teaching. He serves on the editorial board for *MedEdPortal* and *Teaching and Learning in Medicine*. He formerly served as editor of the *Performance Improvement Quarterly*.

David T. Stern, MD, PhD, is vice chair for education and academic affairs at New York University and chief of the medical service at the New York campus of the New York Harbor VA Medical Center. He received his bachelor's degree in anthropology from Harvard University and his medical degree from Vanderbilt Medical School. He completed a residency in internal medicine at Tufts–New England Medical Center. He subsequently served as a fellow in ambulatory care and research at Stanford and the Palo Alto Veterans Affairs Medical Center, and received his PhD from Stanford University School of Education in curriculum and teacher education. He served as director of standardized patients, co-director of the Patient-Doctor course, and founding director of the international office of Global REACH (Research, Education and Collaboration for Health) at the University of Michigan (1994–2008). He served as vice chair for professionalism and faculty affairs at Mount Sinai's Department of Medicine (2008–13). Dr. Stern is the author of over 100 abstracts and papers on the topic, and is editor of *Measuring Medical Professionalism* (Oxford University Press 2006). He has served as a consultant and visiting professor at medical schools nationally and internationally, conducting workshops and seminars on teaching, learning, and evaluating professionalism.

Janelle S. Taylor, PhD, is associate professor and chair of the Department of Anthropology at the University of Washington. A medical anthropologist trained as an ethnographer, she has researched and written about a variety of topics relating to medical technology, medical education, and medical practice. Her publications include *The Public Life of the Fetal Sonogram: Technology, Consumption, and the Politics of Reproduction* (Rutgers 2008) and the co-edited volume *Consuming Motherhood* (Rutgers 2004). She is currently pursuing research on two topics: standardized patient performances in health professions education and issues of recognition and care arising in relation to people with dementia. Both projects use ethnographic methods to explore how people get represented within US biomedicine, and how these processes of representation carry social, cultural, and political as well as clinical consequences.

Cayla R. Teal, PhD, is currently assistant professor of medicine and director of educational evaluation and research in undergraduate medical education at Baylor College of Medicine. As an investigator and consultant, her research experiences have been primarily in applied situations, with an emphasis on educational settings, but also include community-based and volunteer associations, healthcare providers, law enforcement, and mental health facilities. As a mixed-methods educational researcher, she has focused her research agenda on the examination and improvement of cross-cultural communication between providers and patients. She graduated with a BA from William Jewell College in 1989. She earned an MA in community/clinical psychology in 1996 and a PhD in community psychology (with emphases in applied research methods, measurement, and psychometrics) in 2003, both from Wichita State University. Until 2010, Dr. Teal was a health services researcher in the Houston Health Services Research and Development Center of Excellence (at the Michael E. DeBakey VA Medical Center). She also served the center as director of the Health Services Research Post-Doctoral Fellowship Program for fellows with research doctorates and as co-director of the center's education program.

Jill Thistlethwaite, MBBS, PhD, is professor of medical education and a consultant in health professions and interprofessional education, with affiliation to the University of Technology Sydney (UTS) and the University of Queensland, Australia. She trained as a GP/family physician in the university and has been involved in health professional education for more than twenty years. She continues to practice at a health center in Sydney and believes consulting with patients helps keep her feet grounded and in touch with authentic patient experiences. She has a passion for interprofessional education and collaborative practice and is involved with several projects exploring, developing, and assessing interprofessional learning activities for students from multiple health professions. Her most recent book on values-based interprofessional collaborative practice focuses on how personal, professional, and organizations values affect how we work and communicate. When she first moved to Australia in 2003, Dr. Thistlethwaite was struck by how the national health system of a country impinges on how we practice healthcare and make decisions. As a GP, she strives to adopt a shared decision-making model with patients and other professionals.

Britta M. Thompson, PhD, is assistant dean for medical education and director of the Office of Medical Education at the University of Oklahoma College of Medicine. In her role, she oversees activities associated with medical education and simulation, such as faculty development (including directing the Academy of Teaching Scholars), curriculum evaluation and learner assessment, simulation, curriculum development, and instructional technology, as well as the Willed Body Program. Her research interests in medicine include evaluating curricular innovations such as team-based learning, assessing cultural competency education programs, evaluating faculty development programs, and evaluating ways to promote student reflection. She earned her BS from Kansas State University, her MS from the University of Missouri–Columbia, and her PhD in educational psychology from Texas A&M University. After receiving her PhD, she joined the faculty at Baylor College of Medicine in 2004, where she became the director of evaluation and assessment and the director of the Simulation Program. Through her work, she has been awarded several teaching and educational research awards. Her research has resulted in 150 regional and national peer-reviewed and invited presentations and over thirty peer-reviewed articles.

Delese Wear, PhD, is professor of family and community medicine at Northeast Ohio Medical University, where she teaches medical humanities. Her research interests include curriculum theory, humanities education, how cultural issues are conceived and taught in medical education, and all things related to professionalism. She has co-edited several volumes on professionalism, including *Professionalism in Medicine: Critical Perspectives* (Springer 2006, with Julie Aultman). Her most recent work focuses on the theoretical move from the medical humanities to the health humanities in a comprehensive edited collection, *Health Humanities Reader* (Rutgers University Press 2013, with Therese Jones and Lester Friedman).

Claire Wendland, MD, PhD, is associate professor in the Departments of Anthropology, Obstetrics and Gynecology, and Medical History and Bioethics at the University of Wisconsin–Madison. She worked as a practicing physician on the Navajo reservation for many years before turning to medical anthropology. Her publications include *A Heart for the Work: Journeys through an African Medical School* (University of Chicago Press 2010), the first ethnography of medical training in the global South. Her current research considers explanations for maternal death put forward among a wide range of experts working with childbearing women in Malawi.

Virginia Wright-Peterson, PhD, is faculty, Center for Learning Innovation, University of Minnesota-Rochester, and previously was operations manager for the Mayo School of Health Sciences (MSHS), where she provides administrative support for academic and faculty affairs and directly works with several allied health programs. She has over ten years of experience teaching college-level English, humanities, and philosophy in the classroom, online, and in blended learning environments at other institutions. She taught as a Fulbright Scholar in Algeria (2004–5), and served on a military base in Iraq with the American Red Cross (2007–8). She has a BS in accounting from the Carlson School of Business, an MA from University of Minnesota–Duluth, and a PhD from University of Nebraska–Lincoln, both in English. She is leading a blended learning project team at MSHS that is dedicated to moving portions of the current curriculum online to improve the quality of the education delivery and allow for the extension of allied health programs beyond the current walls of the school. She is currently writing a book that reveals the mostly unknown stories of women who made significant contributions to the founding and early years of the Mayo Clinic.

Joseph Zarconi, MD, is system vice president for medical education and chief academic officer at Summa Health System in Akron, Ohio, and cofounded and directs Summa's Institute for Professionalism Inquiry. He is professor of internal medicine and associate dean for clinical education for the Northeast Ohio Medical University (NEOMED). He received his MD degree as a member of the charter class at Northeastern Ohio Universities College of Medicine (now NEOMED), completed residency and chief residency in internal medicine at Akron City Hospital, and completed a nephrology fellowship at the University Hospitals of Cleveland/Case Western Reserve University School of Medicine. He is a practicing nephrologist and has remained active in the teaching of medical students and residents. He has presented at state and national meetings; has coauthored peer-reviewed journal articles and book chapters on topics relating to medical education, narrative medical practice, narrative ethics, and humanism and professionalism in medicine; and is coauthor of two books on narrative in healthcare. Dr. Zarconi is a member of the NEOMED Master Teacher Guild, and has been recognized as a master teacher by the American College of Physicians.

References

Adler, S. R., E. F. Hughes, and R. B. Scott. 2006. Student 'moles': Revealing the hidden curriculum. *Medical Education* 40 (5): 463–64.

Adkoli, B. V., K. U. Al-Umran, M. Al-Sheikh, K. K. Deepak, and A. M. Al-Rubaish. 2011. Medical students' perception of professionalism: A qualitative study from Saudi Arabia. *Medical Teacher* 33 (10): 840–45.

Agrawal, S., P. Szatmari, and M. Hanson. 2008. Teaching evidence-based psychiatry: Integrating and aligning the formal and hidden curricula. *Academic Psychiatry* 32 (6): 470–74.

Al-Bawardy, R., B. Blatt, S. Al-Shohaib, and S. J. Simmens. 2009. Cross-cultural comparison of the patient-centeredness of the hidden curriculum between a Saudi Arabian and 9 US medical schools. *Medical Education Online* 14: 19.

Album, D., and S. Westin. 2008. Do diseases have a prestige hierarchy? A survey among physicians and medical students. *Social Science in Medicine* 66 (6): 182–88.

Alexias, G. 2008. Medical discourse and time: Authoritative reconstruction of present, future and past. *Social Theory and Health* 6 (2): 167–83.

Allport, G. W. 1979. *The nature of prejudice*. 25th anniversary ed. (orig. pub. 1954). Reading, MA: Addison-Wesley.

American Academy of Child and Adolescent Psychiatry (AACAP). 2012. When children have children. http://www.aacap.org/cs/root/facts_for_families/when_children_have_children.

Anderson, D. J. 1992. The hidden curriculum. *American Journal of Roentgenology* 159 (1): 21–22.

Anderson, I. P. S. 2008. The knowledge economy and aboriginal health development. Dean's lecture, Faculty of Medicine, Dentistry and Health Sciences, May 13, 2008, Onemda VicHealth Koori Health Unit, University of Melbourne, Melbourne.

Anderson, S. 2012. Just one more game . . . angry birds, farmville and other hyperaddictive "stupid games." *New York Times*, Apr. 8.

Anderson, W. 2011. Outside looking in: Observations on medical education since the Flexner Report. *Medical Education* 45 (1): 29–35.

Anspach, R. R. 1988. Notes on the sociology of medical discourse: The language of case presentation. *Journal of Health and Social Behavior* 29 (4): 357–75.

Apple, M. 2005. Education, markets, and an audit culture. *Critical Quarterly* 47 (1–2): 11–29.

Arah, O., J. Hoekstra, A. Bos, and K. Lombarts. 2011. New tools for systematic evaluation of teaching quality of medical faculty: Results of an ongoing multi-center survey. *PLoS ONE* 6: 1–10.

Aristotle. 1956. *The Nicomachean ethics*. Trans. by J. A. K. Thomson. London: Penguin.

Aronson, L., B. Niehaus, J. Lindow, P. A. Robertson, and P. S. O'Sullivan. 2011. Development and pilot testing of a reflective learning guide for medical education. *Medical Teacher* 33 (10): e515–21.

Associated Medical Services. 2011a. The genesis and early development of the AMA Phoenix project: A call to caring. http://www.theamsphoenix.ca/amsgenesisjuly2011.pdf.

Associated Medical Services. 2011b. The AMS Health Professional Initiative: Exploring and beginning to build a foundation for sustainable impact: Stage 1 consolidated reports, Associated Medical Services, Toronto. http://www.theamsphoenix.ca/amsstage1reportsmay%202011.pdf.

Association of American Medical Colleges (AAMC). 1998. Medical school objectives project: Report i-learning objectives for medical student education guidelines for medical schools. https://members.aamc.org/eweb/upload/Learning%20Objectives%20for%20Medical%20Student%20Educ%20Report%20I.pdf.

Association of Faculties of Medicine of Canada. n.d. The future of medical education in Canada (FMEC): A collective vision for MD education. http://www.afmc.ca/future-of-medical-education-in-canada/medical-doctor-project/pdf/collective_vision.pdf.

Aston, S. J., W. Rheault, C. Arenson, S. K. Tappert, J. Stocker, J. Orzoff, H. Galitski, et al. 2012. Interprofessional education: A review and analysis of programs from three academic health centers. *Academic Medicine* 87 (7): 949–55.

Aurora, A., and A. True. 2012. What kind of physician will you be? http://www.dartmouthatlas.org/downloads/reports/Residency_report_103012.pdf.

Australian Indigenous Doctors Association. 2012. Aboriginal and Torres Strait Islander medical student numbers jump. Aug. 20: 1–1. http://www.aida.org.au/pdf/news/0012.pdf.

Australian Institute of Health and Welfare. 2011. *Medical labour workforce 2009*. AIHW Bulletin no. 89. Cat. no. AUS 138. Canberra, AIHW.

Baird, P. 2001. The human genome project, genetics and health. *Community Genetics* 4 (2): 77–80.

Baker, L., E. Egan-Lee, M. A. Martimianakis, and S. Reeves. 2011. Relationships of power: Implications for interprofessional education. *Journal of Interprofessional Care* 25 (2): 98–104.

Baker, M., J. Wrubel, and M. W. Rabow. 2011. Professional development and the informal curriculum in end-of-life care. *Journal of Cancer Education* 26 (3): 444–50.

Baldwin, D. C., Jr., S. R. Daugherty, and B. D. Rowley. 1998. Unethical and unprofessional conduct observed by residents during their first year of training. *Academic Medicine* 73 (11): 1195–1200.

Baldwin, D. C., and D. J. Self. 2006. The assessment of moral reasoning and professionalism in medical education and practice. In *Measuring medical professionalism*, ed. D. T. Stern, 75–93. New York: Oxford University Press.

Balmer, D., C. L. Master, B. F. Richards, and A. P. Giardino. 2009. Implicit versus explicit curricula in general pediatrics: Is there a convergence? *Pediatrics* 124: e347–54.

Balmer, D., B. F. Richards, and R. E. Drusin. 2010. Columbia University College of Physicians and Surgeons. *Academic Medicine* 85 (S9): S365–69.

Bandura, A. 1977. *Social foundations of thought and action: A social cognitive theory*. Englewood Cliffs: Prentice Hall.

Beagan, B. L. 2000. Neutralizing differences: producing neutral doctors for (almost) neutral patients. *Social Science and Medicine* 51 (8): 1253–65.

Beagan, B. L. 2003. Teaching social and cultural awareness to medical students: "It's all very nice to talk about it in theory, but ultimately it makes no difference." *Academic Medicine* 78 (6): 605–14.

Bebeau, M. J. 2002. The defining issues test and the four components model: Contributions to professional education. *Journal of Moral Education* 31 (3): 271–95.

Becker, H. S., B. Geer, E. C. Hughes, and A. L. Strauss. 1961. *Boys in white: Student culture in medical school*. Chicago: University of Chicago Press.

Bell, J. 1984. Exposing the hidden curriculum. *Nursing Mirror* 158 (12): 20–22.

Bell, S. K., M. Wideroff, and L. Gaufberg. 2010. Student voices in Readers' Theater: Exploring communication in the hidden curriculum. *Patient Education and Counseling* 80: 354–57.

Belling, C. 2010. Sharper instruments: On defending the humanities in undergraduate medical education. *Academic Medicine* 85 (6): 938–40.

Benbassat J. 2013. Undesirable features of the medical learning environment: A narrative review of the literature. *Advances in Health Science Education. Theory and Practice* 18 (3): 527–36.

Benner, P. 1984. *From novice to expert: Excellence and power in clinical nursing practice*. Menlo Park, CA: Addison-Wesley.

Benner, P., P. Hooper-Kyriakidis, and D. Stannard. 2011. *Clinical wisdom and interventions in acute and critical care: A thinking-in-action approach*. 2nd ed. New York: Springer.

Benner, P., and M. Sutphen. 2007. Learning across the professions: The clergy, a case in point. *Journal of Nursing Education* 46 (3): 103–8.

Benner, P., M. Sutphen, V. Leonard, and L. Day. 2010. *Educating nurses: A call for radical transformation.* Carnegie Foundation for the Advancement of Teaching Series. San Francisco: Jossey-Bass.

Benner, P., C. A. Tanner, and C. A. Chesla. 1996. *Expertise in nursing practice: Caring, clinical judgment, and ethics.* 1st ed. New York: Springer.

Benson, J. 2003. *Third culture personalities and the integration of refugees into the community: Some reflections from general practice.* http://www.mmha.org. au/mmha-productrs/synergy/2003_No2/ThirdCulturePersonalities.

Benson, J., and K. Magraith. 2005. Compassion fatigue and burnout: The role of Balint groups. *Australian Family Physician* 34 (6): 497–98.

Bernabeo, E. C., M. C. Holtman, S. Ginsburg, J. R. Rosenbaum, and E. S. Holmboe. 2011. Lost in transition: The experience and impact of frequent changes in the inpatient learning environment. *Academic Medicine* 86 (5): 591–98.

Bernard, A. W., M. Malone, N. E. Kman, J. M. Caterino, and S. Khandelwal. 2011. Medical student professionalism narratives: A thematic analysis and interdisciplinary comparative investigation. *BMC Emergency Medicine.* http://www.biomedcentral.com/1471-227X/11/11.

Bernstein, R, R. Dibble, T. Hunter, and J. Morris. 2008. *The code: Baseball's unwritten rules and its ignore-at-your-own-risk code of conduct.* Chicago: Triumph Books.

Berwick, D. M., and J. A. Finkelstein. 2010. Preparing medical students for the continual improvement of health and health care: Abraham Flexner and the new "public interest." *Academic Medicine* 85 (9 Suppl): S56–65.

Biggs, J. 1999. *Teaching for quality learning at university: What the student does.* Buckingham, UK: Society for Research into Higher Education and Open University Press.

Billings, M. E., R. Engelberg, J. R. Curtis, S. Block, and A. M. Sullivan. 2010. Determinants of medical students' perceived preparation to perform end-of-life care, quality of end-of-life care education, and attitudes toward end-of-life care. *Journal of Palliative Medicine* 13 (3): 319–26.

Billings, M. E., M. E. Lazarus, M. Wenrich, J. R. Curtis, and R. A. Engelberg. 2011. The effect of the hidden curriculum on residents' burnout and cynicism. *Journal of Graduate Medical Education* 3 (4): 503–10.

Bloom, S. W. 1988. Structure and ideology in medical education: An analysis of resistance to change. *Journal of Health and Social Behavior* 29 (4): 294–306.

Bloom, S. W. 1989. The medical school as a social organization: The sources of resistance to change. *Medical Education* 23 (3): 228–41.

Bolton, G. 2009. Writing values. *Lancet* 374: 20–21.

Bosk, C. 1979. *Forgive and remember.* Chicago: University of Illinois Press.

Bourdieu, P. 1984. *Distinction: A social critique of the judgment of taste.* Cambridge, MA: Harvard University Press.

Bourdieu, P. 1990. *The logic of practice.* Trans. by R. Nice. Stanford, CA: Stanford University Press.

Bourdieu, P., and L. J. D. Wacquant. 1992. *An invitation to reflexive sociology.* Chicago: University of Chicago Press.

Boursicot, K., L. Etheridge, S. Zeryabs, A. Sturrock, J. Ker, S. Smee, and S. Elango. 2011. Performance in assessment: Consensus statement and recommendations from the Ottawa conference. *Medical Teacher* 33 (5): 370–83.

Bradley, F., A. Steven, and D. M. Ashcroft. 2011. Education for safety: The role of hidden curriculum in teaching pharmacy students about patient safety. *American Journal of Pharmaceutical Education* 75 (7): 1–7.

Bradley, J. C., and C. Neylon. 2008. Data on display. *Nature* 455 (7211): 273.

Bragg, S. 2007. "Student Voice" and governmentality: The production of enterprising subjects. *Discourse: Studies in the Cultural Politics of Education* 28 (3): 343–58.

Brainard, A. H., and H. C. Brislen. 2007. Learning professionalism: A view from the trenches. *Academic Medicine* 82 (11): 1010–14.

Branch, W. T., Jr. 2005. Use of critical incident reports in medical education: A perspective. *Journal of General Internal Medicine* 20 (11): 1063–67.

Brooks, V., and J. E. Thistlethwaite. 2012. Working and learning across professional boundaries. *British Journal of Educational Studies* 60 (4): 403–20.

Brosnan, C. 2009. Pierre Bourdieu and the theory of medical education. Thinking "relationally" about medical students and medical curricula. In *Handbook of the sociology of medical education*, eds. C. Brosnan and B. S. Turner, 51–68. London: Routledge.

Brosnan, C. 2010. Making sense of differences between medical schools through Bourdieu's concept of "field." *Medical Education* 44 (7): 64552.

Brottman, M. 2009. Learning to hate learning objectives. *Chronicle of Higher Education: The Chronicle Review.* http://chronicle.com/article/Learning-to-Hate-Learning/49399.

Brown, R. 1996. Tajfel's contribution to the reduction of intergroup conflict. In *Social groups and identities: Developing the legacy of Henri Tajfel*, ed. W. P. Robinson, 169–90. Oxford: Butterworth Heinemann.

Burack, J. H., D. M. Irby, J. D. Carline, R. K. Root, and E. B. Larson. 1999.

Teaching compassion and respect. Attending physicians' responses to problematic behaviors. *Journal of General Internal Medicine* 14 (1): 49–55.

Burger-Lux, M. J., and R. P. Heaney. 1986. For better and worse: The technological imperative in health care. *Social Science and Medicine* 22 (12): 1313–20.

Buss, M. K., D. S. Lessen, A. M. Sullivan, J. Von Roenn, R. M. Arnold, and S. D. Block. 2007. A study of oncology fellows' training in end-of-life care. *Journal of Supportive Oncology* 5 (5): 237–42.

CAIPE: Centre for the Advancement of Interprofessional Education. 2002. http://www.caipe.org.uk/resources/.

Cameron, T., K. Krane, J. Jacobs, and R. Harden. 2012. Mapping medical education curricula. Paper read at 2012 AAMC annual conference.

Campbell, E. G., S. Regan, R. L. Gruen, T. G. Ferris, T. Rao, R. Sowmya, P. D. Cleary, and D. Blumenthal. 2007. Professionalism in medicine: Results of a national survey of physicians. *Annals of Internal Medicine* 147 (11): 795–802.

Carpenter, J., and C. Dickinson. 2011. "Contact is not enough": A social psychological perspective on interprofessional education. In *Sociology of interprofessional healthcare practice*, eds. S. Kitto, J. Chesters, J. Thistlethwaite, and S. Reeves, 55–68. New York: Nova.

Castellani, B., and F. W. Hafferty. 2006. Professionalism and complexity science: A preliminary investigation. In *Medical professionalism: A critical review*, eds. D. Wear and J. M. Aultman, 3–23. New York: Springer.

Charon, R. 2001. A model for empathy, reflection, profession, and trust. *Journal of the American Medical Association* 266 (18): 1897–1902.

Charon, R. 2004. Narrative and medicine. *New England Journal of Medicine* 350 (9): 862–64.

Charon, R. 2006. *Narrative medicine: Honoring the stories of illness*. New York: Oxford University Press.

Charon, R. 2009. American Society for Bioethics and Humanities Lit-Med Listserve.

Charon, R., and N. Hermann. 2012. Commentary: A sense of story, or why teach reflective writing? *Academic Medicine* 87 (1): 5–7.

Choi, C., and A. Pak. 2007. Multidisciplinarity, interdisciplinarity and transdisciplinarity in health research, service education and policy 2: Promoters, barriers and strategies of enhancement. *Clinical Investigative Medicine* 30 (6): E224–32.

Chretien, K., E. Goldman, and C. Faselis. 2008. The reflective writing class blog: Using technology to promote reflection and professional development. *Journal of General Internal Medicine* 23 (12): 2066–70.

Chretien, K. C., S. R. Greysen, J. P. Chretien, and T. Kind. 2009. Online posting of unprofessional content by medical students. *Journal of the American Medical Association* 302 (12): 1309–15.

Christakis, D. A., and C. Feudtner. 1993. Ethics in a short white coat: The ethical dilemmas that medical students confront. *Academic Medicine* 68: 249–54.

Christakis, D. A., and C. Feudtner. 1997. Temporary matters: The ethical consequences of transient social relationships in medical training. *Journal of the American Medical Association* 278 (9): 739–43.

Christensen, C. M. 1997. *The innovator's dilemma: When technologies cause great firms to fail*. Boston: Harvard Business School Press.

Chuang, A. W., F. S. Nuthalapaty, P. M. Casey, J. M. Kaczmarczyk, A. J. Cullimore, J. L. Dalrymple, L. Dugoff, et al. 2010. To the point: Reviews in medical education—taking control of the hidden curriculum. *American Journal of Obstetrics and Gynecology* 203: 316.e1–6.

CIHC: Canadian Interprofessional Health Collaborative. 2010. *A national interprofessional competency framework*. http://www.cihc.ca/files/CIHC_IP-Competencies_Feb1210.pdf.

CITI: Collaborative Institutional Training Initiative. https://www.citiprogram.org/.

Clouser, K. D. 1986. Humanities in a technological education. http://weber-studies.weber.edu/archive/archive%20A%20%20Vol.%201-10.3/Vol.%20 3/3.1Clauser.htm.

Cohen, J. J., B. A. Gabriel, and C. Terrell. 2002. The case for diversity in the health care workforce. *Health Affairs* 21 (5): 90–102.

Contemporary Pediatrics Staff. 2012. Pediatric hospitalists prefer texting to paging. *Contemporary Pediatrics*, Nov. 27. http://contemporarypediatrics. modernmedicine.com/contemporary-pediatrics/news/modernmedicine/ modern-medicine-feature-articles/pediatric-hospitalists (accessed May 19, 2013).

Cooke, M., D. M. Irby, and B. C. O'Brien. 2010. *Educating physicians: A call for reform of medical school and residency*. San Francisco: Jossey-Bass.

Cornbleth, C. 1990. *Curriculum in context*. Bristol, PA: Falmer Press.

Côté, L., and H. Leclère. 2000. How clinical teachers perceive the doctor-patient relationship and themselves as role models. *Academic Medicine* 75 (11): 1117–24.

Cottingham, A. H., A. L. Suchman, D. K. Litzelman, R. M. Frankel, D. L. Mossbarger, P. R. Williamson, D. C. Baldwin, Jr., et al. 2008. Enhancing the informal curriculum of a medical school: A case study in organizational culture change. *Journal of General Internal Medicine* 23 (6): 715–22.

Coulehan, J. 2005. Today's professionalism: Engaging the mind but not the heart. *Academic Medicine* 80 (10): 890–98.

Coulehan, J. 2006. You say self-interest, I say altruism. In *Professionalism and medicine: Critical perspectives*, eds. D. Wear and J. Aultman, 103–28. New York: Springer.

Coulehan, J., and I. A. Granek. 2012. Commentary: "I hope I'll continue to grow": Rubrics and reflective writing in medical education. *Academic Medicine* 87 (1): 8–10.

Coulehan, J., and P. C. Williams. 2001. Vanquishing virtue: The impact of medical education. *Academic Medicine* 76 (6): 598–605.

Council on Graduate Schools. 2009. Best practices in graduate education for the responsible conduct of research. http://www.cgsnet.org/best-practices-graduate-education-responsible-conduct-research.

Cowell, R. N. 1972. The hidden curriculum: A theoretical framework and a pilot study. Ed.d thesis Harvard Graduate School of Education.

Cribb, A. 2000. The diffusion of the health agenda and the fundamental need for partnership in medical education. *Medical Education* 34: 916–20.

Cribb, A., and S. Bignold. 1999. Towards the reflexive medical school: The hidden curriculum and medical education research. *Studies in Higher Education* 24 (2): 195–209.

Cruess, R. L., and S. R. Cruess. 1997a. Professionalism must be taught. *British Medical Journal* 315 (7123): 1674–77.

Cruess, R. L., and S. R. Cruess. 1997b. Teaching medicine as a profession in the service of healing. *Academic Medicine.* 72 (11): 941–52.

Cruess, R. L., and S. R. Cruess. 2009. Principles for designing a program for the teaching and learning of professionalism at the undergraduate level. In *Teaching medical professionalism*, eds. Cruess, R. L., S. R. Cruess, and Y. Steinert, 73–92. New York: Cambridge University Press.

Cruess, S. R., R. L. Cruess, and Y. Steinert. 2008. Role modelling—making the most of a powerful teaching strategy. *British Medical Journal* 336: 718–21.

Cuban, L. 1997. Change without reform: The case of Stanford University School of Medicine 1908–1990. *American Educational Research Journal* 34 (1): 83–122.

Curtis. E., E. Wikaire, K. Stokes, and P. Reid. 2012. Addressing indigenous health workforce inequities: A literature review exploring "best" practice for recruitment into tertiary health programmes. *International Journal for Equity in Health* 11: 13. http://www.equityhealthj.com/content/11/1/13.

Daley, D. 1997. *The Nashville music machine: The unwritten rules of the music business.* Woodstock, NY: Overlook Press.

D'Amour, D., and I. Oandasan. 2005. Interprofessionality as the field of interprofessional practice and interprofessional education: An emerging concept. *Journal of Interprofessional Care* 19 (S1): 8–20.

DaRosa, D. A., K. Skeff, J. A. Friedland, M. Coburn, S. Cox, S. Pollart, M. O'Connell, and S. Smith. 2011. Barriers to effective teaching. *Academic Medicine* 86 (4): 453–59.

D'Eon, M., N. Lear, M. Turner, and C. Jones. 2007. Perils of the hidden curriculum revisited. *Medical Teacher* 29 (4): 295–96.

Deming, N., K. Fryer-Edwards, D. Dudzinski, H. Starks, J. Culver, E. Hopley, L. Robins, and W. Burke. 2007. Incorporating principles and practical wisdom in research ethics education: A preliminary study. *Academic Medicine* 82 (1): 18–23.

Department of Health. 2008a. *Raising the profile of long-term conditions care: A compendium of information.* London: Department of Health.

Department of Health. 2008b. *High quality of care for all. MHS next stage review final report.* London: Department of Health.

Dewey, J. 1938. *Experience and education.* New York: Collier.

Diedrich, L. 2005. AIDS and its treatments: Two doctors' narratives of healing, desire, and belonging. *Journal of Medical Humanities* 26 (4): 237–57.

Donetto, S. 2010. Medical students' views of power in doctor-patient interactions: The value of teacher-learner relationships. *Medical Education* 44 (2): 187–96.

Dosani, N. The top ten things I learned in medical school (but wasn't supposed to). Paper presented to the 2010 Canadian Conference on Medical Education, May 1–5, 2010, St. John, Newfoundland.

Douglas-Steele, D., and E. M. Hundert. 1996. Accounting for context: Future directions in bioethics theory and research. *Theoretical Medicine* 17 (2): 101–19.

Doukas, D., L. B. McCullough, and S. Wear. 2010. Reforming medical education in ethics and humanities by finding common ground with Abraham Flexner. *Academic Medicine* 85 (2): 318–23.

Doukas, D., L. B. McCullough, and S. Wear. 2012. Medical education in medical ethics and humanities as the foundation for developing medical professionalism. *Academic Medicine* 87 (3): 334–41.

Dowell, A., P. Crampton, and C. Parkin. 2001. The first sunrise: An experience of cultural immersion and community health needs assessment by undergraduate medical students in New Zealand. *Medical Education* 35 (3): 242–49.

Doyle, Sir A. C. 1892. The memoirs of Sherlock Holmes: Adventure 1: Silver blaze. http://etc.usf.edu/lit2go/40/the-memoirs-of-sherlock-holmes/573/adventure-1-silver-blaze/.

Dyrbye, L. N., M. R. Thomas, and T. D. Shanafelt. 2005. Medical student distress: Causes, consequences, and proposed solutions. *Mayo Clinic Proceedings* 80 (12): 1613–22.

Eisner, E. W. 1979. *The educational imagination: On the design and evaluation of school programs.* New York: Macmillan.

Eisner, E. W. 1985. *The three curricula that all schools teach: The educational imagination.* New York: Macmillan.

Ellison-Barnes, A., B. Jastrzembski, J. Morris, D. Mallampati, A. Patino, A. Suri, A. Wagner, and D. Ziehr. 2012. CIC systems (improvement) rounds: A "Review of Systems." Personal communication.

Elstein, A. S, L. S. Shulman, and S. A. Sprafka. 1978. *Medical problem solving: An analysis of clinical reasoning.* Cambridge, MA: Harvard University Press.

Englander, R., T Cameron, A. J. Ballard, J. Dodge, J. Bull, and C. A. Aschenbrener. 2013. Toward a common taxonomy of competency domains for the health professions and competencies for physicians. *Academic Medicine* 88 (8): 1088–94.

Entwistle, V., D. Firnigl, M. Ryan, J. Francis, and P. Kinghorn. 2012. Which experiences of health care delivery matter to service users and why? A critical interpretive synthesis and conceptual map. *Journal of Health Services Research and Policy* 17 (2): 70–78.

Epstein, R. M. 1999. Mindful practice. *Journal of the American Medical Association* 282 (9): 833–39.

Epstein, R. M. 2008. Reflection, perception and the acquisition of wisdom. *Medical Education* 42 (11): 1048–50.

Epstein, R. M., and E. M. Hundert. 2002. Defining and assessing professional competence. *Journal of the American Medical Association* 287 (2): 226–35.

Eraut, M. 1994. *Developing professional knowledge and competence.* Washington, DC: Falmer.

Eraut, M. 2004. Transfer of knowledge between education and workplace settings. In *Workplace learning in context*, eds. H. Rainbird, A. Fuller, and A. Munro, 201–21. London: Routledge.

Erickson, K. I., W. R. Boot, C. Basak, M. B. Neider, R. S. Prakash, M. W. Voss, A. M. Graybiel, et al. 2010. Striatal volume predicts level of video game skill acquisition. *Cerebral Cortex* 20 (11): 2522–30.

Esmail, A. 2004. The prejudices of good people. *British Medical Journal* 328 (7454): 1448–49.

Eva, K. W., L. Lohfeld, G. Dhaliwal, M. Mylopoulos, D. A. Cook, and G. R. Norman. 2011. Modern conceptions of elite medical practice among internal medicine faculty members. *Academic Medicine* 86 (10 Suppl): S50–54.

Eva, K. W., J. Rosenfeld, H. I. Reiter, and G. R. Norman. 2004. An admissions OSCE: The multiple mini-interview. *Medical Education* 38 (3): 314–26.

Evetts, J. 2003. The sociological analysis of professionalism. *International Sociology* 18 (2): 395–415.

Ewen, S. C. 2011. Unequal treatment: The possibilities of and need for indigenous Parrhesiastes in Australian medical education. *Journal of Immigrant and Minority Health* 13 (3): 609–15.

Ewen, S.C., O. Mazel, and D. Knoche. 2012. Exposing the hidden curriculum influencing medical education on the health of Indigenous people in Australia and New Zealand: The role of the Critical Reflection Tool. *Academic Medicine* 87 (2): 200–205.

Fernandes, R., W. Shore, J. H. Muller, and M. W. Rabow. 2008. What it's really like: The complex role of medical students in end-of-life care. *Teaching and Learning in Medicine* 20 (1): 69–72.

Feudtner, C., and D. A. Christakis. 1994. Making the rounds. The ethical development of medical students in the context of clinical rotations. *Hastings Center Report.* 24 (1): 6–12.

Feudtner, C., D. A. Christakis, and N. A. Christakis. 1994. Do clinical clerks suffer ethical erosion? Students' perceptions of the ethical environment and personal development. *Academic Medicine* 69 (8): 670–79.

Fine, A. 2010. Social Citizens Discussion Paper. http://www.scribd.com/doc/2626239/Social-Citizens-Discussion-Paper.

Finn, G., J. Garner, and M. Sawdon. 2010. "You're judged all the time!" Students' views on professionalism: A multicentre study. *Medical Education* 44 (8): 814–25.

Fins, J. J., and P. R. del Pozo. 2011. The hidden and implicit curricula in cultural context: New insights from Doha and New York. *Academic Medicine* 86 (3): 321–25.

Fisher, C. B., A. L. Fried, S. J. Goodman, and K. K. Germano. 2009. Measures of mentoring, department climate, and graduate student preparedness in the responsible conduct of psychological research. *Ethics and Behavior* 19 (3): 227–52.

Fiske, P. 2013. Ticket to everywhere. *Nature* (494): 393.

Flexner, A. 1910. Medical education in the United States and Canada: A report to the Carnegie Foundation for the advancement of teaching. *Carnegie Foundation Bulletin No. 4.* New York: Carnegie Foundation for the Advancement of Teaching.

Flinders, D. J., N. Noddings, S. J. Thornton. 1986. The null curriculum: Its theoretical basis and practical implications. *Curriculum Inquiry* 16 (1): 33–42.

Fortin, A. H., F. C. Dwamena, R. F. Frankel, and R. C. Smith. 2012. *Smith's patient-centered interviewing: An evidence-based method.* 3rd ed. New York: McGraw Hill Lange.

Foucault, M. 1972. *The archaeology of knowledge and the discourse on language.* Trans. by A. M. Sheridan Smith. New York: Pantheon.

Foucault, M. 1980. *Power/knowledge: Selected interviews and other writings 1972–1977.* Brighton, Sussex: Harvester Press.

Foucault, M. 1982. The subject and power: Afterword. In *Michel Foucault: Beyond structuralism and hermeneutics*, eds. H. L. Dreyfus and P. Rabinow. Chicago: University of Chicago Press.

Foucault, M. 1994. *The birth of the clinic: An archaeology of medical perception.* New York: Vintage.

Foucault, M. 1995. *Discipline and punish: The birth of the prison.* New York: Vintage.

Foucault, M. 2004. *The birth of biopolitics: Lectures at the College de France 1978–1979.* New York: Palgrave MacMillan.

Frank, E., J. S. Carrera, T. Stratton, J. Bickel, and L. M. Nora. 2006. Experiences of belittlement and harassment and their correlates among medical students in the United States: Longitudinal survey. *British Medical Journal* 333: 682–87.

Frank, J. R., and D. Danoff. 2007. The CanMEDS initiative: Implementing an outcomes-based framework of physician competencies. *Medical Teacher* 29 (7): 642–47.

Freidson, E. 1986. *Professional powers: A study of the institutionalization of formal knowledge.* Chicago: University of Chicago Press.

Freidson, E. 2001. *Professionalism: The third logic.* Chicago: University of Chicago Press.

Freire P. 1970. *Pedagogy of the oppressed.* New York: Herder and Herder.

Freire, P. 2000. *Pedagogy of the oppressed: 30th anniversary edition.* New York: Continuum.

Frenk, J., L. Chen, Z. A. Bhutta, J. Cohen, N. Crisp, T. Evans, H. Fineberg, et al. 2010. Health professionals for a new century: Transforming education to strengthen health systems in an interdependent world. *Lancet* 376 (9756): 1923–58.

Fryer-Edwards, K. 2002. Addressing the hidden curriculum in scientific research. *American Journal of Bioethics* 2 (4): 58–59.

Fullerton, S. M., N. R. Anderson, G. Guzauskas, D. Freeman, and K. Fryer-Edwards. 2010. Meeting the governance challenges of next-generation biorepository research. *Science Translational Medicine* 2 (15): 15cm3. doi: 10.1126/scitranslmed.3000361.

Furnham, F. 1986. Medical students' beliefs about nine different specialities. *British Medical Journal* 293: 1607–10.

Gaiser, R. R. 2009. The teaching of professionalism during residency: Why it is failing and a suggestion to improve its success. *Anesthesia and Analgesia* 108 (3): 948–54.

Gallagher, S. 2009. Philosophical antecedents of situated cognition. In *The Cambridge handbook of situated cognition*, eds. P. A. Robbins and M. Aydede, 35–51. New York: Cambridge University Press.

Ganz, M. 2008. What is public narrative? http://commorg.wisc.edu/syllabi/ganz/What isPublicNarrative5.19.08.htm.

Garden, R. E. 2007. The problem of empathy: Medicine and the humanities. *New Literary History* 38 (3): 551–67.

Garden, R. E. 2010. Telling stories about illness and disability: The limits and lessons of narrative. *Perspectives in Biology and Medicine* 53 (1): 121–35.

Garvey, G., I. Rolfe, and S. Pearson. 2009. Indigenous Australian medical students' perceptions of their medical school training. *Medical Education* 43 (11): 1047–55.

Gaufberg, E. H., M. Batalden, R. Sands, and S. K. Bell. 2010. The hidden curriculum: What can we learn from third-year medical student narrative reflections? *Academic Medicine* 85 (11): 1709–16.

Gaufberg, E. H., D. Hirsh, A. Fabiny, E. Krupat, B. Ogur, S. Pelletier, D. B. Reiff, and D. Bor. 2012. *The future is now: The resilience of humanism*. Poster Abstract. Rendez-vous Meeting. Thunder Bay, Ontario, Canada.

Gershon, I., and J. S. Taylor. 2008. Introduction to "In focus: Culture in the spaces of no culture." *American Anthropologist* 110 (4): 417–21.

Gibson-Graham, J. K. 2006. *The end of capitalism (as we knew it): A feminist critique of political economy*. Minneapolis: University of Minnesota Press.

Gieryn, T. 1983. Boundary work and the demarcation of science from non-science: Strains and interests in professional ideologies of scientists. *American Sociological Review* 48: 781–95.

Gillis, C. M. 2008. Medicine and humanities: Voicing connections. *Journal of Medical Humanities* 29 (5): 5–14.

Ginsburg, G. S., and H. F. Willard. 2009. Genomic and personalized medicine: Foundations and applications. *Translational Research, The Journal of Laboratory and Clinical Medicine* 154 (6): 277–87.

Ginsberg, S. 2012. Duty hours as viewed through a professionalism lens. Unpublished manuscript.

Glouberman, S., and B. Zimmerman. July 2002. Complicated and complex systems: What would successful reform of Medicare look like? Discussion Paper no. 8, Commission on the Future of Health Care in Canada.

Goering S., S. Holland, and K. Fryer-Edwards. 2008. Transforming genetic research practices with marginalized communities: A case for responsive justice. *Hastings Center Report* 38 (2): 43–53.

Goffman, E. 1963. *Stigma*. Englewood Cliffs, NJ: Prentice-Hall.

Gofton, W., and G. Regehr. 2006. What we don't know we are teaching: Unveiling the hidden curriculum. *Clinical Orthopedics and Related Research* 449: 20–27.

Goldie, J. 2012. The formation of professional identity in medical students: Considerations for educators. *Medical Teacher* 34 (9): e641–48.

Goldstein, E. A., R. Maestas, K. Fryer-Edwards, M. D. Wenrich, A. A. Oelschlager, A. M., Baernstein, and H. R. Kimball. 2006. Professionalism in medical education: An institutional challenge. *Academic Medicine* 81 (10): 871–76.

Good, B. J. 2003. *Medicine, rationality and experience: An anthropological perspective*. New York: Cambridge University Press.

Gordon, J., P. Markham, W. Lipworth, I. Kerridge, and M. Little. 2012. The dual nature of medical enculturation in post graduate medical training and practice. *Medical Education* 46 (9): 894–902.

Gramsci, A. 2000. *The Antonio Gramsci reader: Selected writings 1916–1935*, ed. D. Forgacs. New York: New York University Press.

Grandin, T., and S. Barron. 2005. *The unwritten rules of social relationships: Decoding social mysteries through the unique perspectives of autism*. Arlington, TX: Future Horizons.

Grant, J. 1999. The incapacitating effects of competence: A critique. *Advances in Health Sciences Education* 4 (3): 271–77.

Grbic, D., F. W. Hafferty, and P. K. Hafferty. 2013. Medical school mission statements as reflections of institutional identity and educational purpose: A network text analysis. *Academic Medicine* 88 (6): 852–60.

Greene, M. 1995. Art and imagination: Reclaiming the sense of possibility. *Phi Delta Kappa* 76 (5): 378–82.

Groves, T., and E. H. Wagner. 2005. High quality care for people with chronic diseases. *British Medical Journal* 330: 609–10.

Haas, J., and W. Shaffir. 1982. Ritual evaluation of competence: The hidden curriculum of professionalisation in an innovative medical school program. *Work and Occupation* 9 (2): 131–54.

Hafferty, F. W. 1998. Beyond curriculum reform: Confronting medicine's hidden curriculum. *Academic Medicine* 73 (4): 403–7.

Hafferty, F. W. 2000a. In search of a lost cord: Professionalism and medical education's hidden curriculum. In *Educating for professionalism*, eds. D. Wear and J. Bickel, 11–34. Iowa City: University of Iowa Press.

Hafferty, F. W. 2000b. Reconfiguring the sociology of medical education: Emerging topics and pressing issues. In *Handbook of medical sociology*, eds. P. Conrad, C. F. Bird, and A. M. Fremont, 238–56. New York: Prentice Hall.

Hafferty, F. W. 2009. Professionalism and the socialization of medical students. In *Teaching Medical Professionalism*, eds. R. L. Cruess, S. R. Cruess, and Y. Steinert, 53–73. New York: Cambridge University Press.

Hafferty, F. W., and R. Franks. 1994. The hidden curriculum, ethics teaching, and the structure of medical education. *Academic Medicine* 69 (11): 861–71.

Hafferty, F. W., and D. Levinson. 2008. Moving beyond nostalgia and motives: Towards a complexity science view of medical professionalism. *Perspectives in Biology and Medicine* 51 (4): 599–615.

Hafler, J. P., A. R. Ownby, B. M. Thompson, C. E. Fasser, K. Grigsby, P. Haidet, M. J. Kahn, and F. W. Hafferty. 2011. Decoding the learning environment of medical education—a hidden curriculum perspective for faculty development. *Academic Medicine* 86 (4): 440–44.

Hagy, J. 2012. Nine dangerous things you were taught in school. *Forbes*. http://www.forbes.com/sites/jessicahagy/2012/05/02/nine-dangerous-things-you-were-taught-in-school/.

Haidet, P. 2008. Where we're headed: A new wave of scholarship on educating medical professionalism. *Journal of General Internal Medicine* 23 (7): 1118–19.

Haidet, P., J. E. Dains, D. A. Paterniti, L. Hechtel, T. Chang, E. Tseng, and J. C. Rogers. 2002. Medical student attitudes toward the doctor-patient relationship. *Medical Education* 36 (6): 568–74.

Haidet, P., D. S. Hatem, M. L. Fecile, H. F. Stein, H. L. Haley, B. Kimmel, D. L. Mossbarger, and T. S. Inui. 2008. The role of relationships in the professional formation of physicians: Case report and illustration of an elicitation technique. *Patient Education and Counseling* 72 (3): 382–87.

Haidet, P., P. A. Kelly, S. Bentley, B. Blatt, C. L. Chou, A. H. Fortin VI, G. Gordon, et al. 2006. Not the same everywhere. Patient-centered learning environments at nine medical schools. *Journal of General Internal Medicine* 21 (5): 405–9.

Haidet, P., P. A. Kelly, and C. Chou. 2005. Communication, curriculum, and culture study group. Characterizing the patient-centeredness of hidden curricula in medical schools: Development and validation of a new measure. *Academic Medicine* 80 (1): 44–50.

Haidet, P., and H. F. Stein. 2006. The role of the student-teacher relationship in the formation of physicians: The hidden curriculum as process. *Journal of General Internal Medicine* 21 (S1): S16–20.

Halbesleben, J. R., D. S. Wakefield, and B. J. Wakefield. 2008. Work-arounds in health care settings: Literature review and research agenda. *Health Care Management Review* 33 (1): 2–12.

Hall, P. 2005. Interprofessional teamwork: Professional cultures as barriers. *Journal of Interprofessional Care* 19 (S1): 188–96.

Hamburg, M. A., and F. S. Collins. 2010. The path to personalised medicine. *New England Journal of Medicine* 363 (4): 301–4.

Harden, R. M. 2001. AMEE guide no. 21: Curriculum mapping: A tool for transparent and authentic teaching and learning. *Medical Teacher* 23 (2): 123–37.

Harden, R. M., and J. Crosby. 2000. AMEE guide no. 20: The good teacher is more than a lecturer—the twelve roles of the teacher. *Medical Teacher* 22 (4): 334–47.

Harden, R. M., M. Stevenson, W. W. Downie, and G. M. Wilson. 1975. Assessment of clinical competence using objective structured examination. *British Medical Journal* 1 (5955): 447–51.

Harmon, A. Where did you go with my DNA? *New York Times*, Apr. 24, 2010.

Hauer, K. E., D. Hirsh, I. H. Ma, L. A. Hansen, B. Ogur, A. N. Poncelet, E. K. Alexander, and B. C. O'Brien. 2012. The role of role: Learning in longitudinal integrated and traditional block clerkships. *Medical Education* 46 (7): 698–710.

Hauer, K. E., B. C. O'Brien, L. A. Hansen, D. Hirsh, I. H. Ma, B. Ogur, A. N. Poncelet, E. K. Alexander, and A. Teherani. 2012. More is better: Students describe successful and unsuccessful experiences with teachers differently in brief and longitudinal relationships. *Academic Medicine* 87 (10): 1389–96.

Helmich, E., and T. Dornan. 2012. Do you really want to be a doctor? The highs and lows of identity development. *Medical Education* 46 (2): 132–34.

Hilton, S. R., and H. B. Slotnick. 2005. Proto-professionalism: How professionalization occurs across the continuum of medical education. *Medical Education* 39 (1): 58–65.

Hinze, S. W. 1999. Gender and the body of medicine or at least some body parts: (Re)constructing the prestige hierarchy of medical specialities. *Sociological Quarterly* 40 (2): 217–39.

Hirsh, D., E. Gaufberg, B. Ogur, P. Cohen, E. Krupat, M. Cox, and D. Bor. 2012. Educational outcomes of the Harvard Medical School–Cambridge Integrated Clerkship: A way forward for medical education. *Academic Medicine* 87 (5): 1–8.

Hirsh, D., B. Ogur, G. E. Thibault, and M. Cox. 2007. 'Continuity' as an organizing principle for clinical education reform. *New England Journal of Medicine*. 356 (8): 858–66.

Hirsh, D., L. Walters, and A. N. Poncelet. 2012. Better learning, better doctors, better delivery system: Possibilities from a case study of longitudinal integrated clerkships. *Medical Teacher* 34 (7): 548–54.

Hodges, B. 2004. Medical student bodies and the pedagogy of self-reflection, self-assessment, and self-regulation. *Journal of Curriculum Theorizing* 20 (2): 41–51.

Hodges, B. 2006. Medical education and the maintenance of incompetence. *Medical Teacher* 28 (8): 690–96.

Hodges, B. 2009. *The objective structured clinical examination: A socio-history.* Berlin: LAP Lambert.

Hodges, B. D., M. Albert, D. Arweiler, S. Akseer, G. Bandiera, N. Byrne, B. Charlin, et al. 2011. The future of medical education: A Canadian environmental scan. *Medical Education* 45 (1): 95–106.

Hodges, B. D., S. Ginsburg, R. Cruess, et al. 2011. Assessment of professionalism: Recommendations from the 2010 Ottawa conference. *Medical Teacher* 33 (5): 354–63.

Hojat, M., M. J. Vergare, K. Maxwell, G. Brainard, S. K. Herrine, G. A. Isenberg, J. Veloski, and J. S. Gonnella. 2009. The devil is in the third year: A longitudinal study of erosion of empathy in medical school. *Academic Medicine* 84 (9): 1182–91.

Holmboe, E., S. Ginsburg, and E. Bernabeo. 2011. The rotational approach to medical education: Time to confront our assumptions? *Medical Education.* 45 (1): 69–80.

Howard, F., M. F. McKneally, R. G. Upshur Ross, and A. V. Levin. 2012. The formal and informal surgical ethics curriculum: Views of residents and staff surgeons in Toronto. *American Journal of Surgery* 203 (2): 258–65.

Hren, D., M. Marušić, and A. Marušić. 2011. Regression of moral reasoning during medical education: Combined design study to evaluate the effect of clinical study years. *PLoS ONE* 6 (3): e17406.

Huddle T. S. 2005. Teaching professionalism: Is medical morality a competency? *Academic Medicine* 80 (10): 885–91.

Huddle, T. S., and G. R. Heudebert. 2007. Taking apart the art: The risk of anatomizing clinical competence. *Academic Medicine* 82 (6): 536–41.

Hundert, E. M., D. Douglas-Steele, and J. Bickel. 1996. Context in medical education: The informal ethics curriculum. *Medical Education* 30 (5): 353–64.

Hundert, E. M., F. W. Hafferty, and D. Christakis. 1996. Characteristics of the informal curriculum and trainees' ethical choices. *Academic Medicine* 71 (6): 624–42.

Hunt, D. D., C. Scott, S. Zhong, and E. Goldstein. 1996. Frequency and effect of negative comments ("badmouthing") on medical students' career choices. *Academic Medicine* 71 (6): 665–69.

Hunter, K. M., R. Charon, and J. Coulehan. 1995. The study of literature in medical education. *Academic Medicine* 70 (9): 787–94.

Hutzler, L. 2012. Unearthing the rise of ethics in medical education. Unpublished research. http://krieger.jhu.edu/magazine/2012/04/unearthing-the-rise-of-ethics-in-medical-education/.

Indiana University School of Medicine. 2011. *Guidelines for use of online social networks for medical students and physicians-in-training.* Indianapolis: Indiana University School of Medicine.

International Consortium of Longitudinal Integrated Clerkships. Consensus LIC definition. 2007. Cambridge, MA.

Jackson, P. W. 1966. The student's world. *Elementary School Journal* 66 (7): 345–57.

Jackson, P. W. 1968. *Life in Classrooms.* New York: Holt, Rinehart and Winston.

Jarvis-Selinger, S., D. D. Pratt, and G. Regehr. 2012. Competency is not enough: Integrating identity formation into the medical education discourse. *Academic Medicine* 87 (9): 1185–90.

Jaye, C., T. Egan, and S. Parker. 2006. Do as I say, not as I do: Medical education and Foucault's normalizing technologies of self. *Anthropology and Medicine* 13 (2): 141–55.

Jena, A. B., V. M. Arora, K. E. Hauer, S. Durning, N. Borges, N. Oriol, D. M. Elnicki, et al. 2012. The prevalence and nature of postinterview communications between residency programs and applicants during the match. *Academic Medicine* 87 (10): 1434–42.

Johnston, J. L., M. E. Cupples, K. J. McGlade, and K. Steele. 2011. Medical students' attitudes to professionalism: An opportunity for the GP tutor? *Education for Primary Care* 22 (5): 321–27.

Jost, J. T., and D. L. Hamilton. 2005. Stereotypes in our culture. In *On the nature of prejudice: Fifty years after Allport,* eds. J. F. Davidio, P. Glick, and L. A. Rudman, 208–24. Malden, MA: Blackwell.

Kai, J., R. Bridgewater, and J. Spencer. 2008. "'Just think of TB and Asians,' that's all I ever hear": Medical learners' views about training to work in an ethnically diverse society. *Medical Education* 35 (3): 250–56.

Kamaka, M. L. 2001. Cultural immersion in a cultural competency curriculum. *Academic Medicine* 76 (5): 512.

Kansagra, S. M. 2011. *Everything I learned in medical school besides all the book stuff.* Createspace (an Amazon.com company).

Karnieli-Miller O., A. C. Taylor, A. H. Cottingham, T. S. Inui, T. R. Vu, and R. M. Frankel. 2010. Exploring the meaning of respect in medical student education: An analysis of student narratives. *Journal of General Internal Medicine* 25 (12): 1309–14.

Karnieli-Miller O., T. R. Vu, R. M. Frankel, M. C. Holtman, S. G. Clyman, S. L.

Hui, and T. S. Inui. 2011. Which experiences in the hidden curriculum teach students about professionalism? *Academic Medicine* 86 (3): 369–77.

Karnieli-Miller, O., T. R. Vu, M. C. Holtman, S. G. Clyman, and T. S. Inui. 2010. Medical students' professionalism narratives: A window on the informal and hidden curriculum. *Academic Medicine* 85 (1): 124–33.

Kearney, J. 1998. From the inside of a short white coat. *Journal of General Internal Medicine* 13: 647.

Keith-Spiegel, P., and G. P. Koocher. 2005. The IRB paradox: Could the protectors also encourage deceit? *Ethics and Behavior* 15 (4): 339–49.

Kelly, S. D. 2000. Grasping at straws: Motor intentionality and the cognitive science of skilled behavior. In *Heidegger, coping and cognitive science: Essays in honor of Hubert L. Dreyfus*, eds. M. Wrathall and J. Malpas, 161–77. Cambridge, MA: MIT Press.

Khan, S. R. 2011. *Privilege: The making of an adolescent elite at St. Paul's School.* Princeton: Princeton University Press.

Klatt, E. C., and C. A. Klatt. 2011. How much is too much reading for medical students? Assigned reading and reading rates at one medical school. *Academic Medicine* 86 (9): 1079–83.

Knight, J. 2004. Students set up forum to debate hot topics. *Nature* 431 (7007): 390.

Koenig, B. A. 1988. The technological imperative in medical practice: The social creation of a "routine" treatment. In *Biomedicine Examined*, eds. M. Locke and D. Gorden, 465–96. New York: Springer.

Kohn, M., and C. Donley. 2008. *Return to The House of God: Medical residency education 1978–2008.* Kent, OH: Kent State University Press.

Krieger, N. 1994. Epidemiology and the web of causation: Has anyone seen the spider? *Social Science and Medicine* 39 (7): 887–903.

Krupat, E., C. M. Hiam, M. Z. Fleming, and P. Freeman. 1999. Patient-centeredness and its correlates among first year medical students. *International Journal of Psychiatry in Medicine* 29 (3): 347–56.

Krupat, E., S. Pelletier, E. K. Alexander, D. Hirsh, B. Ogur, and R. Schwartzstein. 2009. Can changes in the principal clinical year prevent the erosion of students' patient-centered beliefs? *Academic Medicine* 84 (5): 582–86.

Kuhn, G. J., S. B. Abbuhl, and K. J. Clem. 2008. SAEM taskforce for women in academic emergency medicine. Recommendations from the Society for Academic Emergency Medicine (SAEM) taskforce on women in academic emergency medicine. *Academic Emergency Medicine* 15 (8): 762–67.

Kuper, A., M. A. Martimianakis, P. Karazivan, J. Maniate and S. Reeves. n.d. The culture of medicine and the hidden curriculum: Insights from a Canadian environmental scan. Unpublished manuscript.

Kuper, A., and C. Whitehead. 2012. The paradox of interprofessional education: IPE as a mechanism of maintaining physician power? *Journal of Interprofessional Care* 26 (5): 347–49.

Kuper, A., C. Whitehead, and B. D. Hodges. 2013. Looking back to move forward: Using history, discourse and text in medical education research: AMEE guide no. 73. *Medical Teacher* 35 (1): 85–96.

Lahey, W., and R. Currie. 2005. Regulatory and medico-legal barriers to interprofessional practice. *Journal of Interprofessional Care* 19 (S1): 197–223.

Lamiani, G., D. Leone, E. C. Meyer, and E. A. Moja. 2011. How Italian students learn to become physicians: A qualitative study of the hidden curriculum. *Medical Teacher* 33 (12): 989–96.

Lave, J. 1988. *Cognition in practice: Mind, mathematics and culture in everyday life.* Cambridge, UK, and New York: Cambridge University Press.

Lave, J. 1997. The culture of acquisition and the practice of understanding. In *Situated cognition: Social, semiotic, and psychological perspectives,* eds. D. Kirshner and J. A. Whitson, 17–35. Mahwah, NJ: Lawrence Erlbaum.

Lave, J., and E. Wenger. 1991. *Situated learning: Legitimate peripheral participation.* Cambridge, UK: Cambridge University Press.

Lemke, T. 2001. The birth of bio-politics: Michel Foucault's lecture at the College de France on neo-governmentality. *Economy and Society* 30 (2): 190–207.

Lempp, H., and C. Seale. 2004. The hidden curriculum in undergraduate medical education: Qualitative study of medical students' perceptions of teaching. *British Medical Journal* 329 (7469): 770–73.

Lempp, H., and C. Seale. 2006. Medical students' perceptions in relation to ethnicity and gender: A qualitative study. *BioMed Central Medical Education* 6: 17.

Leo, T., and K. Eagen. 2008. Professionalism education: The medical student response. *Perspectives in Biology and Medicine* 51 (4): 508–16.

Levine, R. B., F. Lin, D. E. Kern, S. M. Wright, and J. Carrese. 2011. Stories from early-career women physicians who have left academic medicine: A qualitative study at a single institution. *Academic Medicine* 86 (6): 752–58.

Liaison Committee on Medical Education [LCME]. 2012. *Functions and structure of a medical school: Standards for accreditation of medical education programs leading to the M.D. degree.* Chicago: LCME.

Liao, J. M., E. J. Thomas, and S. K. Bell. 2013. See one, do one, teach one: Linking the hidden curriculum to patient safety.

Lingard, L. 2009. What we see and don't see when we look at "competence": Notes on a god term. *Advances in Health Sciences Education Theory and Practice* 14 (5): 625–28.

Lingard, L. 2012. Rethinking competence in the context of teamwork. In *The question of competence: Reconsidering medical education in the twenty-first century*, eds. B. D. Hodges and L. Lingard, 42–69. Ithaca: Cornell University Press.

Lingard, L., P. Reznick, I. DeVito, and S. Espin. 2002. Forming professional identities on the health care team: Discursive constructions of the "other" in the operating room. *Medical Education* 36 (8): 728–34.

Litzelman, D. K., and A. H. Cottingham. 2007. The new formal competency-based curriculum and informal curriculum at Indiana University School of Medicine: Overview and five-year analysis. *Academic Medicine* 82 (4): 410–21.

Lucey, C., and W. Souba. 2010. The problem with the problem of professionalism. *Academic Medicine* 85 (6): 1018–24.

MacIntyre, A. 1984. *After virtue: A study in moral theory*. 2nd ed. Notre Dame, IN: University of Notre Dame Press.

Madigosky, W. S., L. A. Headrick, K. Nelson, K. R. Cox, and T. Anderson. 2006. Changing and sustaining medical students' knowledge, skills, and attitudes about patient safety and medical fallibility. *Academic Medicine* 81 (1): 94–101.

Mahood, S. 2011. Medical education. Beware of the hidden curriculum. *Canadian Family Physician* 57 (9): 983–85.

Mann, K., J. Gordon, and A. MacLeod. 2009. Reflection and reflective practice in health professions education: A systematic review. *Advances in Health Sciences Education: Theory and Practice* 14 (4): 595–621.

Martimianakis, M. A. 2008. Reconciling competing discourses: The University of Toronto's equity and diversity framework. In *Whose university is it, anyway? Power and privilege on gendered terrain*, eds. A. Wagner, S. Acker, K. Mayuzumi, 44–60. Toronto: Sumach.

Martimianakis, M. A., J. M. Maniate, and B. D. Hodges. 2009. Sociological interpretations of professionalism. *Medical Education* 43 (9): 829–37.

Martinson, B. C., M. S. Anderson, and R. de Vries. 2005. Scientists behaving badly. *Nature* 435 (7043): 737–38.

Martinson, B. C., A. L. Crain, R. de Vries, and M. S. Anderson. 2010. The importance of organizational justice in ensuring research integrity. *Journal of Empirical Research on Human Research Ethics* 5 (3): 67–83.

Mayson, J., and W. Hayward. 1997. Learning to be a nurse: The contribution of the hidden curriculum in the clinical setting. *Nurse Practitioner New Zealand* 12 (2): 16–22.

McCormick, J. B., R. R. Sharp, A. L. Ottenberg, C. R. Reider, H. A. Taylor, and B. S. Wilfond. 2013. The establishment of research ethics consultation services (RECS): An emerging research resource. *Clinical Translational Science* 6 (1): 40–44.

McLean, M., F. Cilliers, and J. Van Wyk. 2008. AMEE guide no. 36: Faculty development: Yesterday, today and tomorrow. *Medical Teacher* 30: 555–84.

Merton, R. K. 1957. *Social theory and social structure.* Glencoe, IL: Free Press.

Merton, R. K., G. Reader, and P. Kendall. 1957. *The student physician: Introductory studies in the sociology of medical education.* Cambridge, MA: Harvard University Press.

Michalec, B. 2012. The pursuit of medical knowledge and the potential consequences of the hidden curriculum. *Health (London)* 16 (3): 267–81.

Miéville, C. 2009. *The city and the city.* New York: Ballantine.

Miller, J. B., D. C. Schaad, R. A. Crittenden, N. E. Oriol, and C. MacLaren. 2003. Communication between programs and applicants during residency selection: Effects of the match on medical students' professional development. *Academic Medicine* 78 (4): 403–11.

Monrouxe, L. 2010. Identity, identification and medical education: Why should we care? *Medical Education* 44 (1): 40–49.

Monrouxe, L., and C. E. Rees. 2012. "It's just a clash of cultures": Emotional talk within medical students' narratives of professionalism dilemmas. *Advances in Health Science Education* 17 (5): 671–701.

Monrouxe, L., C. E. Rees, and W. Hu. 2011. Differences in medical students' explicit discourses of professionalism: Acting, representing, becoming. *Medical Education* 45 (6): 585–602.

Mueller, P. S., and C. C. Hook. 2013. Technological and treatment imperatives, life-sustaining technologies, and associated ethical and social challenges. *Mayo Clinical Proceedings* 88 (7): 641–44.

Muzzin, L. 2001. Powder puff brigades: Professional caring vs. industry research in the pharmaceutical sciences curriculum. In *The hidden curriculum in higher education*, ed. E. Margolis, 135–54. New York: Routledge.

National Human Genome Research Institute. 2003. International consortium completes human genome project. http://www.genome.gov/11006929.

National Institutes of Health. n.d. Extramural support: Grants and funding. http://grants.nih.gov/grants/research_integrity/.

National Institutes of Health. 2008. Policy for sharing of data obtained in NIH supported or conducted Genome-Wide Association Studies (GWAS). http://grants.nih.gov/grants/guide/notice-files/NOT-OD-07-088.html.

Neufeld, V. R., R. F. Maudsley, R. J. Pickering, J. M. Turnbull, W. W. Weston, M. G. Brown, and J. C. Simpson. 1998. Educating future physicians for Ontario. *Academic Medicine* 73 (11): 1133–48.

Newton, B., L. Barber, J. Clardy, E. Cleveland, and P. O'Sullivan. 2008. Is there a hardening of the heart during medical school? *Academic Medicine* 83: 244–49.

Nicholson, J. M., and J. P. Ioannidis. 2012. Research grants: Conform and be funded. *Nature* 492 (7427): 34–36.

Noddings, N. 1984. *Caring: A feminine approach to ethics and moral education.* Berkeley: University of California Press.

O'Brien, B. C., A. Poncelet, L. Hansen, D. Hirsh, B. Ogur, E. Alexander, E. Krupat, and K. E. Hauer. 2012. Students' workplace learning in two clerkship models: A multi-site observational study. *Medical Education* 46 (6): 613–24.

Office of Human Subjects Research Protections (OHRP). n.d. Guidance on research involving coded private information or biological specimens. http://www.hhs.gov/ohrp/policy/cdebiol.html.

Ogur, B., and D. Hirsh. 2009. Learning through longitudinal care—narratives from the Harvard Medical School–Cambridge Integrated Clerkship. *Academic Medicine* 84 (7): 844–50.

Ogur, B., D. Hirsh, E. Krupat, and D. Bor. 2007. The Harvard Medical School–Cambridge Integrated Clerkship: An innovative model of clinical education. *Academic Medicine* 82 (4): 397–404.

Open Science Federation. n.d. http://opensciencefederation.com.

Ownby, A. R., F. W. Hafferty, J. P. Hafler, and B. M. Thompson. 2011. *Teaching faculty how to decode and navigate the hidden curriculum.* Denver, CO: Association of American Medical Colleges (AAMC).

Oxford English Dictionary. 2nd ed. 1989. Oxford: Clarendon.

Paice, E., and J. Firth-Cozens. 2003. Who is a bully then? *British Medical Journal Careers* 12: s127–28.

Palmer, P. J. 2004. A hidden wholeness: The journey toward an undivided life. San Francisco: John Wiley, Jossey-Bass.

Parsons, T. 1958. *Essays in sociological theory.* Rev. ed. Glencoe, IL: Free Press.

Partridge, B. 1983. The hidden curriculum of nursing education. *Lamp* 40 (8): 30.

Patenaude, J., T. Niyonsenga, and D. Fafard. 2003. Changes in students' moral development during medical school: A cohort study. *Canadian Medical Association Journal* 168 (7): 840–44.

Perkins, M. B., P. S. Jensen, J. Jaccard, P. Gollwitzer, G. Oettingen, E. Pappadopulos, and K. E. Hoagwood. 2007. Applying theory-driven approaches to understanding and modifying clinicians' behavior: What do we know? *Psychiatric Services* 58 (3): 342–48.

Perloff, R., B. Bonder, G. Ray, E. B. Ray, and L. A. Siminoff. 2006. Doctor-patient communication, cultural competence, and minority health: Theoretical and empirical perspectives. *American Behavioural Scientist* 49 (6): 835–52.

Perry, A. G., and P. A. Potter. 2006. *Clinical nursing skills and techniques*. 6th ed. St. Louis, MO: Elsevier.

Peterkin, A. D., and A. A. Prettyman. 2009. Finding a voice: Revisiting the history of therapeutic writing. *Medical Humanities* 35 (2): 80–88.

Peterson, A., A. Bleakley, R. Brömer, and R. Marshall. 2008. The medical humanities today: Humane health care or tool of governance? *Journal of Medical Humanities* 29 (1): 1–4.

Petrie, M., and G. Rugg. 2011. *The unwritten rules of PhD research*. New York: McGraw Hill, Open University Press.

Pettinari, C. J. 1988. *Task, talk and text in the operating room: A study in medical discourse*. Advances in Discourse Processes Series. Westport, CT: Praeger.

Phillips, N., and C. Hardy. 2002. *Discourse analysis: Investigating processes of social construction*. London and New York: Sage.

Phillips, S. P., and M. Clark. 2012. More than an education: The hidden curriculum, professional attitudes and career choice. *Medical Education* 46 (9): 887–93.

Plaza, C. M., J. L. R. Draugalis, M. K. Slack, G. H. Skrepnek, and K. A. Sauer. 2007. Curriculum Mapping in Program Assessment and Evaluation. *American Journal of Pharmaceutical Education* 71 (2): Article 20.

Polanyi, M. 1974. *Personal knowledge: Towards a post-critical philosophy*. Chicago: University of Chicago Press.

Pololi, L. H., P. Conrad, S. Knight, and P. Carr. 2009. A study of the relational aspects of the culture of academic medicine. *Academic Medicine* 84 (1): 106–14.

Pololi L. H., L.A. Cooper, and P. Carr. 2010. Race, disadvantage and faculty experiences in academic medicine. *Journal of General Internal Medicine* 25 (12): 1363–69.

Pololi, L. H., S. M. Knight, K. Dennis, and R. M. Frankel. 2002. Helping medical school faculty realize their dreams: An innovative, collaborative mentoring program. *Academic Medicine* 77 (5): 377–84.

Pololi, L. H., E. Krupat, J. T. Civian, A. S. Ash, and R. T. Brennan. 2012. Why are a quarter of faculty considering leaving academic medicine? A study of their perceptions of institutional culture and intentions to leave at 26 representative U.S. medical schools. *Academic Medicine* 87 (7): 859–69.

Popkewitz, T. S., and M. Brennan. 1998. *Foucault's challenge: Discourse, knowledge, and power in education*. New York: Teachers College Press.

Prensky, M. 2001a. Digital natives, digital immigrants. *On the Horizon* 9 (5): 1–6.

Prensky, M. 2001b. Digital natives, digital immigrants, part II: Do they really think differently? *On the Horizon* 9 (6): 1–6.

Prentice, R. 2012. *Bodies in formation: An ethnography of anatomy and surgery education.* Durham, NC: Duke University Press.

Prideaux, D., P. Worley, and J. Bligh. 2007. Symbiosis: A new model for clinical education. *Clinical Teacher* 4 (4): 209–12.

Quaintance, J. L., L. Arnold, and G. S. Thompson. 2008. Development of an instrument to measure the climate of professionalism in a clinical teaching environment. *Academic Medicine* 83 (10 Suppl): S5–8.

Quaintance, J. L., L. Arnold, and G. S. Thompson. 2010. What students learn about professionalism from faculty stories: An "appreciative inquiry" approach. *Academic Medicine* 85 (1): 118–23.

Rabinow, P., and N. Rose. 2006. Biopower today. *Biosocieties* 1 (2): 195–217.

Rabow, M. W., C. Evans, and R. N. Remen. 2013. Professional formation and deformation: repression of personal values and qualities in medical education. *Family Medicine* 45 (1): 13–18.

Rabow, M., J. Gargani, and M. Cooke. 2007. Do as I say: Curricular discordance in medical school end-of-life care education. *Journal of Palliative Medicine* 10 (3): 759–69.

Rabow, M. W., R. N. Remen, D. X. Parmelee, and T. S. Inui. 2010. Professional formation: Extending medicine's lineage of service into the next century. *Academic Medicine* 85 (2): 310–17.

Rabow, M. W., J. Wrubel, and R. N. Remen. 2007. Authentic community as an educational strategy for advancing professionalism: A national evaluation of the healer's art course. *Journal of General Internal Medicine* 22 (10): 1422–28.

Ranjbar, V. 2012. Risk assessment as a paradox: When actions of an IRB become incompatible with ethical principles. *Accountability in Research* 19 (5): 273–84.

Ratanawongsa, N., A. Teherani, and K. E. Hauer. 2005. Third-year medical students' experiences with dying patients during the internal medicine clerkship: A qualitative study of the informal curriculum. *Academic Medicine* 80 (7): 641–47.

Rees, C. E. 2004. The problem with outcomes-based curricula in medical education: Insights from educational theory. *Medical Education* 38 (6): 593–98.

Reeves, S. 2011. Using the sociological imagination to explore the nature of interprofessional interactions and relations. In *Sociology of interprofessional healthcare practice*, eds. S. Kitto, J. Chesters, J. Thistlethwaite, and S. Reeves, 9–22. New York: Nova.

Reeves, S. 2013. Interprofessional education—reflecting upon the past, scanning the future. http://macyfoundation.org/news/entry/interprofessional-education-scott-reeves.

Reeves, S., A. Fox, and B. D. Hodges. 2009. The competency movement in the health professions: Ensuring consistent standards or reinforcing conventional domains of practice? *Advances in Health Sciences Education* 14 (4): 451–53.

Remen, R. N., J. F. O'Donnell, and M. W. Rabow. 2008. The healer's art: Education in meaning and service. *Journal of Cancer Education* 23 (1): 65–67.

Resnick, B. 2013. Will we ever learn the benefits of teams? *Journal of the American Geriatrics Society* 61 (6): 1019–21.

Rich, E., and A. Miah. 2009. Prosthetic surveillance: The medical governance of healthy bodies in cyberspace. *Surveillance and Society* 6 (2): 163–77.

Rogers, D. A., M. L. Boehler, N. K. Roberts, and V. Johnson. 2012. Using the hidden curriculum to teach professionalism during the surgery clerkship. *Journal of Surgical Education* 69 (3): 423–27.

Rosch, E. 1975. Cognitive representations of semantic categories. *Journal of Experimental Psychology: General* 104 (3): 192–233.

Rosch, E., and C. B. Mervis. 1975. Family resemblances: Studies in the internal structure of categories. *Cognitive Psychology* 7 (4): 573–605.

Rose, N. 1998. *Inventing ourselves: Psychology, power and personhood.* Cambridge, UK: Cambridge University Press.

Rothman, D. J. 1997. *Beginnings count: The technological imperative in American health care.* New York: Oxford University Press.

Royal College of Physicians of London. 2005. *Doctors in society: Medical professionalism in a changing world.* London: Royal College of Physicians of London.

Saha, S., M. C. Beach, and L. A. Cooper. 2008. Patient centeredness, cultural competence and healthcare quality. *Journal of the National Medical Association* 100 (11): 1275–85.

Schein, E. H. 2004. *Organizational culture and leadership.* 3rd ed. San Francisco: Jossey-Bass.

Schon, D. A. 1987. *Educating the reflective practitioner: Toward a new design for teaching and learning in the professions.* San Francisco: Jossey-Bass.

Schwartz, B., and K. Sharpe. 2011. *Practical wisdom: The right way to do the right thing.* New York: Riverhead.

Self, D. J., and D. C. Baldwin, Jr. 1994. Moral reasoning in medicine. In *Moral development in the professions,* eds. J. R. Rest and D. F. Narvaez. 147–62. Hilsdale, NJ: Lawrence Earlbaum.

Sewell, G., and N. Phillips. 2010. Introduction. Joan Woodward and the study of organizations. In *Technology and organization: Essays in honour of Joan*

Woodward, eds. N. Phillips, G. Sewell, and D. Griffiths. Bingley, UK: Emerald Group.

Sharp, R. R. 2002. Teaching old dogs new tricks: Continuing education in research. *American Journal of Bioethics* 2 (4): 55–56.

Shortell, S. M. 1974. Occupational prestige differences within the medical and allied health professions. *Social Science and Medicine* 8 (1): 1–9.

Silko, L. M. 1977. *Ceremony*. New York: Penguin.

Simanton, E. 2012. Sanford School of Medicine at the University of South Dakota. Personal communication.

Simon, P. 1964. Sound of silence. New York: Columbia Records.

Skelton, A. 1997. Studying hidden curricula: Developing a perspective in the light of postmodern insights. *Curriculum Studies* 5 (2): 177–93.

Smedley, B. D., A. Y. Stith, and A. R. Nelson. 2002. *Unequal treatment: Confronting racial and ethnic disparities in health care*. Washington, DC: National Academy Press.

Smith, K. L., R. Saavedra, J. L. Raeke, and A. O'Donell. 2007. The journey to creating a campus-wide culture of professionalism. *Academic Medicine* 82 (11): 1015–21.

Snyder, B. R. 1971. *The hidden curriculum*. New York: Knopf.

Solomon M. Z., L. O'Donnell, B. Jennings, V. Guilfoy, S. M. Wolf, K. Nolan, R. Jackson, D. Koch-Weser, and S. Donnelley. 1993. Decisions near the end of life: Professional views on life-sustaining treatments. *American Journal of Public Health* 83 (1): 14–23.

Souba, C. 2010. The language of leadership. *Academic Medicine* 85: 1609–18.

Souba, W., D. Way, C. Lucey, D. Sedmak, and M. Notestine. 2011. Elephants in academic medicine. *Academic Medicine* 86 (12): 1492–99.

Spindler, S. 1992. *Doctors to be*. Doctors at large. London: BBC.

Squier, S. 2007. Beyond nescience: The intersectional insights of health humanities. *Perspectives in Biology and Medicine* 50 (3): 334–47.

Steinecke, A, and C. Terrell. 2010. Progress for whose future? The impact of the Flexner Report on medical education for racial and ethnic minority physicians in the United States. *Academic Medicine* 85 (2): 236–45.

Steinert, Y., R. L. Cruess, S. R. Cruess, J. D. Boudreau, and A. Fuks. 2007. Faculty development as an instrument of change: A case study on teaching professionalism. *Academic Medicine* 82 (11): 1057–64.

Steinert, Y., K. Mann, A. Centeno, D. Dolmans, J. Spencer, M. Gelula, and D. Prideaux. 2006. A systematic review of faculty development initiatives designed to improve teaching effectiveness in medical education: BEME guide no. 8. *Medical Teacher* 28 (6): 497–526.

Steinert, Y., P. J. McLeod, M. Boillat, S. Meterissian, M. Elizov, and M. E. Macdonald. 2009. Faculty development: A "field of dreams"? *Medical Education* 43 (1): 42–49.

Stern, D. T. 1996. *Hanging out: Teaching values in medical education*. Dissertation. Palo Alto, CA: Stanford University.

Stern, D. T. 1998a. Practicing what we preach? An analysis of the curriculum of values in medical education. *American Journal of Medicine* 104 (6): 569–75.

Stern, D. T. 1998b. In search of the informal curriculum. When and where professional values are taught. *Academic Medicine* 73 (10 Suppl): S23–30.

Stern, D. T. 2006. *Measuring medical professionalism*. New York: Oxford University Press.

Stern, D. T, and M. D. Papadakis. 2006. The developing physician—becoming a professional. *New England Journal of Medicine* 355 (17): 1794–99.

Sternod, B. M. 2011. Role models or normalizing agents? A genealogical analysis of popular written news media discourse regarding male teachers. *Curriculum Inquiry* 41 (2): 267–92.

Strasser, R., and D. Hirsh. 2011. Longitudinal integrated clerkships: Transforming medical education worldwide? *Medical Education* 45 (6): 436–37.

Suchman, A. L., P. R. Williamson, D. K. Litzelman, R. M. Frankel, D. L. Mossbarger, and T. S. Innui. 2004. Toward an informal curriculum that teaches professionalism. Transforming the social environment of a medical school. *Journal of General Internal Medicine* 19 (5): 501–4.

Sullivan, W. M. 2005. *Work and integrity: The crisis and promise of professionalism in America*. 2nd ed. Carnegie Foundation for the Advancement of Teaching Series. San Francisco: Jossey-Bass.

Sullivan, W. M., and M. S. Rosin. 2008. *A new agenda for higher education: Shaping a life of the mind for practice*. Carnegie Foundation for the Advancement of Teaching Series. San Francisco: Jossey-Bass.

Swick, H. M., P. Szenas, D. Danoff, and M. E. Whitcomb. 1999. Teaching professionalism in undergraduate medical education. *Journal of the American Medical Association* 282 (9): 830–32.

Tajfel, H., and J. Turner. 1979. An integrative theory of inter-group conflict. In *The social psychology of intergroup relations*, eds. W. G. Austin and S. Worchel, 33–47. Monterey, CA: Brooks/Cole.

Tamboukou, M. 2003. Genealogy and ethnography: Fruitful encounters or dangerous liaisons? In *Dangerous encounters: Genealogy and ethnography*, eds. M. Tamboukou and S. E. Ball, 1–36. New York: Peter Lang.

Tavare, A., and F. Godlee. 2012. Helping research institutions handle misconduct. *British Medical Journal* 345: e5402.

Taylor, J. S. 2003. Confronting "culture" in medicine's "culture of no culture." *Academic Medicine* 78 (6): 555–59.

Taylor, J. S. 2011. The moral aesthetics of simulated suffering in standardized patient performances. *Culture, Medicine, and Psychiatry* 35 (2): 134–62.

Teherani, A., D. M. Irby, and H. Loeser. 2013. Outcomes of different clerkship models: Longitudinal integrated, hybrid, and block. *Academic Medicine* 88 (1): 1–9.

Thompson, B. M., C. R. Teal, J. C. Rogers, D. A. Paterniti, and P. Haidet. 2010. Ideals, activities, dissonance, and processing: A conceptual model to guide educators' efforts to stimulate student reflection. *Academic Medicine* 85 (5): 902–8.

Thornicroft, G., H. Lempp, and M. Tansella. 2011. The place of implementation science in the translational medicine continuum. *Psychological Medicine* 42 (10): 2015–21.

Thornicroft, G., D. Rose, and A. Kassam. 2007. Stigma: Ignorance, prejudice or discrimination? *British Journal of Psychiatry* 190: 192–93.

Todhunter, S., S. R. Cruess, R. L. Cruess, M. Young, and Y. Steinert. 2011. Developing and piloting a form for student assessment of professionalism. *Advances in Health Sciences Education* 16 (2): 223–38.

Trautmann, J. 1982. The wonders of literature in medical education. *Mobius* 2 (3): 23–31.

Trowler, P., and P. Knight. 1999. Organizational socialization and induction in universities: Reconceptualizing theory and practice. *Higher Education* 37: 177–95.

Tsai, S. L., M. J. Ho, D. Hirsch, and D. E. Kern. 2012. Defiance, compliance or alliance? How we developed a medical professionalism curriculum that deliberately connects to cultural context. *Medical Teacher* 34: 614–17.

Tsang, A. K. L. 2011. Students as evolving professionals: Turning the hidden curriculum around through the threshold concept pedagogy. *Teaching and Learning Journal* 4: 1–11.

Turbes, S., E. Krebs, and S. Axtell. 2002. The hidden curriculum in multicultural medical education: The role of case examples. *Academic Medicine* 77 (3): 209–16.

Turner, J. C. 1982. Towards a cognitive redefinition of the social group. In *Social identity and intergroup relations*, ed. H. Tajfel, 15–40. Cambridge, UK: Cambridge University Press.

Turner, J. C. 1996. Henri Tajfel: An introduction. In *Social groups and identities: Developing the legacy of Henri Tajfel*, ed. W. P. Robinson, 1–23. Oxford: Butterworth Heinemann.

Turunen, T., and J. Rafferty. 2013. Insights beyond neo-liberal educational practices: the value of discourse analysis. *Educational Research for Policy and Practice* 12 (1): 43–56.

Twenge, J. M. 2009. Generational changes and their impact in the classroom: Teaching generation me. *Medical Education* 43 (5): 398–405.

Veatch, R. M. 2002. White coat ceremonies: A second opinion. *Journal of Medical Ethics* 28 (1): 5–6.

Veazey Brooks, J., and C. S. Bosk. 2012. Remaking surgical socialization: Work hour restrictions, rites of passage, and occupational identity. *Social Science and Medicine* 75 (9): 1625–32.

Verby, J. E., J. P. Newell, S. A. Andresen, and W. M. Swentko. 1991. Changing the medical school curriculum to improve patient access to primary care. *Journal of the American Medical Association* 266 (1): 110–13.

Viggiano, T. R., W. Pawlina, K. D. Olsen, and D. A. Cortese. 2007. Putting the needs of the patient first: Mayo Clinic's core value, institutional culture, and professionalism covenant. *Academic Medicine* 82 (11): 1089–93.

Wachtler, C., and M. Troein. 2003. A hidden curriculum: Mapping cultural competency in a medical programme. *Medical Education* 37 (10): 861–68.

Wakefield, A. B., C. R. M. Boggis, and M. Holland. 2006. Team working but no blurring thank you! *Learning in Health and Social Care* 5 (3): 142–54.

Wald, H. S., J. M. Borkan, J. S. Taylor, D. Anthony, and S. P. Reis. 2012. Fostering and evaluating reflective capacity in medical education: Developing the REFLECT rubric for assessing reflective writing. *Academic Medicine* 87 (1): 41–50.

Wald, H. S., S. P. Reis, A. D. Monroe, and J. M. Borkan. 2010. The loss of my elderly patient: Interactive reflective writing to support medical students' rites of passage. *Medical Teacher* 32 (4): 178–84.

Walker, L., H. Starks, K. M. West, and S. M. Fullerton. 2011. dbGaP data access requests: A call for greater transparency. *Science Translational Medicine* 3 (113): 113–34.

Walters, L., J. Greenhill, J. Richards, H. Ward, N. Campbell, J. Ash, and L. W. T. Schuwirth. 2012. Outcomes of longitudinal integrated clinical placements for students, clinicians and society. *Medical Education* 46 (11): 1028–41.

Wear, D. 1997. Professional development of medical students: Problems and promises. *Academic Medicine* 72 (12): 1056–62.

Wear, D. 1998. On white coats and professional development: The formal and the hidden curricula. *Annals of Internal Medicine* 129 (9): 734–37.

Wear, D. 2009. A perfect storm: The convergence of bullet points, competencies, and screen reading in medical education. *Academic Medicine* 84 (11): 1500–1504.

Wear, D., and J. M. Aultman. 2005. The limits of narrative: Medical student resistance to confronting inequality and oppression in literature and beyond. *Medical Education* 39 (10): 1056–65.

Weaver, R., K. Peters, J. Koch, and I. Wilson. 2011. "Part of the team": Professional identity and social exclusivity in medical students. *Medical Education* 45 (12): 1220–29.

Wendland, C. 2010. *A heart for the work: Journeys through an African medical school.* Chicago: University of Chicago Press.

Wendland, C., J. S. Taylor, and F. W. Hafferty. 2013. Medical work as cultural practice. In *Behavioral and social science in medicine: Principles and practice of biopsychosocial care,* eds. S. R. Waldstein, M. F. Muldoon, J. M. Satterfield, et al. New York: Springer.

Wenger, E. 1998. *Communities of practice: Learning, meaning, and identity.* New York: Cambridge University Press.

White, J., K. Brownell, J. F. Lemay, and J. M. Lockyer. 2012. What do they want me to say? The hidden curriculum at work in the medical school selection process: A qualitative study. *BioMed Central Medical Education* 12: 17.

Whitehead, C. 2007. The doctor dilemma in interprofessional education and care: How and why will physicians collaborate? *Medical Education* 41: 1010–16.

Whitehead, C. R. 2011. The good doctor in medical education 1910–2010: A critical discourse analysis. PhD thesis, University of Toronto. http://hdl.handle.net/1807/32161.

Whitehead, C., B. D. Hodges, and Z. Austin. 2013a. Dissecting the doctor: From character to characteristics in North American medical education. *Advances in Health Sciences Education and Practice,* 18(4): 687–99.

Whitehead, C., B. D. Hodges, and Z. Austin. 2013b. Captive on a carousel: Discourses of "new" in medical education 1910–2010. *Advances in Health Sciences Education and Practice* 18 (4): 755–68.

Wilkerson, L., and D. M. Irby. 1998. Strategies for improving teaching practices: A comprehensive approach to faculty development. *Academic Medicine* 73 (4): 387–96.

Willis, P. 1981. *Learning to labor: How working-class kids get working-class jobs.* New York: Columbia University Press.

Wilson, J. W., and K. M. S. Ayers. 2004. Using significant event analysis in dental and medical education. *Journal of Dental Education* 68 (4): 446–53.

Wislar, J. S., A. Flanagin, P. B. Fontanarosa, C. D. Deangelis. 2011. Honorary and ghost authorship in high impact biomedical journals: A cross sectional survey. *British Medical Journal* 343: 6128.

W. K. Kellogg Foundation. 2004. *Using logic models to bring together planning, evaluation, and action: Logic model development guide.* Battle Creek, MI: W. K. Kellogg Foundation.

Woloschuk, W., P. H. Harasym, and W. Temple. 2004. Attitude change during medical school: A cohort study. *Medical Education* 38 (5): 522–34.

Wood, D. F. 2006. Bullying and harassment in medical schools. *British Medical Journal* 333: 665–66.

Woolf, K., H. W. Potts, S. Patel, and I. C. McManus. 2012. The hidden medical school: A longitudinal study of how social networks form, and how they relate to academic performance. *Medical Teacher* 34 (7): 577–86.

Worley, P., D. Prideaux, R. Strasser, A. Magarey, and R. March. 2006. Empirical evidence for symbiosis medical education: A comparative analysis of community and tertiary-based programs. *Medical Education* 40 (2): 109–16.

Wright, S. M., A. Gozu, K. Burkhart, H. Bhogal, and G. A. Hirsch. 2012. Clinicians' perceptions about how they are valued by the academic medical center. *American Journal of Medicine* 125 (2): 210–16.

Wright, S., D. E. Kern, K. Kolodner, D. E. Howard, and F. L. Brancati. 1998. Attributes of excellent attending-physician role models. *New England Journal of Medicine* 339: 1986–93.

Yarborough, M., K. Fryer-Edwards, G. Geller, and R. R. Sharp. 2009. Transforming the culture of biomedical research from compliance to trustworthiness: Insights from nonmedical sectors. *Academic Medicine* 84 (4): 472–77.

Yarborough, M., and L. Hunter. 2013. Teaching research ethics better: Focus on excellent science, not bad scientists. *Clinical and Translational Research* 6 (3): 201–3.

Index

Page references in *italics* refer to boxes or figures.